MAKE YOUR MEDICINE SAFE

How to Prevent Side Effects from the Drugs You Take

D1573385

JAY SYLVAN COHEN, M. D.

AVON BOOKS ◆ NEW YORK

AVON BOOKS, INC.
1350 Avenue of the Americas
New York, New York 10019

Copyright © 1998 by Jay Sylvan Cohen, M.D.
Published by arrangement with the author
Visit our website at **http://www.AvonBooks.com**
Library of Congress Catalog Card Number: 98-92458
ISBN: 0-380-79075-0

First Avon Books Printing: September 1998

AVON TRADEMARK REG. U.S. PAT. OFF. AND IN OTHER COUNTRIES, MARCA
REGISTRADA, HECHO EN U.S.A.

Printed in the U.S.A.

WCD   10 9 8 7 6 5 4 3 2

For Barbara and Rory

Make Your Medicine Safe is meant to provide educational and scientific information about prescription and nonprescription medications to the public. This book focuses on specific drugs and issues, and it is neither complete nor exhaustive in its listing of drugs, disorders, or side effects, nor meant to be a substitute for personal medical care. *Make Your Medicine Safe* is not intended in any way to direct the personal usage of any medication or dosage without the approval of your physician. *Each person, each medical disorder, and each drug is different, and a medical assessment by a physican should always be obtained before any changes in medication dosages are made.* The intention of this book is to provide you with new, little known information about medications that will allow *you and your physician together* to make better informed drug and dosage decisions, and as a result, to markedly reduce your risk of side effects.

Contents

Part 4: Drugs for Lowering Cholesterol and Controlling Hypertension

Part 5: Medications for Pain and Inflammation

Part 6: Medications for Allergies and Motion Sickness

Part 7: Other Medications

Part 8: How to Improve the System

Introduction

I have never met a patient who didn't want to take the very small-est amount of medication needed to treat his or her condition. I've never met a physician who wanted to prescribe more than the least amount of medicine necessary to treat a patient.

When you receive a prescription, you probably believe that you are receiving the very lowest dosage necessary to treat your ill-ness. When physicians prescribe medications according to the guidelines in the *Physicians' Desk Reference* (PDR) or other med-ical references, they generally believe they are using the very low-est effective doses of these drugs. Unfortunately, this frequently isn't the case.

As the data for each of the medications discussed in this book will demonstrate, a great deal of information about medications, especially about effective drug doses below those recommended by manufacturers, is unknown to most physicians and patients. Considering that most medication side effects are directly related to dosage, these data are essential for the most knowledgeable and safest use of prescription and nonprescription drugs. Yet little of this data is contained in the leading drug references utilized by physicians and consumers.

In addition, a large segment of the population is medication-sensitive—that is, sensitive to the standard, often one-size-fits-all initial dosaging that manufacturers recommend to physicians and physicians prescribe to patients.

It is the purpose of *Make Your Medicine Safe* to explain the relationship between the medication sensitivities of people like you, the failure of the medical establishment to define and utilize the very lowest, safest drug dosages, and the excessively high incidence of medication side effects. *Make Your Medicine Safe* will then provide you with the scientific data that demonstrate the effectiveness of lower, safer drug dosages. These dosages will offer you and your physician new alternatives in the selection of medications and dosages that can lessen the risk of your experiencing medication side effects.

PART 1

Drugs, Doses, and Side Effects

ONE

⚘

Side Effects—Why They Occur and How to Prevent Them

Many adverse reactions probably arise from failure to tailor the dosage of drugs to widely different individual needs.

—*Goth's Medical Pharmacology*, a standard medical school textbook for decades*

THE DOSAGE MAKES THE DIFFERENCE

Why do you get side effects from medications? Is it the drug? The doctor? Your body's sensitivity? It may be one or all of the above, but in many cases it's none of them.

It's the dose.

The medicine in the dosage you were prescribed is simply too strong for your individual system. That same dosage may be perfect for someone else, too low for another, but for you it is excessive, resulting in unwanted side effects.

How can you avoid medication side effects? Simple—be sure to take the right dose. But that's easier said than done, because present-day medicine spares little time in trying to individualize the dose of a drug to the individual's characteristics.

Most medications are initially prescribed in one or two dosages for everyone. Imagine if that's how coffee and alcohol were dispensed. It wouldn't work very well, would it? Well, neither does this approach to dispensing medications. That's why the side ef-

---

*Citations for all quotes and studies can be found in the Notes section.

3

fect rate is so high. That's why a specific term, *iatrogenic illness*, has been coined to describe treatment-related injury. And what's the most common cause of iatrogenic illness? Medication side effects.

Surprisingly, the medical literature is filled with information about lower, effective drug doses than are commonly prescribed with most medications. But you won't find mention of these lower, safer doses in the *Physicians' Desk Reference* (PDR), *The Pill Book*, or most other drug references. Your physician won't likely know about these lower doses, either.

That's what *Make Your Medicine Safe* is about—providing you with scientifically based data on lower, safer, effective doses of medication for more than 100 of America's top-selling drugs. This will allow you and your physician to individualize your treatment and thereby prevent or minimize undesirable and unnecessary dose-related side effects.

LOWER DOSES WORK

When I first began prescribing Prozac in 1989, I found that many patients did exceedingly well with it, but others developed disagreeable, often intolerable side effects. For example, when I prescribed Prozac to a 32-year-old depressed woman, within days she developed severe jitteriness, sudden and intense hot flashes and sweating, episodes of panic, and insomnia—symptoms she had never experienced before. These side effects were severe, so she discontinued the medication.

I had given her only the manufacturer-recommended initial dose, 20 mg. The woman was in good health and had no prior history of medication side effects. Nevertheless, 20 mg of Prozac was too much for her system.

The woman still needed treatment for her depressive disorder. Because Prozac had worked so well in other patients, and because the other antidepressants available then were even more prone to causing side effects, we agreed to stick with the Prozac but at a lower dose. This took some doing because Prozac was produced only as a 20-mg capsule, and 20 mg was the manufacturer-recommended initial dose *for everyone*. But by twisting open the capsules and dumping out half of the powder, the woman fashioned 10-mg pills—to which she responded beautifully.

This wasn't an isolated case. As many as half of my Prozac patients required and responded to lower-than-recommended doses. According to a 1997 journal article, I wasn't the only physician who had encountered such problems:

> *It soon became apparent that many patients found the 20-mg dose [of Prozac] to be either too activating or associated with gastrointestinal side effects. Physicians started dissolving the 20-mg capsules in orange juice to create a suspension, which allowed lower doses. Eventually 10-mg capsules and a liquid formulation became available.*

But although many of my patients did well at lower doses, I was uncomfortable. I felt like I was flying blind with no guidelines or data to support my prescribing of 5 or 10 mg a day of Prozac. Prozac's manufacturer made no mention of any doses below the recommended 20 mg a day in its product information, including its write-up in the *PDR*. Yet so many patients were reacting badly to the recommended dosage but doing great at lower doses, how could it be that the manufacturer hadn't noticed such glaring responses during its pre-release testing? It didn't make sense.

When I finally got around to going to the medical library, I discovered that the manufacturer had indeed noticed. In a study conducted *before* Prozac's approval by the FDA and release for general usage, a dosage of only 5 mg a day was nearly as effective as 20 mg and caused fewer side effects. No wonder so many people were reacting at 20 mg, yet doing well at 5 or 10 mg a day.

Why didn't the manufacturer include this vital information in Prozac's package insert? Why wasn't the 5-mg dosage—75% less than the manufacturer-recommended amount yet demonstrably effective with fewer side effects—made available? These issues are discussed in later chapters this book, but for now the basic fact is that Prozac *wasn't* produced at 5 or even 10 mg a day. It was 20 mg a day for everyone. And the result was and remains a continuing very high rate of side effects with this medication.

Indeed, although many subsequent studies have confirmed the effectiveness of low-dose Prozac for many people (see Chapter 6), still today none of this low-dose data is contained in Prozac's package insert, the PDR, or other medical references. And except for those with kidney or liver disease, or elderly persons with other illnesses or taking other medications, 20 mg a day remains the manufacturer-recommended starting dose for everyone.

This means that despite the present availability of a wealth of data on the effectiveness of Prozac at doses of 5 and 10 mg a day, and even 2.5 mg a day, probably at least 90% of patients prescribed Prozac by their physicians are started at 20 mg.

DIFFERENT PEOPLE, DIFFERENT DOSAGES

This one-size-fits-all approach ignores interindividual variation, one of the most basic principles of medical pharmacology: different people display widely differing responses to the same dose of the same drug. How much variation? According to the AMA: "In normal subjects, the extent of interindividual variability ranges from 4- to 40-fold depending on the particular drug and population." This means that the range of response from one individual to the next may vary 400% to 4,000%! Such variation isn't rare. It's the norm. It occurs with any drug.

That's why some people respond to 2.5 or 5 mg a day of Prozac, while others require 80 mg. With Sinequan, doses range from 10 to 400 mg a day, although one of my patients developed intolerable side effects at just 5 mg.

Actually, you are already well acquainted with interindividual variation. You've seen it demonstrated in you and your friends with coffee and alcohol. Some of us can't tolerate a single cup of coffee, while others can drink it by the pot and remain unaffected. Some of us can barely handle a glass of wine, yet others can drain a bottle or more and show no visible effects.

It's because of this same wide range of reactions to medications that the pharmacology reference *The Hazards of Medication* states: "Always administer the smallest amount of the least potent drug that will achieve the desired therapeutic effect." Unfortunately, most medications are neither manufactured nor prescribed with interindividual variation in mind. Often, the smallest amount—i.e., the lowest effective dosage—is neither defined nor manufactured. The result is side effects. This is why the incidence of medication-induced iatrogenic illness is so unnecessarily high.

WHY LOW-DOSE DATA ISN'T READILY AVAILABLE

When you receive a prescription, you probably assume that you are receiving the very lowest amount of medication necessary to treat your condition. When physicians prescribe medications according to the guidelines in the PDR or other medical references, they generally assume they are using the very lowest effective doses of these drugs. When consumers consult *The Pill Book* and other popular drug references, they believe that the dosages listed reflect the very lowest effective dosage for each drug. Unfortunately, this frequently isn't the case.

The omission of vital information about effective lower drug dosages is not limited to Prozac. Similar omissions are common with antidepressant, antihistamine, anti-ulcer, antihypertensive, anti-inflammatory, anti-anxiety, cholesterol-lowering, sleep-enhancing, and many other types of drugs. As a 1996 journal article put it: ''The research data lags behind—rather than leads—experience in everyday clinical practice.'' In other words, we often discover the truly lowest, safest doses *after* a drug is released, rather than before. Unfortunately, it is the limited, pre-release research that goes into the PDR and other drug references, and this information rarely changes even after subsequent experience and study demonstrate the effectiveness and improved safety of lower doses. That's why the PDR still recommends an initial 20 mg a day of Prozac for most people and makes virtually no mention of the impressive data on lower dosages.

Why is this information omitted? Because drug manufacturers aren't required to include all of their data in their product information. For example, Ornade, a popular allergy medication, doesn't tell us whether the drug is eliminated by the liver or kidneys, vital information in prescribing for some patients, especially the elderly.

WHY YOU GET SIDE EFFECTS

Medications have become such an integral part of our culture that we sometimes forget that they are foreign substances, potent chemicals designed to influence our bodies. As *Goodman and Gilman's The Pharmacological Basis of Therapeutics* puts it: "Any drug, no matter how trivial its therapeutic actions, has the potential to do harm."

Medications are always double-edged swords. Side effects occur because most medications go to cells in nearly all parts of the body—liver, lungs, kidneys, heart, skin, intestines, muscles, joints, brain—potentially affecting any and all of them. A drug may be called an antihistamine or a cholesterol-lowering medication, for example, but this doesn't mean that it has only this effect. All medications exert multiple effects throughout the human system.

An adverse drug reaction is defined as "any response to a drug that is noxious and unintended." Approximately 80% to 85% of side effects are dose-related—that is, directly related to the dose of a medication. The remaining 15% to 20% of adverse effects are allergic reactions (usually manifested by itching, swelling, or a rash) or other reactions not related to dosage. The dose-related side effects are the focus of this book.

Why do people get side effects? In most cases, not because the medication is wrong, but because the dose is too high. At a lower dose, many individuals do fine on the very same drug.

Technically speaking, the dose of a medication that is effective and the dose that causes side effects are different variables. The difference between these two variables is called the therapeutic window, the range of doses at which a medication may be effective without causing side effects. Sometimes the therapeutic window is wide, as in the case of Tylenol. Sometimes it is narrow, as with lithium and Coumadin. Sometimes side effects are unavoidable, as with many cancer drugs. The therapeutic window of a drug varies with different people. This interindividual variation occurs with every medication or other chemical substance.

Because medications can affect so many internal systems, and because the great majority of side effects are directly related to the doses used, a flexible, individualized approach to dosing is the key to minimizing the risks of side effects. Side effects don't have to be inevitable. They can be avoided.

As a 1994 journal article stated, "It is estimated that half of adverse drug reactions could be avoided, and in general when drugs are used correctly, toxicities are minimized." I can't say it any better.

WHY LOWER, SAFER, EFFECTIVE DOSAGES OFTEN AREN'T DEVELOPED OR PUBLICIZED

Why aren't lower, safer doses made available as a matter of course? Because the Food and Drug Administration (FDA) doesn't require it. Because for manufacturers, extensively testing a wide range of very precise dosages would consume a lot of time and money.

FDA regulations require pharmaceutical companies to develop drug doses that are "safe and effective," a vague term that leaves a lot of latitude to the manufacturers. FDA regulations do not require the determination of the very lowest, safest doses.

From a manufacturer's point of view, the goal is to develop doses that are the most useful for the largest proportion of the population and to do so as quickly as possible to beat the competition in securing a stake in the market. Considering that the sales of prescription drugs to pharmacies in 1996 was $85.35 billion—and this doesn't include sales to hospitals and nursing homes that account for perhaps even more—the incentive to beat the competition is powerful.

So the time allotted for determining the dosage of a new drug is brief, testing a limited number of possibilities. In the case of Seldane, dosages of 20, 40, 60, and 120 mg were tested. Notice that each dose is 50% or 100% larger than the previous. Fine-tuning—for example, testing doses of 30, 50, 70 mg—wasn't done. Doses of 25, 35, 45, 55, 65, and 75 mg should also have been considered—the difference between 50 and 55 mg is 10%, not an insignificant amount—but they weren't. This is typical. Indeed, although effectiveness was shown with the 20 and 40 mg doses, the company selected 60 mg twice a day as the recommended dosage *for everyone*.

The problem is that the drug manufacturer's goal is different from yours. You want to take the least amount of medication necessary for your illness and your system. The manufacturer's goal is to find a dose that is reasonably safe yet strong enough to be effective in a large percentage of the population; otherwise physicians won't be persuaded to switch to the new drug from ones with which they're already familiar.

For example, an initial dose of a new drug that's beneficial for 40% to 50% of research subjects may be just right for you and half of the rest of the population, but from the manufacturer's point of view this dose will be less competitive and financially successful than a higher dose that benefits 75%—even if the latter causes more side effects. So the company will most likely market the higher dose, which will be prescribed to everyone, including you and the others who would respond at the much lower dose (with fewer side effects).

The result is that many individuals receive higher doses than they actually need—which becomes obvious when side effects develop. Remember, most side effects are directly related to dose; unnecessarily high doses expose patients to increased risks. This may explain why, of about 37,000 adverse drug reactions reported to the FDA in 1985, 72% involved "usual doses of drugs." These "usual" doses obviously were too high for the patients involved (see below).

Problems with Manufacturer-Recommended Drug Doses

In February 1996, the *Journal of Clinical Psychiatry* published a letter to the editor I'd sent about a case reported by Dr. Ronald Pies, an expert in psychopharmacology (psychiatric drugs). The case was of a woman who developed unusual side effects to the sleep medication Ambien (zolpidem). The manufacturer-recommended usual dose is 10 mg before bedtime, but to avoid potential side effects Dr. Pies had first prescribed a 5-mg dose. This amount made the woman tired, but didn't provide sound sleep. He increased the dose to the standard 10 mg, at which the woman experienced sensations that her body and bed were moving. In reporting this case Dr. Pies noted, "While pre-release data show that zolpidem is both safe and well tolerated, several reports of tolerance, withdrawal symptoms, and hallucinatory phenomena have appeared."

My response to this case report was that if the initial 5-mg dose of Ambien made the woman tired, she probably needed only a slightly higher dosage to promote sleep. Thus, it wasn't surprising that increasing the dose 100% caused side effects. An increase to 7.5 mg, a 50% bump, may well have been sufficient; indeed a 25% increase to 6.25 mg, if it were possible, might have been enough. Overall, I pointed out that physicians frequently forget that small increases in dosage may produce powerful effects, and that drug manufacturers all too often provide us with pills that make it difficult to avoid large increases when only small ones may be necessary.

Dr. Pies responded to my comments. He didn't hesitate to agree.

This method of choosing drug doses is the norm throughout the pharmaceutical industry. For instance, the manufacturer-recommended initial dose of the cholesterol-lowering drug Mevacor is 20 mg per day for most patients. Yet studies after Mevacor's release showed that a dose of 10 mg per day was highly effective (and considerably less expensive) for a large percentage of patients (see Chapter 11). For eight years after Mevacor was released, the PDR contained very little information about this lower, safer 10-mg dosage. Beginning in 1996, some guidelines were added, recommending the lower dose mainly for those requiring small reductions in cholesterol. Twenty mg per day remains the usual initial dosage, including for the elderly. But if you are concerned about avoiding side effects and if you know that Mevacor can cause serious ones that are dose-related, at which dose would you prefer your physician to prescribe initially? If the lower dose doesn't work, it can easily be increased.

You see, the issue here isn't whether 10 mg or 20 mg is a better dose of Mevacor—they both have their uses. The issue is *safety* and *flexibility*—and most of all, *your right to make informed choices*. You and your physician should be made aware of *all* of the options so that you can work together in selecting and, when necessary, adjusting drug doses according to your specific needs and tolerance.

THE PHASES OF DRUG DEVELOPMENT: THEIR LIMITATIONS AND CONSEQUENCES

The current method of drug research is done in four phases. Phase 1 involves animal research. Phase 2 is the phase in which potential dosages are selected. This phase is usually brief and confined to a few small studies. In my opinion, as presently performed, Phase 2 research is woefully inadequate. I'm not alone in reaching this conclusion; a 1994 study said:

> *Often, a commercial sponsor does not want the Phase 2 to be prolonged, and hence, the extra time needed to explore the full dose range and various dose intervals to obtain good dose and concentration information may not be committed. . . . On too many occasions failure to define dose-concentration-response relationships leads to unacceptable toxicity or adverse effect rates, marginal evidence of effectiveness, and a lack of information on how to individualize dosing.*

Phases of New Drug Research

Phase 1: New drug studied in animals.
Phase 2: Drug dosage determined in a few brief, small studies with human subjects.
Phase 3: Safety and effectiveness studies with hundreds or

thousands of people over periods as brief as six weeks or as long as one year or more.

Phase 4: The largest and longest phase by far, Phase 4 is the collective experience with a new drug after it is approved by the FDA and released for usage in the general population. New side effects or other problems are almost always discovered, and new beneficial usages may also be found.

Phase 3 encompasses larger studies involving hundreds or perhaps thousands of subjects for periods of as short as 6 to 8 weeks, but sometimes as long as 6 to 12 months, with the purpose of proving the safety and effectiveness of the drug at the already selected dosages.

Even under the best of circumstances, these three phases of prerelease research can identify only the most obvious side effects of a new drug. Most consumers and physicians aren't aware of this. That's why *Melmon and Morrelli's Clinical Pharmacology* warns:

> *It would disappoint the patients and the [medical] profession to realize how truly little of the important medical consequences is known about [a new drug] at the time it becomes a salable product. What should be more important to all of us is how lax we are in detecting available data that could optimize our use of drug products.*

Yet this is the information that is codified in the PDR and other drug references. This is the information that dictates the dosages your physician prescribes to you. Even if later studies show the effectiveness and superior safety of lower doses, these doses may never be added to the package insert or PDR.

Further limiting our knowledge of a new drug is the fact that it must be proven effective for only one disorder to obtain FDA approval. After approval, physicians may use a new drug for many other illnesses, and although the required dosages may differ for some of these other conditions, the manufacturer-recommended dosage remains the same in the package insert and PDR. Yet it is to the PDR that physicians most often turn for dosage information.

For example, Zoloft, which was the eleventh most prescribed drug in the United States in 1996, and most other antidepressants were first approved for treating major depression, a severe depressive disorder. But after its release, physicians have prescribed Zoloft for other types of depression, many of them far milder than major depression. These milder conditions often require lower doses (12.5–25 mg/day) than the manufacturer-recommended 50 mg to 100 mg per day for initiating treatment for major depression, yet not a word is said about this in the PDR. Today the manufacturer-recommended initial dosage remains a blanket 50 mg to 100 mg per day, and that's what most doctors, unaware of these diagnostic distinctions, prescribe for their patients, regardless of the mildness or severity of the patient's depression.

Most of my patients on Prozac had mild forms of depression, but the manufacturer recommended a one-size-fits-all initial dosage of 20 mg per day, which was also based on treating major depression. Is it any wonder that so many of my patients reacted badly to the drug?

Similar deficiencies are true for virtually all classes of drugs. As the chairman of the department of gastroenterology of a nationally renowned clinic told me: "All of the recommended doses of the drugs we use [e.g., Zantac, Axid, Tagamet, Pepcid, Prilosec, Prevacid] are much higher than necessary for many individuals. As many as 30% or 40% would do just as well at doses a third to a half as large. But the drug companies produce their medications for the broad population, using doses that are high enough to cover the largest number possible. Consequently, many people get overmedicated."

THE DOSAGES IN THE PDR AND *THE PILL BOOK* MAY NOT BE MEANT FOR YOU

Physicians rely heavily on the PDR. According to surveys, nine out of ten physicians first turn to the PDR as their source of drug and dosing information. It's the book physicians rely upon most when prescribing a drug they're not familiar with.

The problem is that when physicians prescribe medications according to the guidelines in the PDR, they generally believe the recommendations are for the lowest effective doses of these drugs. When patients use the PDR, *The Pill Book*, or other drug references to learn about their medications, they believe the information offered is complete and up-to-date. They also believe that the data on side effects is accurate. This isn't necessarily the case.

In fact, the PDR is nothing more than a compilation of hundreds of medication package inserts, indexed and organized as a book and sent free to every physician each year—"the most effective and subtle form of ongoing drug advertising ever conceived," according to one expert. But this doesn't mean that the information within is comprehensive or current. In fact, some of the information in the PDR is unchanged from when the drug was originally approved—in some cases, decades ago.

For example, in a study published in the 1997 *Annals of Emergency Medicine*, twenty drugs were reviewed for the reliability of their overdose management guidelines in the PDR. The results:

> *We found serious discrepancies in overdose treatment advice in the PDR compared with a consensus of current toxicology references. Altogether, four of five [meaning, 16 of the 20] PDR entries were deficient, and almost half advised ineffective or frankly contraindicated therapies. Despite FDA approval, the use of PDR overdose advice in a serious poisoning case could result in unnecessary morbidity or mortality.*

The reason for such terrible inaccuracy is that the PDR overdose guidelines, like much of its other information, is outdated and doesn't offer the best, most up-to-date methods. The fact that a new edition of the PDR is published every year is somewhat misleading because a new edition doesn't mean that each drug entry has been updated. A few are, but the main changes in each annual PDR are the addition of descriptions of new drugs that have been released the previous year.

Other deficiencies of the PDR are numerous and sometimes equally harmful. In 1996, Dr. Paul Insel and I published an article in the *Archives of Internal Medicine* listing eight other areas of substantial deficiency in the PDR.

And the PDR isn't used solely by physicians. It's also available in major bookstores, where hundreds of thousands of copies are sold annually to consumers seeking drug information. The problem is that the purchasers, as well as many physicians, aren't aware of the PDR's many deficiencies. They're not aware that the PDR's recommended doses aren't necessarily the lowest effective doses of many drugs. And they're almost certainly not aware that the side effect rates are based on limited, pre-release studies and often are outdated and understated.

Compounding the problem, many of the medication references written for physicians and the public derive their data from the PDR, so the PDR's inaccuracies and omissions are passed along. Like the PDR, many professional drug references including the *American Medical Association Drug Evaluations* and *Drug Facts and Comparisons*, and popular consumer references such as *The Pill Book* and many others often fail to mention much of the low-dose data contained in the medical literature. This is the case with Prozac, Pravachol, Motrin, Ambien, Lescol, Dalmane, Mevacor, Voltaren, Wellbutrin, Zoloft, and Serzone, to name just a few.

In a few cases, references such as the annual AMA drug evaluations series and the American Hospital Formulary Service series do contain some low-dose information, but the PDR and *The Pill Book*, which are by far the most used by physicians and consumers, respectively, don't. For example, in the treatment of high blood pressure (hypertension), hydrochlorothiazide (HCTZ) is frequently prescribed. Years ago, physicians started patients with high doses of HCTZ, but more recently it has become widely known that these doses are unnecessary and actually harmful, so lower doses are recommended by most medical references. However, *The Pill Book* and several listings in the PDR (Oretic, HydroDIURIL) still recommend the higher doses of HCTZ.

Another top-selling antihypertensive drug, Lopressor, is recommended by the manufacturer starting at 100 mg a day. But because of its many side effects, several authorities suggest initiating treatment at half this amount, or 50 mg a day. In fact, the *AMA Drug Evaluations Annual 1994* specifically mentions the wide range of individual variation with Lopressor and also recommends starting at 50 mg a day. But *The Pill Book* defines the "usual dose" of Lopressor as "100 to 450 mg per day."

Most important, no drug reference that I've seen addresses the fundamental issues underlying the persistent problem of medication-related iatrogenic illness. This is why I've spent seven years writing this book.

FINDING THE RIGHT DOSE FOR YOU

The dosages recommended by drug manufacturers may work fine for some people. With some drugs, they may work fine for you. But if you're like most people, you've probably encountered medication side effects at one time or another. In these instances, the dose of the medication was too high for you. And if you've had a side effect from your medication—even one that the medical profession considers minor, such as dizziness, anxiety, heartburn, diarrhea, insomnia, or a headache—you probably don't want to have another, particularly if it's entirely avoidable.

Whether you've had trouble with side effects once or many times, with the information provided in this book you can avoid many drug-related problems. Virtually any drug can be fitted to the individual, just as we learn to fit our alcohol or coffee consumption to our own specific tolerances. Indeed, careful dose adjustment is already routine medical practice with a few types of drugs—hormones and insulin, for example—but these are the exceptions.

Yet individual dose titration can be done with any drug, usually without undue effort. Under the guidance of your physician or pharmacist, you can split or cut tablets and caplets. Capsules can also be fashioned into lower doses.

Using these methods, people who have had reactions to standard doses of a drug can often benefit from the very same medication when started low enough. If the dose is too low, then it can be gradually increased—with no harm done.

A unique example of the unlimited possibilities of the low-dose approach can be seen with the anti-inflammatory drug colchicine, a medication that has many uses but is often essential for individuals with a rare but serious genetic condition, familial Mediterranean fever. Colchicine at a full dosage of 1 mg to 1.8 mg a day often causes severe abdominal cramps and diarrhea. By starting with a lower dosage such as 0.3 mg to 0.6 mg a day, most people can gradually adjust to colchicine. But for those who are unusually sensitive to the drug's adverse effects, the *United States*

Pharmacopeia describes a stepwise method that few physicians would ever conceive:

> *The regimen used . . . consisted of administering 1 mcg (0.001 mg) diluted in sodium chloride solution on the first day, doubling the dose each day until the tenth day, when 500 mcg (0.5 mg) was given, then increasing the dose to 750 mcg (0.75 mg) per day after 3 months and to 1 mg per day after another 3 months.*

In other words, colchicine treatment was started at 1 microgram—that's 1/1,000th of the ultimate target dose of 1 mg. Over time the full dose was ultimately achieved.

Low doses are sometimes all that you may need. Other times, as with colchicine, low doses allow your body to gradually adjust to a new medication without triggering intolerable side effects as a step toward ultimately reaching a higher therapeutic dose. Either way, starting with low doses offers many advantages in many medical situations.

USING PREVIOUS SIDE EFFECTS AS A GUIDE

You can avoid many of the side effects of drugs if your physician takes into consideration your history of reactions and tolerances before prescribing a new medication to you. By doing so, you and your doctor can minimize the risk of future drug reactions.

For example, knowing that antihistamines make you sleepy or decongestants give you insomnia can provide vital clues (see pages 19–22). Family tendencies may also serve as useful indicators. When I've discussed antidepressant therapy with patients, some have mentioned siblings or parents who've done well on a specific drug. If the medication is appropriate for the condition and the patient's side effect profile, I usually start with it—usually with good results.

If nonprescription antihistamines such as Benadryl or Dramamine make you drowsy, you should be prescribed nonsedating drugs whenever possible. If all that's available for your condition is a medication that is likely to cause sedation, it should be started at a very low dose.

❧

Medications That Often Cause Sedation

If you are sensitive to medications that cause sedation, drowsiness, or fatigue, you should avoid the drugs listed here. If they must be used, they should be used at very low doses initially.

ANTIHISTAMINES:

    Benadryl (diphenhydramine)
    Dramamine (dimenhydrinate)
    Antivert, Bonine, Dramamine II (meclizine)
    Marezine (cyclizine)
    Atarax, Vistaril (hydroxyzine)
    Tavist (clemastine)
    Nonprescription cold, cough, allergy, sinus, and sleep remedies that contain antihistamines may be highly sedating to susceptible individuals.

ANTI-ANXIETY MEDICATIONS:

All may cause sedation, but these may be particularly sedating to sensitive individuals:

    Valium (diazepam)
    Serax (oxazepam)
    Klonopin (clonazepam)
    Others (see Chapter 7)

SLEEP REMEDIES:

All prescription (e.g., Halcion, Dalmane, Restoril) and nonprescription (e.g., Sominex) sleep remedies may produce increased and/or prolonged effects in susceptible individuals.

ANTIDEPRESSANTS:

Those frequently causing sedation include:

Elavil (amitriptyline)
Adapin, Sinequan (doxepin)
Desyrel (trazodone)
Paxil (paroxetine)
Ludiomil (maprotiline)

BETA BLOCKERS:

All may cause drowsiness or lethargy in susceptible individuals, including Inderal, Tenormin, Lopressor.
Prescription pain remedies containing opiates such as codeine, Percodan, Percocet, Vicodan

PHENOTHIAZINES:

All may cause sedation, but these may be particularly sedating to sensitive individuals:

Phenergan (promethazine): Frequently used for motion
   sickness and nausea
Thorazine (chlorpromazine)
Mellaril (thioridazine)

MUSCLE RELAXANTS:

Flexeril (cyclobenzaprine)
Parafon Forte (chlorzoxazone)
Soma (carisoprodol)
Robaxin (methocarbamol)

✍

Medications That Often Cause Nervousness, Agitation, or Insomnia

If you are sensitive to medications that cause edginess, nervousness, anxiety, or insomnia, you should avoid the drugs listed here. If they must be used, they should be taken at very low doses initially.

DECONGESTANTS:

The most common decongestants used in nonprescription cold, cough, and sinus remedies are pseudoephedrine and phenylpropanolamine. These and similar drugs can cause edginess or agitation in medication-sensitive individuals. Well-known preparations containing decongestants are Sudafed, Drixoral, Afrin, and nondrowsy formulas of Contac, Allerest, Sinarest, and many others (see Chapter 16).

ANTIDEPRESSANTS:

Some antidepressants can cause anxiety, agitation, or insomnia even in people not prone to these symptoms.

  Prozac (fluoxetine)
  Zoloft (sertraline)
  Paxil (paroxetine)
  Wellbutrin (bupropion)
  Effexor (venlafaxine)
  Tofranil (imipramine)
  Norpramin (desipramine)
  Vivactil (protriptyline)
  Nardil (phenelzine)

DIET PILLS:

Most prescription and nonprescription diet pills

RITALIN

(methylphenidate), in adults

PHENOTHIAZINES:

Although the mechanism is different than direct stimulants, some phenothiazines are prone to causing agitation-like symptoms.

    Compazine (prochlorperazine): frequently used for nausea
    Haldol (haloperidol)
    Stelazine (trifluoperazine)
    Prolixin (fluphenazine)

If coffee or decongestants such as Sudafed or prescription or nonprescription diet remedies make you edgy or anxious, you should receive nonenergizing drugs whenever possible. If the only choice is a medication that may cause anxiety or insomnia, it should be prescribed at a very low initial dose.

Similar strategies can be employed if you have a history of drug-related headaches, abdominal pain, heartburn, palpitations, ringing in the ears (tinnitus), weight gain, blurred vision, constipation or diarrhea, joint or muscle pain, a drop or rise in blood pressure, or any of the long list of other dose-related side effects. These adverse experiences, if imparted to your physician, can help the two of you avoid medications that may cause similar problems and choose a safer, less side-effect prone course of treatment.

MAXIMIZING THE BENEFITS AND MINIMIZING THE RISKS OF MEDICATION TREATMENT

Preventive medicine means thinking ahead. It means paying heed to the facts and using them to avoid problems and obtain maximum benefit. In this instance, the basic facts are:

1. that we are all different;
2. that the variation between individuals in response to any medication may be considerable;
3. that drug dosages usually aren't researched, manufactured, or prescribed with adequate consideration of the wide differences in individual response;
4. that the side effect rate is unacceptably high, as acknowledged by the medical establishment;
5. that 80% to 85% of adverse reactions to medications are dose-related—in other words, the problem isn't the drugs itself, but the dosage of the drug. People are often overmedicated.

Just because the pharmaceutical industry makes its decisions about drug dosages based on statistical averages derived from limited studies and aimed at large populations, this doesn't mean that you and your physician must follow their guidelines. The manufacturer-recommended doses and guidelines may be fine for some people, but these doses may not be appropriate for you. Pharmacologists repeatedly emphasize that each time a physician prescribes a medication to a patient, it's an entirely unique situation involving a singular combination of factors. Or as *Goth's Medical Pharmacology* puts it, "Biologic variation in drug effect is an important reason to individualize dosage and adjust treatment to the requirements of a given patient."

With the information about lower, safer, effective drug doses contained in this book, you and your physician can fashion an individually tailored treatment plan. If you have had previous problems with side effects or have are sensitive to alcohol, coffee, or other drugs, or simply want to start with the very lowest, safest dosage of a new medication, this will often entail starting with a dose of medication less than that recommended by the manufacturer. If this dose proves insufficient, increase it slowly until the desired effect is attained. The process is simple and safe.

In essence, this method offers you the opportunity to test your system with a range of drug doses, starting with a low dose and gradually increasing it until you find a dose that fits. It also provides an extra margin of safety against becoming overmedicated, which of course is the basis of the side effect problem. By using the lower doses suggested in this book, you stand a good chance of getting good results with few problems—the essence of preventive medicine.

THE FINAL HURDLE—DEALING WITH YOUR PHYSICIAN

Because many physicians follow the PDR recommendations instead of individualizing medication dosages to fit people like you, the problem of side effects goes on and on, as evidenced by a case reported in a leading journal. The psychiatrist of a 29-year-old-woman recognized that she was a slow metabolizer (a person unable to rapidly eliminate medications from her system and therefore prone to side effects), but the information didn't help her with other doctors:

> Over the years she had considerable difficulties in explaining to prescribing physicians that she was a slow metabolizer of antidepressants and its implications for drug dosage. After many problems with side effects on various antidepressants, she decided to drop all drug therapy.

As this case illustrates, many physicians are unfamiliar with their patients' tendencies toward side effects or with adjustment of medication dosages to fit the individual—even when the patient warns the physician about the problem. One reason for such unawareness is that there's little information to be found on the subject. Few drugs come with any practical guidelines about individual responses. In general, doctors stay with what they know, as evidenced by their continuing to prescribe standard dosages of drugs such as Dalmane, Tagamet, Prozac, Coumadin, Mevacor, Xanax, and many others long after multiple studies have demonstrated the benefit of lower doses.

A typical dosage recommendation that doctors receive is offered by the 1997 PDR dosage guidelines for Voltaren (diclofenac), a top-selling anti-inflammatory drug:

> Diclofenac [Voltaren], like other NSAIDs, shows interindividual differences in both pharmacokinetics and clinical response. Consequently, the recommended strategy for

initiating therapy is to use a starting dose likely to be effective for the majority of patients and to adjust dosage thereafter based on observation of diclofenac's beneficial and adverse effects.

But if you have had problems with anti-inflammatory drugs or are generally sensitive to medications, you may have side effects in response to a dose that's "effective for the majority." Of course, by then it's too late. You develop side effects—and *then* your physician lowers the dosage. The goal of this approach is to prescribe a standard manufacturer-recommended dosage to cover most patients, with adjustments for side effects after the fact. This is the method offered by most pharmaceutical manufacturers and followed by most physicians.

Obviously, if you prefer to minimize the risk of side effects, rather than starting at the standard dosage and adjusting afterward, you should start with a lower dosage and, if necessary, gradually increase it until you reach the specific amount your body needs. The goal of this individualized approach is to prevent side effects and ensure that you receive no more medication than is absolutely necessary.

The low-dose method makes further sense because if you are prone to side effects with a specific medication, your system may adapt to it without problems if it is started at a lower, less provocative dose. In time, your tolerance may increase and you may be able to handle higher doses, if necessary.

For example, antihypertensive drugs (for treating high blood pressure) at standard dosages often cause side effects, leading many patients to stop taking them. For this reason, some specialists use flexible doses, starting low and increasing the dosage only by degrees.

One specialist told me of two women who'd repeatedly reacted to standard doses of antihypertensive drugs prescribed by their general physicians. Ultimately they were referred to the specialist. "These patients, both very sensitive, insisted at starting at one-fourth and one-half dosages," he told me. "If you want them to be cooperative, you've got to work with them. At these lower starting doses, they had no reactions. In time, both were able to tolerate and benefit from full doses."

It's too bad that these two patients, like so many others, had to endure side effect after side effect until by pure chance they found a physician who understood the problem. Not everyone is so lucky. Most physicians don't understand these issues, and you may have to work to convince your doctor to start with a dose lower than recommended in the PDR. It's not entirely his or her fault. The needed data isn't there.

Your physician is a scientist, and science isn't very good with subtle, variable phenomena. As Dr. Kenneth Foster of the University of Pennsylvania said, "We know why planes fly and how people get AIDS, but science is very much less reliable when it comes to [individual, less quantifiable situations]. That's because the signals are subtle, and science isn't good at detecting subtle signals."

The consequence is that most physicians don't realize that often there are effective, lower-dose alternatives to the standard limited range of doses provided by drug manufacturers in the PDR. This is why it's not enough for me to say, "Use the lowest dose," because that's what many physicians believe they are already doing. This is why it's not enough for you to say, "I'm prone to side effects" or "I want to use the very lowest, safest dose in order to avoid side effects," because physicians possess no reliable reference offering the data they need to guide them in knowledgeably and accurately prescribing lower doses. This is where the information in *Make Your Medicine Safe* can be helpful, for it is the first drug reference that enables you and your physician to consider lower doses that may better fit you.

Physicians are trained to give credence to scientific data. Many are less inclined to embrace a patient's subjective complaints. Your report of side effects may not impress your doctor, except perhaps to raise the possibility that you're a hypochondriac. On the other hand, a well-organized history backed by scientific data is more likely to be persuasive. If you present it in this manner, your doctor will more than likely listen.

For example, suppose your doctor is going to prescribe a sleep medication such as Dalmane for you at the standard dose of 30 mg, a dose that often causes oversedation and next-day hangovers, especially in those sensitive to sedating drugs. But instead of unquestioningly accepting this prescription, you present him with your neatly filled-out questionnaire (pages 27–29) listing those medications you have had reactions to. Most important, you show him the data in this book citing five authorities recommending 15 mg, a 50% lower dose, as the preferred starting dose of Dalmane not just for the ill or elderly or medication sensitive, but for everyone.

When you then ask, ''Can we start at the lower dose?'' he will likely give your request serious consideration. After all, he knows that starting at 15 mg is not only safer, but if it proves too mild, it can easily be increased.

Without data they can trust, physicians are skeptical of un-proven doses that may be inadequate for the disorders they treat. They want to be successful in their efforts. If you can offer them reliable data, a host of possibilities suddenly emerge.

So the next time you visit your physician, take this book with you. Tell him or her if you have had problems with side effects or are concerned about them. If he is planning to prescribe a medication, consult the data contained in this book. Clear and specific information is the key. That's what this book provides— clear, scientifically supported data, the key to allowing you and your doctor to consider a more flexible approach to the use of medications.

Questionnaire on Medication Side Effects and Sensitivities

1. Are you unusually sensitive to any prescription or non-prescription medications? If yes, please list and describe them.

2. Are you sensitive to any foods, odors, cosmetics, cigarette smoke, soaps, chemicals, or any other substances? Please list and describe these sensitivities.

3. How does alcohol affect you? Check one:
 ___Easily affected ___Moderately affected
 ___Not affected

4. Are you sedated or fatigued by any of these drugs? If so, please describe:
  Benzodiazepines (e.g., Valium, Xanax, Librium)

Cold or allergy remedies or antihistamines (e.g., Contac, Benadryl, Tavist)

Other drugs

5. Are you energized by stimulants? If so, please describe:

Coffee, tea, chocolate, or other caffeine-containing substances

Prescription or nonprescription appetite suppressants

Cold or allergy remedies, decongestants (e.g., Sudafed)

Others

6. Have you ever reacted to epinephrine (adrenaline)? Epinephrine is often contained in dentists' pain-numbing injections. Typical reactions include palpitations, sweating, anxiety, headaches.

7. Have you had any side effects such as impaired memory or coordination, blurred vision, headaches, indigestion, constipation, palpitations, rashes, swelling, ringing in the ears (tinnitus) or other reactions to any other prescription or nonprescription medications? Please describe these reactions.

8. Overall, with medications would you describe your system as:

___Very sensitive   ___Normally sensitive

___Not particularly sensitive to medications

KEY

If you answered yes to one or two of the above questions, or listed one or two side effects, you most likely demonstrate an average susceptibility to medication side effects. Like you, many people have encountered one or two adverse reactions. Although you may do fine with standard, manufacturer-recommended drug dosages in many instances, you may prefer to start at lower dosages just to be on the safe side.

If you answered yes to three or more of these questions, or have listed three or more medications that have caused side effects, you may be more sensitive to medications than average. Because you may be highly susceptible to experiencing medication side effects, you should start with lower drug dosages whenever possible.

If you answered yes to almost all of the questions, especially question 2, you may have a multiple chemical sensitivity syndrome (see Chapter 3). You should consider starting any medication at a low dosage, whenever possible.

If you haven't answered yes to any of the above questions or listed any medication side effects, you are not particularly sensitive to medications. Standard doses may usually be used unless you prefer to start at lower dosages just to be extra careful to prevent medication-related side effects.

TWO

~

The Scope of the
Side-Effect Problem

*Patients, to a greater extent than physicians, are unaware
of the limitations of the premarketing phase of drug development in defining even relatively common risks of new
drugs.*

—*Goodman and Gilman's The Pharmacological
Basis of Therapeutics*, 1990

If you've experienced a medication side effect, you've got a lot
of company. Statistics on side effects vary considerably. Various
studies have reported that from less than 10% to more than 40%
of patients experience drug-related side effects, with 15% to 20%
being perhaps the most likely incidence. That's a lot of people
when you consider that about 80 million people use medications
regularly. This means that about 12 to 20 million will encounter
side effects. And these numbers don't include people who use
medications intermittently. When prescribed medications such as
antibiotics or anti-inflammatory drugs for short-term usage, some
of these people will also get side effects.

Many of these side effects will be mild, but all will be unpleasant and some will be serious, even fatal. Serious medication side
effects aren't rare—they account for approximately one in twenty
hospital admissions. In the elderly population, this number soars
to as high as one in five.

These figures may seem high, but actually I'm being conservative. Others offer higher numbers. According to a study released at a 1995 American Medical Association conference:

> *Bad effects from prescriptions created about 115 million visits to the doctor last year, and sent an estimated 8.75 million people to the hospital. That's almost three of every 10 people admitted.*

The hospital doesn't necessarily provide refuge. In the United States, hospitalized adults receive on average about ten drugs, so it's not surprising that 15% to 30% of hospitalized patients report one or more side effects. Three percent experience side effects that are considered severe, and three of every thousand hospital patients die as the result of adverse drug effects.

According to a 1995 study that evaluated the incidence and severity of medication-related adverse effects in New York State:

> *If the numbers from New York are extrapolated to the country as a whole, over a million patients are injured [due to medications] in hospitals each year, and approximately 180,000 die annually as a result of these injuries. Therefore, the iatrogenic injury rate dwarfs the annual automobile accident mortality of 45,000 and accounts for more deaths than all other accidents combined.*

Side effects are also costly. The estimated medical expenditure for handling side effects is $3 billion annually, and this figure doesn't includes the costs of missed work, reduced performance, lawsuits, and increased malpractice rates.

ARE THE RATES OF SIDE EFFECTS UNDERESTIMATED?

As daunting as these statistics may be, the true incidence of side effects may be much higher. Many authorities agree that a substantial number of adverse drug reactions are either missed entirely or inaccurately attributed to the patient's disease or the development of some additional illness. Indeed, as *Melmon and Morrelli's Clinical Pharmacology* puts it: "It is likely that only a fraction of the ADRs [adverse drug reactions] are actually being detected; many are missed completely, and others are attributed to the natural progress of the patient's disease or development of a new illness.''

Experience has taught me that specific, focused questions are required to uncover many side effects. Agitation, impaired memory, weight gain, low-grade sedation, headaches, blurred vision, ringing in the ears (tinnitus), mild tremors, and a host of other side effects can be quite subtle. You may not be aware that these reactions may be related to the medication you're taking.

A few years ago a woman came to me with complaints of severe depression and anxiety. We quickly controlled the depression, but in trying to control her anxiety with the usual medications, we ran into problem after problem. Ultimately I put her on a very low dose of a stronger drug, perphenazine (Trilafon). She responded extremely well and was delighted with her overall improvement. When she returned for a follow-up visit a month later, I asked if she was experiencing any side effects.

"Not at all,'' she replied happily.

I was equally pleased because we'd worked closely for several months to get her stabilized. Still, knowing the medications I'd prescribed, I wasn't satisfied without asking about a few of the subtle side effects that perphenazine can cause. When I asked if she'd noted any tendency toward smacking her lips or moving her tongue around more often than usual, her brow furrowed.

She said, "Now that you mention it, I do seem to be constantly running my tongue against my teeth. I just assumed it was some nervous habit I've developed."

It wasn't. In fact it was a drug-induced reaction, tardive dyskinesia, usually seen at high doses but occasionally at low doses of perphenazine and related drugs (Haldol, Stelazine). The reaction is due to medication-related changes in the brain; it's similar to the constant, involuntary lip smacking seen in some elderly people. As a drug reaction, it can become severe and permanent if overlooked too long. We stopped the medication, the reaction disappeared, and we found an alternate way of controlling her anxiety.

Sexual dysfunctions are side effects that are also frequently overlooked. For example, when Prozac was first released in 1989, its package insert listed the incidence of decreased libido (reduced sexual drive) at 1.6%, male impotence at 1.7%, and other sexual dysfunctions (such as delayed orgasm or failure to experience orgasm) at 1.9%. But that's not what other doctors and I heard from our patients. Letters to the editors of medical journals claimed much higher incidences of these problems, and a 1992 study demonstrated a rate as high as 34%. That's one in three Prozac users.

Years after Prozac's release, new studies by Prozac's manufacturer found decreased libido in 7% and abnormal ejaculation in 11%—a total of 18%, an incidence more than three times higher than the original report. Yet clinical physicians, when asked, still provide far higher estimates—from 30% to 60%. In fact, Prozac's tendency to delay orgasms has been used by some therapists as part of the treatment for premature ejaculation.

Why the wide discrepancies? Because the results of measuring side effects depends on the method used. A 1997 study showed that when determined by spontaneous reports of patients, 9% of subjects reported Prozac-related sexual dysfunctions. But when those taking the drug were asked directly or on a questionnaire, the incidence jumped to 50%. Similar gaps were found with other drugs: of those taking Paxil, 11% spontaneously reported sexual side effects, while 47% reported them when asked directly. With Zoloft, the numbers were 19% versus 39%, respectively.

When asked about this discrepancy between the manufacturer's rate of Prozac-induced sexual dysfunctions versus contradictory reports in the literature, Dr. Alan Gelenberg, the editor of the *Journal of Clinical Psychiatry*, commented, "I think all the published figures are underestimates because we don't usually ask." I think he's right.

If doctors don't ask about side effects, they miss them, and the estimated rates of medication-related side effects, already unacceptably high, may be considerably higher than recognized. And because most side effects are dose-related, this is another reason for you (and your physician) to consider using the very lowest effective dosages of medications whenever initiating treatment.

PROBLEMS CAUSED BY INACCURATE SIDE EFFECT DATA

A friend of mine, a writer, did me the favor of reading a rough draft of this manuscript. When she finished, she told me: "I once took Prozac for chronic depression. After being on it awhile, I noticed that my sexual drive had disappeared. I asked my doctor whether the Prozac could be responsible. He assured me it wasn't. Nevertheless, the change in my libido was unusual. My suspicions were confirmed when I stopped the medication and my drive returned to normal.''

As this woman's experience illustrates, when physicians rely on the PDR, as the vast majority do, they may receive incomplete, inaccurate, or outdated side effect information. This in turn may cause them to dismiss or overlook side effects that present real problems for patients. Worse, they may consider the side effect a new condition and then prescribe more medications to treat that.

The side effect data contained in package inserts and the PDR are obtained from studies done *before* a drug's release. These data are often deficient for a variety of reasons:

1. Many studies are of short duration (six to eight weeks), far shorter than the medication will be used with patients in the general population.
2. Research subjects are often younger and healthier than typical patients.
3. The total number of research subjects is usually limited to 1,000 to 3,000.
4. Studies have traditionally excluded subjects with other illnesses and/or taking other medications, favored males over females, and rarely been representative of specific ethnic or other groups.

In other words, pre-release studies have often been done with subjects and for time frames that bear little resemblance to the reality of everyday medical practice.

When research subjects are healthier and younger than typical patients, they tolerate higher doses with fewer side effects. Thus, not only may the manufacturer-recommended doses derived from these studies be inaccurately high for average patients, but the reported rates of side effects may be inaccurately low. New FDA guidelines requiring greater representation of women, minorities, and the elderly in pre-release studies will improve matters, but most of the drugs we use today were researched under the old, less rigorous, more error-prone standards. It will be decades before these older drugs are gradually replaced by newer, better-researched alternatives.

Under the new guidelines, study subjects may still not be representative of the general population. By necessity, studies often exclude women of child-bearing age, people taking other medications or with other illnesses, or elderly persons with significant health problems. Yet in everyday practice, these people do require treatment. Studies often obtain subjects by advertising for volunteers, a group that may differ in many ways from typical office patients. And new drug studies usually focus on one disease, whereas physicians often prescribe medications for conditions other than those indicated by the manufacturer.

Even when the studies are designed well, there are reasonable limits to the applicability of pre-release research when a new drug is prescribed to you. For example, one man took the stomach acid–inhibiting drug Prevacid (lansoprazole). The pre-release studies conformed to the new FDA guidelines and involved about 10,000 subjects. In these studies, Prevacid demonstrated a high degree of effectiveness and a reportedly very low rate of side effects. Yet, in using this drug at the lowest available dose, this individual experienced severe side effects within hours of the first dose. When it comes to the individual, the specific drug response is difficult to anticipate.

There are other reasons that the recommended dosages and side effect profile of a new drug must not be considered the final word, no matter how thorough the pre-release research. A specialist in internal medicine who has conducted a lot of research offered these caveats: "Many studies are done on volunteers who are reluctant to complain about side effects because their treatment is free, or they're hoping for a cure where other methods have failed, or they don't want to disappoint the doctors. I never believe the rates of side effects provided by the manufacturers. As far as I'm concerned, the jury is still out on any newly released drug."

Thus, approval by the FDA does not guarantee that a medication is safe for you. As *Goth's Medical Pharmacology* states: "It would seem that with all these safeguards, approval of a drug by the FDA would be free of hazard. Unfortunately, there are many unusual side effects, idiosyncrasies, and allergies that are observed only after extensive use by large numbers of patients."

Yet it is this limited pre-release side effect data that goes into package inserts and the PDR. And, this data usually remains unchanged even when later experience reveals new side effects or higher rates of side effects than already recognized. Instead, this new information often escapes physicians' attention because it is usually reported in only one or two medical journals, and doctors read only a small percentage of the many hundreds of journals that are published.

PHASE 4, THE FINAL PHASE OF DRUG RESEARCH—AND YOU ARE PART OF IT

When do we actually obtain sufficient information about the best dosages of a new drug? About the true incidence of side effects? The American Medical Association (AMA) addresses this question:

> *The full range of adverse reactions may not be known until a drug has been used: 1. in patients with a wide variety of diseases, disorders, or conditions; 2. in hundreds of thousands of patients . . . ; 3. only long after exposure to the drug.*

In other words, the true range and frequency of a medication's side effects is actually determined *after* the drug is released, during the time when millions of people like you unknowingly participate in the broadest, longest, and most comprehensive, final phase of drug discovery (see pages 12–13).

As mentioned in Chapter 1, Phases 1, 2, and 3 of new drug research are conducted before a drug is approved by the FDA. But the pharmaceutical industry and the FDA know that the most important test of any new medication actually occurs after its release, when it's used in the general population. Indeed, there's an official appellation for this phase: Phase 4.

Phase 4, by involving the populations of entire countries or continents for an unlimited number of years, dwarfs all of the previous phases. To some degree, this is unavoidable. Pre-release research, even when conscientiously done, has its limits, and excessive study might delay the availability of a potentially new and important remedy.

The problem, of course, is that much of the data gleaned during Phase 4 comes at the expense of patients like you. Because the amount of time and study devoted to finding the best medication doses in Phase 2 is inadequate, many medications, including relatively new drugs such as Mevacor, Serzone, Redux, Zoloft, Prilosec, Claritin, Norvasc, and others, are released at dosages higher than necessary for many people. The result is an unnecessarily high rate of overall side effects or the occurrence of serious, sometimes fatal side effects. If the Phase 2 study of these drugs had been more complete, many drugs would be recommended at lower doses, and many problems discovered in Phase 4—on you and other patients—would not occur.

Unfortunately, because Phase 2 usually isn't adequately done, the general population pays the price in Phase 4. In the case of Prozac, Dr. Charles Popper told the *Clinical Psychiatry News*: "Prozac, for example, has been available for several years, but reports continue to appear in the literature about its side effects." Meaning, of course, that they have been discovered after occurring in patients.

Perhaps the most glaring recent examples of this problem are the weight-loss drugs Redux and fen-phen. Fen-phen is a combination of weight-loss drugs (Pondimin and Ionamin) that have been available for decades. Redux was a new drug that was supposedly thoroughly studied as well as prescribed for several years in Europe before its approval in the United States. But both of these remedies quickly went from fads to failures, and in 1997 they were withdrawn from the market because of higher than expected rates of a severe, irreversible, often fatal side effect, primary pulmonary hypertension, and a totally unexpected new problem, heart valve damage, in a high percentage of study subjects. Both fen-phen and Redux were one-size-fits-all preparations. Would lower doses have caused fewer problems? Very possibly, based on a previous incident with the antidepressant Wellbutrin.

After Wellbutrin was first released, it was withdrawn from the market because of an unacceptable incidence of seizures. A couple of years later it reappeared at a lower, safer dosage. It has since been widely used as an effective antidepressant, and in 1997 it was re-released under the name Zyban as a medication for assisting smoking cessation.

What's really scary about the fen-phen debacle is that the medication in fen-phen responsible for the dangerous side effects, Pondimin (fenfluramine), had been available and used for years by weight-loss specialists. Until the fen-phen craze, the overall usage of Pondimin was relatively small—meaning that it was prescribed to thousands instead of millions annually. It is very possible that Pondimin, prescribed long-term, had been causing primary pulmonary hypertension and heart valve damage in hundreds or thousands of people for years without being noticed.

The fact is that problems with many medications go undetected for years or decades. Because a great many drug-induced side effects aren't reported, the true magnitude of a problem may not be readily apparent. This is why fifteen years elapsed after Valium's release before its greater than expected potential for addiction became common knowledge.

Fifteen years after Xanax's release, the word is still spreading about its addictive qualities. Meanwhile, many physicians continue to employ extremely high doses of Xanax that unnecessarily expose patients to drug dependency.

The entire history of birth control pills has been one of repeated lowerings of the doses of hormones because of successive findings associating oral contraceptives with increased rates of thrombophlebitis, pulmonary embolisms, heart disease, and possibly breast cancer. Other Phase 4 discoveries have included the relatively recent association of estrogens, used for decades by millions of women, with an increased risk of breast cancer. And of tamoxifen, the drug taken by many women with breast cancer, with an increased risk of cancer of the uterus.

A 1994 study found that a thyroid hormone used for many years by millions of people weakened the bones of patients over fifty. The report suggested using the very lowest possible doses of this hormone.

Even digoxin, a heart medication that has been standard for decades, has recently been shown to be effective and safer at lower than usually prescribed dosages in treating heart failure. In a 1997 article in the *Journal of the American College of Cardiology*, the authors stated: ''We conclude that moderate dose digoxin provides no additional . . . benefit for patients with mild to moderate heart failure over low dose digoxin. Because higher doses of digoxin may predispose to [arrhythmias], lower dose digoxin should be considered in patients with mild to moderate heart failure."

It's impossible, of course, to uncover all possible side effects before a drug is released. Some long-term problems are inevitable. But because most side effects, short-term or long-term, are dose-related, the lower the dose, the lower the risk of long-term problems. This is why the AMA advises: "When prescribing newly released drugs, particular attention must be given to dosage and adverse effects."

NEW PHASE 4 DATA ABOUT DOSES AND SIDE EFFECTS USUALLY TRAVELS SLOWLY

The widely reported rise and fall of fen-phen and Redux from 1995 to 1997 were exceptions. With most medications including top sellers such as Prozac, Halcion, Desyrel, Xanax, and Capoten, as new side effects or higher rates of previously recognized side effects have been identified during Phase 4, the information has filtered far more slowly, if at all, into package inserts and the PDR, and into your doctor's awareness. The result is that the side effect rates in many package inserts and PDR descriptions become increasingly obsolete and inaccurate—but few people, including physicians, are aware of this obsolescence. As a consequence, if you develop a side effect, your physician may not recognize it, the PDR may not list it, and the reduction you require to a lower dose may not be made.

As one pharmacist told me, "Very few physicians go to the trouble of adjusting drug dosages to fit their patients. In most instances when side effects occur, most physicians just switch from one drug to another, then another, then another, until they either find one that works at the manufacturer-recommended dosage or until they or the patient gives up."

The chairman of the department of psychiatry of a large HMO told me, "I'm frequently consulted regarding patients who've developed side effects to three or four medications, all at standard recommended doses. When I take a careful medication history, I find that these patients are sensitive to a wide range of drugs, and often that their mother or sister or other blood relative is also sensitive. Most of them do fine at one-fourth or one-half doses of one of the same drugs they'd reacted to previously.''

I asked this doctor why the physicians kept prescribing standard doses, despite their patients' recurrent reactions.

He shrugged. "Because that's how we're trained. There's no data available to suggest otherwise, so it doesn't occur to these physicians that doses lower than those recommended in the PDR might actually work for some people."

A QUESTION OF BALANCE

The statistics about side effects presented in this chapter are enough to make anyone take pause. However, I don't want to lose sight of the fact that medications are also our foremost and most formidable healing tools. The drugs developed in the last sixty years have worked wonders and changed human history. They have played indispensable roles in the vast improvements in childbirth, longevity, and the general level of health and comfort wherever modern medical care is available. If you talk with the elderly, they marvel at the health of today's youth and how much more slowly people seem to age. In both cases medications have played a major role.

When I was a small child, I had chronic ear infections, bled from my ears, and was hospitalized for weeks with mastoiditis, a condition rarely seen today. Once home, I developed pneumonia. Penicillin, available only a few years earlier, saved my life. I still vaguely remember the doctor visiting my home every day for a week to give me the dreaded healing shot. Perhaps these experiences had something to do with my interest in pharmacology and my generally positive attitude about medications and their potential.

Because *Make Your Medicine Safe* takes a critical look at drug development and usage, I want to emphasize that the overwhelming percentage of medications discussed in this book are good drugs that have provided more benefit than harm. Indeed, the development of drugs such as Prozac, Tagamet, Prilosec, Motrin, and Claritin have represented major advances in medication therapy. Even Valium, Xanax, and Halcion, despite their problems, are vast improvements over their highly addictive and often lethal predecessors, the barbiturates.

At the same time, if you have experienced drug-related side effects, you know that medications can cause problems that are at the very least unpleasant, and sometimes highly distressing or downright dangerous. The fact is that medications, despite often doing much good, are also our most frequent agents of treatment-induced injury, drug dependency, and accidental death.

It is my hope that if the principles offered in *Make Your Medicine Safe* are adopted, physicians will prescribe medications more flexibly and individuals like you will obtain better results with fewer side effects. And the heretofore intractable problem of medication-related iatrogenic illness will dramatically diminish.

THREE

❧

Why People Respond
Differently to Medications and
What to Do About It

The ultimate hazard is variability of patient response.

—E. W. Martin, *The Hazards of Medication*

THE WIDE RANGE OF INDIVIDUAL
VARIATION IN DRUG RESPONSE

Medical science and common sense agree: different people respond differently to the same amount of medication. The scientific term for this, as mentioned previously, is interindividual variation.

Interindividual variation isn't an esoteric concept. It's a well-known principle to which medical textbooks devote entire chapters. It's also widely known that with any given medication, the range of interindividual variation may range from 4- to 40-fold—that is 400% to 4,000%. Such variation isn't rare. It's the rule.

Every time a doctor pens a prescription and every time a patient swallows a pill, interindividual variation plays an important, sometimes crucial, role. Yet in the everyday world of drug development and medical practice, interindividual variation is frequently overlooked. The consequences are obvious, as *Goth's Medical Pharmacology* points out: "The frequency at which adverse reactions occur demonstrates the need to understand the causes of differences among patients in drug response."

For example, Tylenol (acetaminophen) is a drug with an approximately 6-fold range of variation (i.e., a variation of 600%), meaning that some patients will require about six times more medication to obtain the same effect as others. To obtain the very same degree of pain relief, some people require the 1,000-mg extra-strength dose, others the regular 650-mg dose, and still others only a single 325-mg regular-strength Tylenol tablet. A few people don't obtain pain relief at any of these doses; that's because they actually require 1,500 or 2,000 mg, which exceeds the manufacturer's recommendation (and should not be taken without a physician's guidance). This variation explains why some individuals obtain little pain relief from even Tylenol's maximum-strength preparations. Meanwhile, if you are sensitive to Tylenol, you might develop side effects with the very same dose.

Over the years, several people have told me that they don't tolerate aspirin. In every case, they'd taken the usual two tablets, 650 mg. Because aspirin also demonstrates effectiveness at 325 mg (the label of regular Bayer aspirin recommends 325 *or* 650 mg), I've asked them if they'd tried taking just one or even half a regular-strength aspirin tablet. None had. Because two regular-strength aspirin is the standard dose, it never occurred to them that anything less might be effective. Yet if two aspirins cause side effects, one may be plenty.

An example of this was one patient's response to low-dose aspirin following hernia surgery. The wound healed properly, but continued severe pain necessitated the use of extra-strength Tylenol plus a narcotic pain reliever for weeks. Because persistent inflammation was believed to be the source of the lingering pain, anti-inflammatory drugs were considered but had previously caused many side effects with this person.

Yet the patient didn't want to remain dependent on a narcotic. He knew he was generally sensitive to medications because of many previous drug-related side effects at standard dosages, so he started with a very low dose of Ecotrin, an enteric-coated form of aspirin that protects the stomach better than regular or buffered aspirin. The dose was just one regular 325-mg pill three times a day with meals, or 975 mg per day. Within a day his pain was cut in half. Further rapid improvements in his symptoms indicated that this low dose was providing not only pain relief but also probably an anti-inflammatory effect, an effect usually obtained only at aspirin doses of 2,500 to 4,000 mg a day. Yet at a third to a fourth of this amount, he obtained this response.

Drugs like Tylenol and aspirin are believed to exhibit about a 6-fold range of interindividual variation, so you can imagine the impact of a 40-fold range of variation on drug response. For example, the PDR tells us that with the antidepressant Norpramin (desipramine), a 36-fold difference in blood levels were obtained with individuals taking identical doses of this drug. Yet most patients are started at a standard dose of 50 to 100 mg per day, only a 2-fold range of dosage, which explains why many people react adversely to these standard doses, yet do fine when started at 10 or 25 mg.

In summary, interindividual variation is the reason that some people do well at standard medication doses, while others react again and again.

WHY DIFFERENT PEOPLE GET DIFFERENT SIDE EFFECTS

People also differ in the types of side effects that they may encounter from the very same dose of the same drug. For instance, the anti-anxiety drug Valium (diazepam) can be highly sedating for many individuals. Even at 1 mg, half the smallest tablet, Valium sedates people sensitive to this effect. In contrast, individuals who aren't sensitive to sedation often obtain excellent anti-anxiety responses with the standard 5-mg dose, and a few people tolerate as much as 10 mg without experiencing drowsiness. On the other hand, in a small percentage of people Valium produces the opposite effect, an idiosyncratic reaction characterized by heightened agitation and irritability. In others, Valium may not cause sedation, but headaches, dizziness, lack of coordination, or depression.

The range of variability in sensitivity to side effects can differ greatly from person to person and from drug to drug. For example, a person sensitive to the sedating tendency of one medication may display no such reaction to others. For example, a physician recently told me of patient who is highly sensitive to the usually mild sedating tendency of Paxil, an antidepressant. Overwhelmed by drowsiness at the PDR-recommended dose, 20 mg, she does well at half that amount, 10 mg a day. This same woman, however, encounters no sedation with Valium, requiring the standard 5-mg dose to control anxiety.

Similar interindividual variability may occasionally be seen with drugs causing identical side effects. Although many patients who develop agitation with Prozac will encounter the same problem with Zoloft, some react this way with one of these drugs but not the other. Similarly, some develop intense gastric pain with one anti-inflammatory drug, yet not with another.

Most people will ultimately develop side effects to one medication or another. Some individuals, however, experience side effects with a wide range of medications, sometimes enduring so many adverse drug reactions that they become fearful of medications and may refuse to take even medically necessary drugs. Such people simply drop out of treatment, denying themselves medication that might preserve their well-being or longevity. These people are medication-sensitive. They may react to a broad spectrum of medications at standard dosages, but have no problem at pediatric or even lower doses of drugs. Based on the input of physicians, I suspect about 10% or 15% of the population may be medication-sensitive. These people are slow metabolizers, meaning that their bodies' ability to metabolize and eliminate medications is deficient, making them prone to drug reactions.

Although most side effects fall into the categories listed in the PDR, *The Pill Book*, and other standard references, some side effects are unique to just a few individuals. One physician I know becomes depressed with 400 mg of Motrin. Another spaces out with dextromethorphan, a common ingredient in cough remedies such as Robitussin. Another becomes drowsy with Claritin, a "nonsedating" antihistamine. Just because a side effect isn't listed in the package insert or a drug reference doesn't mean that it never develops.

DRUG ACTIVITY AND BREAKDOWN: THE CYTOCHROME P450 ENZYMES

When you take a medication orally, the substance is subjected to the digestive process. Then varying amounts of it are absorbed into the bloodstream, which carries the drug to the liver, which begins the metabolic breakdown of some of the drug. The remainder remains in the bloodstream, where a portion may be bound to blood proteins. The rest is dispersed throughout the body, with some of the drug going to the intended target and some going to other tissues. As the drug circulates, the liver and kidneys continue to metabolize and/or excrete the drug until very little remains in the system.

At each step of this process, there is considerable variation from one individual to another in how much and how quickly the drug is absorbed, bound to blood protein, and carried to the targeted organ or other organs, as well as how fast the drug is metabolized and excreted. Recently, medical science has developed the technology to begin to unravel the factors influencing each of these functions, and although much remains to be learned, our knowledge has expanded tremendously.

Perhaps no area has received more scrutiny than the enzymes involved in drug metabolism, breakdown, and elimination. Enzymes are molecules that catalyze and regulate the transformation of one substance into another. They're essential for building new molecules and dismantling old, flawed, or foreign ones. Enzymes exist in all cells, but the special enzymes involved in drug metabolism are located primarily in the liver (and to a lesser extent in the intestines, kidneys, lungs, and skin).

Perhaps the most important enzymes involved in drug breakdown are those belonging to the cytochrome P450 (CYP) group, a large family of enzymes that metabolize molecules originating both internally (hormones, prostaglandins, etc.) and externally (medications, pollutants, foods). The activity of the CYP enzymes can be influenced by many factors, including some drugs and foods. For example, Prozac and Zoloft are two of several drugs that inhibit the ability of enzymes CYP2C9 and CYP2C10 to metabolize the anticoagulant Coumadin (warfarin), thereby increasing the amount of Coumadin in the blood. If you are taking Coumadin and you are prescribed Prozac, Zoloft, or several other drugs, your risk of serious internal bleeding (hemorrhage, stroke) may increase unless your Coumadin dosage is lowered and then tested to ensure that it remains at the proper blood level.

Food and pollutants that influence CYP enzyme activity include cabbage and the hydrocarbons from smoking, which can accelerate the metabolism of Coumadin, Luvox (fluvoxamine), Tofranil (imipramine), and verapamil (Calan, Verelan, Isoptin), thereby hastening their breakdown and diminishing their effectiveness.

Some drug interactions are researched before a new drug is released, but many others, including most food interactions, aren't. Occasionally the result is catastrophic. When the antihistamine Seldane was released in 1985, the inhibitory effect of several drugs and grapefruit juice on Seldane metabolism wasn't well understood. Because these agents blocked the ability of enzyme CYP3A4 to metabolize Seldane, the result was an increase in Seldane blood levels, which caused hundreds, perhaps thousands, of serious cardiac arrhythmias and several deaths (Chapter 16).

Some chemicals accelerate their own metabolism by CYP enzymes. This explains why people who drink alcohol frequently often develop an increased tolerance to it.

Similarly, starting treatment with a medication at a low dosage may stimulate the body's ability to metabolize the drug, thus allowing for a gradual increase in dosage with reduced risks of side effects—in effect, giving the body an opportunity to accommodate to the new drug. This low-dose, stepwise method is precisely how some physicians start medications for treating depression (Chapter 6) and high blood pressure (Chapter 12), drugs that when started at standard recommended doses are notorious for high incidences of side effects and patients quitting therapy.

ENZYME DEFICIENCIES, GENETICS, AND SLOW METABOLIZERS

Deficiencies or variations (polymorphisms) in the forms of specific cytochrome P450 and other enzymes involved in drug metabolism play a key role in the broad range of interindividual variation in drug response. The variations from person to person in a given enzyme may number in the hundreds. For example, the metabolic efficiency of the CYP2D6 enzyme ranges from ultrafast to normal to reduced to completely lacking. This is a result of the widely varying activity of at least sixteen different known forms of this enzyme found in different people. Those with a deficient or relatively inactive form of CYP2D6 are often slow metabolizers of drugs such as codeine, dextromethorphan, and several antihypertensive, antidepressant, and antipsychotic medications.

Similar variations from slow to ultrafast metabolism may occur with each of the dozens of CYP and other drug-metabolizing enzymes. Many of these variations are genetically determined and display great variability from person to person and drug to drug. This explains why different people may be sensitive to different drugs or drug groups. It also explains why similar drug sensitivities may be seen among members of the same family, such as with mothers and daughters or brothers and sisters.

Because of the large number of genes and enzymes involved in drug metabolism, the variables from person to person are huge. And although we are presently limited in our ability to preventively identify the slow metabolizers of most drugs, we do know that slow metabolizers aren't unique. Quite the opposite, states the highly respected *Melmon and Morrelli's Clinical Pharmacology*: "Genetic polymorphisms [variations from the usual patterns] in enzymes and other proteins are the rule rather than the exception, and genetic diversity is a large source of interindividual, interethnic, and racial differences in drug response." This means that variations in enzyme activities exist in a large proportion of the population. This in large part explains the wide range of variation seen in response to medications.

ETHNIC AND RACIAL DIFFERENCES IN DRUG SENSITIVITIES

Enzyme deficiencies can vary greatly between different ethnic and racial groups. For example, as a group, Caucasians are more sensitive than Asians to the sedation and impaired coordination commonly seen with the antihistamine Benadryl. In contrast, 30% of Asians are slow metabolizers of Elavil and other tricyclic antidepressants; among Caucasians it's only 5% to 10%.

With Xanax, the data show that Asians develop higher blood levels of this drug than Caucasians taking identical doses, suggesting that some (but not all) Asian patients may display a heightened response and a greater risk of side effects with standard Xanax doses.

Similar variability is seen in people with hypertension (high blood pressure) and in the response to treatment with antihypertensive drugs. Hypertension is a common condition, yet in all age groups and both genders, it occurs even more frequently in African Americans than in Caucasians or Hispanics. The difference isn't small: the incidence of hypertension is about 40% greater among African Americans. The result is a higher incidence of the ultimate ravages of hypertension—kidney failure, cardiac disease, and strokes.

Treatment is also more difficult. Whereas most Caucasians respond well to many types of medications for controlling hypertension, a large proportion of Afro-American and Afro-Caribbean patients demonstrate reduced effectiveness with many of these same drugs. However, Afro-Americans often respond equally well or better to one group of antihypertensive drugs, the thiazide diuretics, than some Caucasians. Thus, while physicians can choose from three or four types of medications in treating other patients, the initial medication treatment of hypertension in African Americans nearly always includes a thiazide diuretic.

The most studied instance of ethnic variation in the metabolism of a specific medication involves isoniazid, an anti-tuberculosis drug. Slow metabolizers of isoniazid were first recognized nearly forty years ago. Subsequent study has revealed that about half of the members of most European and North American populations are deficient in the enzyme metabolizing isoniazid. Eighty three percent of Egyptians and 90% of Moroccans are similarly deficient, yet only 5% of Canadian Eskimos. The enzyme that metabolizes isoniazid also metabolizes other drugs, including several sulfa preparations, some benzodiazepines (the Xanax and Valium group), caffeine, and others. People with sensitivities to one of these may be sensitive to all.

Knowing how different ethnic groups react to specific medications can be helpful in allowing you and your physician to make knowledgeable drug and dosing decisions. At the same time, although a particular ethnic group may display general tendencies toward certain medications, considerable interindividual variability will still be seen between members of that group. For example, about 10% of Caucasians have a deficiency or less active form of the cytochrome P450 enzyme 2D6, making them slow metabolizers of debrisoquine, a drug used for high blood pressure. These people metabolize debrisoquine 10 to 200 times more slowly than the 90% of Caucasians with normal CYP2D6 enzymes.

Your response or that of any individual cannot be assumed based solely on ethnic, gender, age, or family-related factors. A thorough *individual* medication history is always the most reliable guide, and a thoughtful and flexible approach to medication dosing must always be the rule in order to avoid or minimize drug-related side effects.

ALCOHOL, ETHNICITY, AND THE ACETALDEHYDE SYNDROME

People assume that the term *firewater* that Native Americans gave to alcohol was from the psychological disinhibiting effects of the drug. However, the term may in fact derive from the flushing sensation and red blush to their faces and skin that alcohol frequently caused. The red flush is part of the acetaldehyde syndrome, a reaction to alcohol that may include other side effects such as increased heart rate, dizziness, headache, nausea, and shortness of breath.

The acetaldehyde syndrome is caused by the relative lack of a liver enzyme that is involved in the metabolism of alcohol. People with a deficiency or a less active form of this enzyme metabolize alcohol slowly, causing acetaldehyde to accumulate in the blood, provoking the characteristic reaction.

Acetaldehyde syndrome occurs only in a small percentage of Caucasians but in a much higher proportion of Native Americans. About 90% of Asians demonstrate the syndrome. Previously it was believed that the low incidence of alcoholism in Asian societies was due to cultural factors, but it is now believed that chemistry may be an equally important factor. A 1972 study showed that while alcohol caused a relaxing sensation in most Caucasians subjects, the same amount of alcohol caused visible flushing and other side effects in most Asian subjects.

Studies have suggested a genetic link to acetaldehyde syndrome. If one or both of your parents is sensitive to alcohol, you also are more likely to be sensitive than someone without alcohol-sensitive parents.

Most important, alcohol-related acetaldehyde syndrome appears to be related to other drug sensitivities. If you are sensitive to alcohol, you may be similarly sensitive to aspirin, antihistamines, cough syrups, narcotics, and some anesthetics. You may also be more susceptible to the toxic effects of insecticides.

A similar mechanism probably is involved with those who like alcohol too much, who can't stop after the first drink. In this alcoholism-vulnerable population, the tendency also sometimes runs in families and therefore is likely at least in part genetically determined. People with normal responses to alcohol can usually take it or leave it, but this population appears to experience an altered brain response that causes a craving difficult to control, especially after a drink or two. We don't know if the mechanism involves metabolic enzymes, an alteration in brain response, or some other variable, nor have we identified the actual genetic factors underlying this tendency, but in time these will surely be identified.

GENDER DIFFERENCES IN DRUG SENSITIVITIES

In previous decades women were often excluded from medication research because of concerns about the impact of new or untested drugs on the fetus during pregnancy. Even with improved methods of birth control, the occasional failure of these methods created a risk that was considered unacceptable. This is one reason that our knowledge about the differences in drug response between males and females has lagged.

Another reason is that until recently, medicine has been a male-dominated profession. In medical school I had few female teachers, and in my class of one hundred and twenty students, there were only seven women. During my internship in 1972, one of my rare female attending physicians was an endocrinologist who complained that male physicians had a hard time appreciating the physical and psychological rigors of female menopause. This lack of appreciation influenced how they treated their female patients. A similar male-dominated perspective surely influenced research decisions as well.

This has begun to change. Centers for women's studies have sprung up at medical centers and universities. Specialists in women's medicine can be found in most cities. In research, serious attention is now being paid to the factors that separate the genders. It's generally known that differences in size, drug absorption and metabolism, hormonal and genetic factors, and other unidentified causes, account for differences in medication response between men and women. Current and future research will focus on unraveling the mechanisms underlying these factors.

Perceptive practicing physicians usually learn through trial and error that many women require different, usually lower, doses than men. Yet dosage guidelines in the PDR and other drug references rarely differentiate between the genders. For example, the description of the anti-inflammatory drug Orudis (ketoprofen) in the 1997 PDR states that not only may elderly people obtain a more potent effect at the same dosage as younger adults, but this increase in medication potency (and probably side effect potential, too) may be greater in elderly women than in elderly men. Yet the Orudis dosage recommendations (located two pages and six columns away from this data) don't reflect this difference; indeed, they don't even mention it.

Recent research has also shown that women may respond differently than men to some medications. A 1997 study in *Nature Medicine* demonstrated that women obtained more relief with some pain medications and less relief with others than men. Study author Dr. Jon Levine commented: "Biologically, men and women don't obtain relief in the same way. It may be that the brain circuitry regulating pain relief differs between the sexes— or that sex hormones facilitate or interfere with pain drugs."

Similarly, until this decade little attention was paid to illnesses that occur disproportionately in women, or many common illnesses may run their course differently in women than in men. For example, rheumatoid arthritis strikes women about twice as often and is usually more aggressive than in men, yet the recommended drug dosages for this condition make few concessions to gender differences in size and metabolism, despite the high degree of toxicity of many of the drugs used for this chronic disease. Fibromyalgia and chronic fatigue syndrome are disorders that also occur more frequently in women, and both of these conditions are associated with an increased incidence of medication sensitivities as well as a condition known as multiple chemical sensitivity syndrome.

Women are also twice as likely as men to develop a biochemical depression, but differences in the characteristics and course of this illness are just now gaining attention. Studies have now shown that women may metabolize antidepressant drugs differently, but this information has not as yet led to dosing guidelines reflecting these differences.

To expedite the process of defining gender differences, new FDA regulations require greater representation of women in drug trials. In addition, several universities have undertaken studies to define specific methods of treatment, including drugs and dosages, that may be safer and more effective for women than those previously applied to both sexes.

From an empirical point of view, females seem to account for the majority of medication-sensitive individuals. In my own work, women have been far more likely to exhibit medication sensitivities than men, and they often give histories of medication sensitivities in their mothers or sisters, raising the likelihood of genetic factors. But my experience has been skewed by the fact that the majority of my patients were female.

Other practitioners have related similar experiences to me. As a specialist in women's medicine told me, ''I see a lot of women who are unusually sensitive to medications. While the majority handle standard doses just fine, a surprising number do better and get fewer side effects with lower doses.'' Another physician added, ''If their mothers are sensitive to a drug, many of my female patients are sensitive, too.''

Being a slow metabolizer may be important beyond drug dosages. A 1996 study in *JAMA* found that postmenopausal women with deficiencies in the enzyme n-acetyltransferase, which metabolizes the carcinogenic aromatic amines from tobacco smoke, have an increased risk of developing breast cancer. The risk is dose-dependent—it increases with greater tobacco usage. For example, postmenopausal women who smoked more than a pack a day were found to have more than a 4-fold (400%) increased risk. On the other hand, women smokers with normal n-acetyltransferase activity showed no increased risk of breast cancer, nor did any women who were premenopausal.

The findings from this study may have wider implications. People who are slow metabolizers of different kinds of carcinogens, such as toxins, pollutants, or chemicals in household products, may have a greater risk for some types of cancers, just as people who are slow metabolizers of medications run a greater risk of developing side effects at standard .drug dosages. After all, the mechanism is the same—to the body, medications, pollutants, and carcinogens are all foreign substances that in excess can cause harm or death, quickly or slowly.

As more research is completed, our knowledge of gender variation in disease states, biochemical processes, and drug metabolism will provide much-needed information about the differences between men and women. These data will be welcome, but we must remember that whatever general trends are revealed, individual women will differ considerably from one another in their sensitivities to specific medications. In the end, the role of gender may be important, but not as much as your own personal experience with medications and side effects.

MEDICATION SENSITIVITIES, CHRONIC ILLNESS, AND MULTIPLE CHEMICAL SENSITIVITY SYNDROME (MCSS)

A tendency to react to many medications—to be medication-sensitive—may sometimes be associated with other disorders. People with severe or long-term illnesses may become sensitive to medications that hadn't caused them problems before. In some, this may be related to liver or kidney dysfunction, but in others it may occur without detectable organ impairment. Current liver tests are better indicators of liver cell damage than cell function. For example, liver cells may show no damage, but their ability to metabolize medications or other foreign substances may be compromised. Deficits in cytochrome P450 or other enzymes aren't revealed by standard blood tests, yet their deficiencies may surely be felt when drug breakdown is impaired and higher medication levels accumulate in the blood and tissues.

In some people a generalized medication sensitivity may occur as part of a broader disorder known as a multiple chemical sensitivity syndrome (MCSS). MCSS is characterized by heightened sensitivities to odors such as perfumes, insecticides, cigarette smoke, volatile petroleum products such as gasoline, car and diesel exhaust, and barbecue starter, and sometimes newly developed food allergies. People with MCSS are often highly sensitive to medications and frequently report adverse effects at standard or even low doses.

Some people have MCSS without any accompanying medical problems, but in others it is accompanied by a medical disorder. And in others an unrecognized disorder ultimately appears. The symptoms of MCSS can vary widely from individual to individual. No common thread has been found diagnostically, and no specific tests have been developed to confirm the diagnosis. Because MCSS has been difficult to establish unequivocally as a specific disorder, many physicians remain skeptical that it exists at all, instead believing it to be a form of hypochondriasis, although studies have shown no increased association of MCSS with psychiatric disorders.

The most compelling data about MCSS have come from studies showing a strong association of this syndrome with chronic fatigue syndrome and with fibromyalgia, a rheumatoid condition characterized by mild to severe tenderness or burning sensations in the muscles or soft tissue. In these disorders, about a third of sufferers develop a multiple chemical sensitivity syndrome. Interestingly, fibromyalgia, chronic fatigue syndrome, and MCSS all occur most frequently in women, especially among the relatively young (ages 25 to 45) and well-educated. Young, well-educated women are also the most frequent victims of rheumatoid arthritis, systemic lupus, and multiple sclerosis, in each of which multiple sensitivities have been reported.

MCSS is also seen in some asthma patients. Many sufferers of Gulf War syndrome also have developed MCSS—about 25%, according to the most recent data.

One theory regarding MCSS and chronic disorders is that over time, the ability of the enzymes involved in the breakdown of medications and other foreign substances become overburdened and impaired, thereby reducing their ability to protect the body from the adverse effects of foreign chemicals, including medications. This would fit with our current knowledge about how inborn, genetically determined deficiencies in these same enzymes can cause specific medication reactions in a large percentage of the population.

In the meantime, people with severe MCSS may become quite disabled, and the lack of knowledge or medical support can be demoralizing. Fortunately, support groups can be found on the Internet, and MCSS Referral and Resources (410-362-6400) provides information about this perplexing condition. This organization has also performed considerable research on porphyria, a rare disorder that is often overlooked but can cause a varying array of physical and psychological symptoms, as well as hypersensitivities to many medications.

INTRAINDIVIDUAL VARIATION

We have already seen that you may respond differently than others to the same dose of the same medication. Equally true is the fact that you may demonstrate different responses at different times to the very same dose of the same drug. This is called *intra*individual variation.

It's well known that in childhood and old age, people display widely differing sensitivities to medications. What's less recognized are the changes occurring between young adulthood and late middle age. The time span from 20 to 65 is a dynamic period physiologically, and medication tolerances and sensitivities can shift dramatically. "Hardly any people realize that as they progress from age 20 to age 75, their kidney function decreases by 50%, even if they remain perfectly healthy," states Dr. Michael Ziegler, professor of medicine at the University of California, San Diego. "These patients need only half the dose of drugs that are excreted by the kidneys. This is a constant which so eludes physicians that we have built into our hospital pharmacy computer an estimate of patients' creatinine clearance based on their serum creatinine, sex, and age so that we can flag patients who are likely being overdosed."

This reduction in kidney function and other physiological processes doesn't develop suddenly after age 70, but gradually during the thirties, forties, fifties, and sixties, meaning that an individual's tolerance to medications may be declining and his vulnerability to side effects increasing. It has been my professional experience that many people at 40, 50, and 60 sometimes develop problems with medications they took without incident decades earlier.

Many people over 40 are already acquainted with intraindividual variation via their reduced tolerances to alcohol or caffeine as compared with when they were 20. The same may apply to illegal drugs. Typically, marijuana usage drops considerably after a person is age 35. Although this may be related to settling down and having children, it may also be due in part to intraindividual variation. I've seen several patients with pronounced physical reactions (palpitations, nausea, anxiety attacks) to doses of marijuana that fifteen years earlier wouldn't have affected them. Now older, they'd become more sensitive to the physical influences of the drug.

Intraindividual variation is part of the ongoing, ever-changing evolution of our systems from infancy to old age. Until recently, adulthood has been mistakenly viewed as a kind of prolonged physiological plateau. This assumption explains why the medication doses recommended in the PDR and most other drug references make few distinctions between 20-, 40-, and 60-year-olds.

Age isn't the only factor responsible for intraindividual variation. Illness, stress, extreme diets, dehydration, the concomitant use of other medications including nonprescription drugs, the lack of exercise, the overuse of alcohol, and other changes can alter our responses to medications. Many of my female patients taking Prozac or other antidepressants have reported a diminution of the effect of their medication when they're premenstrual. A mild temporary increase in dose during this time is usually effective in balancing the physiological shift.

People seem surprised when their tolerances to coffee, alcohol, and medications change, or when they suddenly develop a side effect to a medication they've used uneventfully many times previously. They feel no different than before, but their bodies have nonetheless changed.

The reality is that decade by decade, life event by life event, your physiology is constantly changing, and these changes can make you vulnerable to overmedication and dose-related side effects. This is why it's important for you to notice your intraindividual variations—i.e., your changing sensitivities and tolerances to chemical substances such as alcohol, caffeine, prescription and nonprescription medications—and to communicate this information to your physician. Changes in sensitivities to these substances can provide warnings about increased risks with other drugs producing similar side effects. Heeding these warnings may mean the difference between a beneficial or harmful medication response.

RECOGNIZING INDIVIDUAL VARIATIONS TO MEDICATIONS BEFORE THEY CAUSE SIDE EFFECTS

When I began writing this book in 1990, the first data about specific enzymes of the cytochrome P450 group were emerging, but the everyday application of such information seemed decades away. Just four years later this statement appeared in an issue of *Science*:

> Doctors may soon be able to tailor treatments to match drug doses with individual differences in metabolism and to avoid giving people drugs that disagree with them. Researchers in Berlin found that people who are unusually sensitive to particular drugs can be identified by a few simple DNA tests. . . . Blood tests may soon be available to allow people to find out their cytochrome P450 "profile." Those who find out that they are poor metabolizers should then know how to avoid certain drugs.

Another sign of things to come: The 1997 PDR is the first edition in which I've seen data pertaining to cytochrome P450 enzymes and their effect on a given drug. So maybe the day of determining the enzyme pattern of every person, perhaps with the blood from a simple finger prick in a doctor's office, isn't so far off.

Today, however, we are still mired in the traditional method of prescribing medications by trial and error, and unfortunately, our prescribing methods usually ignore the wealth of information we are accumulating about the diversity in drug-metabolizing enzymes and individual response. Prescribing drugs in one or two standard doses to fit a very broad and diverse population ignores the fact that genetically determined enzyme variations are "the rule."

The range of interindividual and intraindividual variation is wide. Specific degrees of medication sensitivity vary from individual to individual and from drug to drug. That's why a careful, individualized medication history is so important, particularly because medication sensitivities aren't always black and white. The degree of a specific medication sensitivity can be highly variable, from slight to severe, depending upon the degree of inactivity or outright deficiency of the medication-metabolizing enzyme. Also, many people are sensitive to one or two drugs, yet display normal tolerances to the rest. Other folks are sensitive to just about everything. And people with no histories of medication sensitivities will nevertheless display shifts in their drug tolerances as they proceed from young adulthood to midlife to retirement to old age. And because many enzyme deficiencies are genetic, you should find out about medication sensitivities in blood relatives, especially if one of them has taken medication similar to a type that's being considered for you.

Your physician should consider all of these issues before prescribing a drug at a specific dosage. He or she can obtain all of the information needed about your susceptibility to side effects with just a few pointed questions. As one physician told me, "The patients know. The ones who tell me they're sensitive are sensitive, and the ones who tell me they're not, aren't."

But does your physician have the knowledge to understand and apply these issues? Perhaps not, according to *Melmon and Morrelli's Clinical Pharmacology*: "Many physicians are not aware of this source [genetic] of variation and are reluctant to accept that, for certain drugs, genetic factors are important and should be incorporated in their dosage considerations. Unawareness of these common variabilities will continue to result in. . . . the overtreatment of [slow metabolizers]. A substantial number of patients will be affected."

If you like your physician but he or she is unfamiliar with these issues, help your doctor out. Show your physician your filled-out questionnaire from Chapter 1, the information in this chapter on interindividual variation, and the data in this book regarding the medication that's being considered for you. As mentioned previously, most physicians mean well, but the data they need to confidently prescribe lower than standard doses is generally lacking. This book has been written to fill this void.

Your physician's willingness to address your concerns, to take an interest in your medication history and family tendencies, and to discuss drugs and dosages will say a lot about his or her knowledge of issues such as interindividual variation and enzyme deficiencies, as well as his or her open-mindedness and willingness to treat you and other patients as individuals.

FOUR
~

Medication Sensitivities and Side Effects in the Elderly

The normal aging process makes people more sensitive to some drugs and less able to eliminate drugs from the body. Too, usual doses may be too strong for older bodies.

—General Accounting Office Study, as reported in the Associated Press, 1995

WHY A "LOW DOSE" ISN'T ALWAYS LOW ENOUGH

One Christmas I attended a party. Someone asked about my research on medications. An endocrinologist (a physician specializing in endocrine/hormonal conditions), laughing but not really amused, recounted a recent incident in which his mother had been grossly overmedicated by her internist.

"He's a good doctor," the endocrinologist assured us. "But boy, did he snow her!"

The endocrinologist's mother was having difficulty sleeping. She's in her seventies, and the internist, wary of Halcion, Dalmane, and other standard sleep remedies because of their addictive tendencies and ability to cause confusion and memory deficits in elderly patients, prescribed Elavil (amitriptyline). Because Elavil, an antidepressant, is very sedating, some physicians prescribe it in low dosage as a nonaddictive sleep medication for elderly patients. But what is "low dosage"?

In the 1994 PDR, the recommended geriatric dose of Elavil is 50 mg a day (10 mg three times a day and 20 mg at bedtime), but that's for treating severe depression, not insomnia—yet this isn't made clear in the dosage recommendations. For using Elavil for insomnia, the PDR offers no guidelines, despite the fact that Elavil is commonly used for this purpose.

Being cautious, the internist prescribed only 25 mg, 50% less than the recommended total daily dose of Elavil, to help this elderly woman sleep. According to most sources, this is a low dose, but not for the endocrinologist's mother.

"She was delirious," he said of her condition after a few days on the Elavil. "She didn't know where she was. She was completely out of it."

The endocrinologist stopped the Elavil. His mother's mental functioning returned to normal, but her insomnia returned, too. Now what? He decided to continue with Elavil—much of the internist's reasoning was sound—but with the smallest pill available, 10 mg. Now, she sleeps fine without any medication side effects.

Why didn't he discontinue the Elavil altogether? Because he recognized that the problem wasn't the drug, but the dose. He also knew that there are no perfectly safe sleep medications, especially with a medication-sensitive elderly woman. His mother would likely be sensitive to many drugs. Adjusting the Elavil dose, rather than discontinuing it and experimenting anew with another, solved the problem.

THE HIGH INCIDENCE OF SIDE EFFECTS IN THE ELDERLY

If you are over 65, your chances of developing side effects from a prescription or nonprescription drug are far greater than those of the general population. As reported in medical journals over many years, adverse drug reactions with elderly patients constitute a serious medical problem in themselves. Many articles have been written on this subject, including one entitled "Rational Drug Therapy in the Elderly, or How Not to Poison Your Elderly Patients," which states: "Illness caused by medications is arguably the most significant treatable geriatric health problem." The high incidence of serious side effects and hospitalizations due to medications bear this out. As stated in *Melmon and Morrelli's Clinical Pharmacology:* "Mismedication of the elderly has become a critical health care issue. . . . Although Americans aged 60 years or greater make up about 17% of the U.S. population, they account for 39% of all hospitalizations and 51% of deaths from drug reactions." Dr. Sidney Wolfe, in his *Worst Pills, Best Pills II: The Older Adult's Guide to Avoiding Drug-Induced Death or Illness*, adds: "The risk of an adverse drug reaction is about 33% higher in people aged 50 to 59 than it is in people aged 40 to 49. It becomes two to three times higher as people get even older."

If the statistics aren't enough—and some believe they don't represent the true scope of the problem—it must also be remembered that even so-called mild side effects, which rarely get reported, can be serious in the elderly. For example, a side effect such as light-headedness may have minor consequences in younger patients, but if it causes a senior citizen to have an automobile accident or to fall and break a hip, it can lead to prolonged disability or death.

For this reason the potential for side effects must be weighed heavily whenever medications are prescribed to elderly individuals, and no side effect should be taken lightly.

WHY THE ELDERLY ARE HIGHLY SENSITIVE TO MEDICATIONS

Although our society tends to think of the elderly as a fairly homogeneous group, this is not the case. The elderly represent a highly diverse group—more diverse, perhaps, than any other segment of the population.

The elderly offer the same physical variations in size, weight, gender, and ethnicity as other age groups. In addition, the elderly also present many age-related changes in body chemistry and physiology. These changes profoundly alter the way the elderly process and eliminate medications.

For example, a relative increase in body fat means that elderly individuals may store a greater proportion of a dose of some medications, thus decreasing the rate at which they can be eliminated. Valium is one of many medications that is readily stored in the body's fat deposits, from which it is gradually released back into the system to exert its effects. Whereas younger adults require an average of 20 hours to eliminate half of a dose of Valium, in the elderly it may require 40 to 80 hours to eliminate half of the same dose. Valium's affinity for and slow release from fat tissues is why it and other fat-soluble drugs can accumulate, a danger that is magnified in the elderly.

In addition, an age-related reduction of blood proteins means that less medication is bound up, thereby freeing more medication to exert its effects. Reductions in the size of and blood flow to the liver of older people reduce the speed of drug metabolism and elimination. Blood flow and the rate of drug clearance are also reduced in the kidneys, which excrete many medications.

All of these can contribute to higher and more prolonged levels of medication in the bloodstream and tissues of the elderly. Routine blood tests for the kidneys and especially the liver are not always highly accurate measures of these organs' level of function. The blood measurements may still register in the normal range, yet an elderly individual may have markedly reduced liver or kidney functioning. This is why, for example, the *United States Pharmacopeia* warns that with the anti-inflammatory drug colchicine, "Geriatric patients, even those with normal renal and hepatic function, may be more susceptible to cumulative toxicity with colchicine."

Furthermore, receptor sensitivity—the sensitivity of the tissues affected by a medication—may be heightened in elderly individuals, meaning that even with normal blood levels of a drug, the body's responses may be enhanced. With increased blood levels due to the bodily changes mentioned above, drug responses may be even more exaggerated, and so too the risks of side effects. For example, adverse reactions that cause kidney damage, hearing loss, a drop in blood pressure, mental confusion or disorientation, and dizziness occur more commonly in the elderly.

In addition to all of these physiological changes, the elderly, just like other age groups, manifest a wide range of individual variation in their innate, genetically determined sensitivities to medications. Medically, the elderly are also more likely to have preexisting illnesses or to be taking other medications, factors that add further uncertainty when adding a new drug to the mix. All of these factors add up to a degree of variability in drug response that is immense.

It's not surprising that medication sensitivities are common among the elderly. So, too, are unusual, idiosyncratic reactions such as becoming agitated by medications that usually sedate. As one pharmacist told me, "I see a lot of sensitive patients, especially among the elderly as their ages pass 70 and march toward 80. By that time, they're all hypersensitive. And once they've become sensitive, they're that way across the board. One aspirin makes them drowsy. I recently had one who became psychotic on regular doses of tetracycline [an antibiotic]. Before Prozac was finally released in a liquid form, I was opening the 20 mg capsules and mixing Prozac solutions of 2 mg to 5 mg, most of it for elderly patients."

ARE ELDERLY PATIENTS PRESCRIBED TOO MUCH MEDICATION?

Elderly patients present a dilemma for physicians. Given that medications should be prescribed as cautiously and sparingly as possible to elderly patients, the fact is that the elderly experience more illnesses, as well as more chronic and severe illnesses, than any other age group. Hypertension, insomnia, arthritis, depression, heart disease, diabetes, and a host of other afflictions affect longevity and/or the quality of life of a large proportion of the elderly population.

Should doctors ignore the destructiveness or pain caused by such conditions? Should they ignore the need for medication therapy because of the possibility of side effects? Of course not, but they should be thorough in their evaluations and cautious in their selections of drug doses, utilizing very low initial doses whenever possible.

Some authorities believe that, on the whole, the medical profession doesn't demonstrate such caution, and as a consequence the amount of medication prescribed to the elderly is excessive. Studies indicate that the average elderly patient is taking approximately three drugs, prescription and nonprescription, at any given time. And although people over 65 years of age constitute about 12% of the population, it is estimated that in developed countries the elderly consume 30% of the prescription and 40% of the nonprescription drugs.

For emergency physicians and hospital nurses it's a daily ritual to admit elderly patients who arrive with bags crammed with medications. The result is cases such as this one reported by Dr. Robert Berkow, coauthor of the *Merck Manual of Geriatrics*:

> *She was a vocal woman with several complaints, and every time she complained, someone prescribed a medication. She was taking a dozen different drugs, some of which were reacting with each other and disorienting her. She was dying. We got her off most of the medications and restored her electrolyte balance, but it took three months of nursing-home care before she was back home.*

Repeated encounters with elderly patients taking too many medications led one emergency physician to suggest this solution: "The way to cut down on adverse reactions in the elderly is to require physicians to limit their number of prescriptions to four for people over age 65. We get 80-year-olds in the ER on nine different medications—there's no pharmacist or pharmacologist in the world who could tell you the effect on the body of nine different drugs at the same time."

He's not exaggerating. In a 1995 article on the dangers of side effects in the elderly, Dr. Leonard Schulkind stated, "Elderly patients often have multiple medical problems, and the physician prescribes a drug for each problem. And next thing you know, you see their patients in the emergency room. We have a saying: Any patient taking more than two or three medications isn't good; four or five and you have to worry about serious drug interactions."

THE PROBLEM WITH STANDARD GERIATRIC DOSES

Too many medications represents one kind of overmedication. Another is one medication at too high a dosage. For some elderly persons, the standard recommended doses that doctors employ may be too high.

Indeed, a 1990 study found 9% of hospital admissions of elderly patients were caused by drug reactions at the "*usual doses of medications commonly prescribed for elderly patients* [my italics]." In other words, the usual doses were too high for tens of thousands of elderly individuals who ended up in the hospital.

And this statistic, daunting as it is, doesn't include the adverse reactions that didn't require hospitalization, but were unpleasant, unsettling, or medically dangerous nonetheless.

But don't all medications come with lower geriatric dosages? Surprisingly, no. According to the Public Citizen Health Research Group, a 1985 survey of 425 of the drugs most used by the elderly revealed that only 212—less than half—offered geriatric doses. And although FDA has since taken steps to remedy this deficiency, many top-selling drugs are still recommended at the very same doses for elderly patients as for younger adults. Notable examples include Zantac, Prilosec, Motrin, Naprosyn, and Seldane.

Sometimes PDR drug descriptions do mention the differences in drug response in elderly individuals, yet the dosage guidelines make no allowances for these differences. For example, the 1997 PDR description of the anti-inflammatory drug Orudis and extended-release Oruvail (ketoprofen) states that not only may elderly people obtain a more potent effect at the same dosage as younger adults, but the increase may be greater in elderly women than in elderly men. Yet the recommended dosages contain no suggestions reflecting this potential difference.

Even when geriatric dosages are provided, safety isn't guaranteed. That's because even with medications that come with geriatric recommendations, the geriatric dose often is limited to a single size. The next higher dose is usually the full adult dose, sometimes 100% higher. Examples here include Ambien, Paxil, Halcion, and Dalmane. Yet, as mentioned above, the range of individual variation in drug response among the elderly is extremely wide. Thus, a single one-size-fits-all geriatric dose may be appropriate for some elderly individuals but too strong for others, especially those who are medication-sensitive.

For example, the manufacturer-recommended dose of the popular sleep medication Dalmane (flurazepam) is 15 mg for elderly persons. Since Dalmane is manufactured as a capsule in only two sizes, 15 and 30 mg, there's no adjusting the dose downward for more sensitive, more sickly, or multiple-medication-taking older patients. The only possible adjustment is upward, doubling the amount to the full, manufacturer-recommended adult dose, 30 mg.

Worse, many authorities recommend the so-called geriatric 15-

mg dose of Dalmane as the preferred initial dose for all adults, so if 15 mg is the preferred starting dose for young, healthy adults, clearly 15 mg may be too much for medication-sensitive elderly persons. Yet that's what the manufacturer has recommended for over twenty years, and that's what doctors prescribe. Not surprisingly, at standard recommended doses Dalmane causes a high incidence of side effects, particularly in the elderly.

The problems with Dalmane aren't unique to this drug. Similar inadequacies are common to many different drug groups.

FASHIONING QUALITY TREATMENT FOR ELDERLY INDIVIDUALS

Because the elderly represent perhaps the most heterogeneous of all age groups, it's difficult to know how one specific person will respond to a given drug at a given dosage. One thing we do know: with elderly individuals, medication sensitivities are frequent. Exaggerated or unusual reactions are commonplace. And the side effect rate is high, higher than any other age group.

If these realities cause you concern, you're not alone. A 1994 study found that elderly patients are most concerned about drug effectiveness and safety. Are these concerns warranted? Certainly.

So what should you do? In acute, serious situations that require quick and effective treatment, without hesitation go with the recommended doses. But in the more common less serious situations, it may be safer to start with lower initial doses until your sensitivity to a new drug is determined. If the dose is too low, it should be raised gradually, if possible, rather than immediately jumping to double or triple the initial dose.

Most of all, you and your physician shouldn't always rely on the doses recommended by manufacturers, as in the PDR. Often these doses are the same as those for younger adults. Even when manufacturers provide geriatric doses, these shouldn't be considered definitive; although the PDR may not mention it, in many incidences even lower doses may have been proved effective in some elderly subjects in clinical trials. With other medications, lower than recommended doses were never studied at all, so the very lowest effective dose has never been defined. As *Melmon and Morrelli's Clinical Pharmacology* states: "Recently approved drugs usually have not been given to many elderly patients during phase III [pre-release] testing. Data concerning dosing and adverse reactions in elderly patients are often lacking, even for many established drugs.''

In other words, you may respond at a dose that's lower than usually recommended or prescribed, but you'll never know unless treatment begins with a lower dose. This approach may require a bit more time and deliberation, but the payoff is that by starting at the lowest effective dose, your chances of developing side effects may be greatly reduced. This is especially true if you have a history of medication sensitivities or have other illnesses or are already taking other medications.

Recent changes in FDA policies regarding the research of new drugs with elderly subjects should improve matters, but because of the limited time frames and limited numbers of pre-release studies, there will always be an inevitable gap between what we know about a new drug initially and what we know about it five or ten years down the road. And even then there will always be a gap between our general knowledge of a medication and that medication's function in the individual. For these reasons, careful dosaging is always extremely important. That's why many authorities, such as *Goth's Medical Pharmacology*, the *United States Pharmacopeia, Worst Pills, Best Pills II*, and the journal *Drug Safety*, recommend as a general rule the use of lower doses in the elderly.

Remember, the vast majority of medication-induced side effects are directly related to the dose of medication prescribed. This is especially true in the elderly. So if you are concerned about side effects, talk to your physician. Together, you should be able to fashion a treatment approach that recognizes the alterations in medication response attributable to aging and that makes sense for you as an individual. The result will be a better relationship with your physician, a better result with the medications that are prescribed, and a greater chance of avoiding becoming another statistic in the tide of side effects sustained by the elderly population.

As Dr. Robert Kane of the University of Minnesota School of Public Health stated in an article about side effects: ''There are things that older people can do to help themselves, and I think they should do them.''

FIVE

The Uses and Limitations of Low-Dose Medication Therapy

Clinical trials by physician-scientists are done on groups of patients. . . . Clinicians, however, do not treat groups of patients. Rather, they treat individuals.

—Melmon and Morrelli's Clinical Pharmacology: Basic Principles in Therapeutics, 1993

INDICATIONS FOR THE LOW-DOSE APPROACH

As the following chapters will demonstrate in detail, you may benefit from lower medication doses in a broad range of situations. Most prescriptions are written for symptomatic relief, conditions of mild severity, and other non-life-threatening problems. These include most cases of allergies, headaches, stomach problems, anxiety, depression, hypertension, motion sickness, muscle and back pain, inflammation, menstrual discomfort, insomnia, coughs and colds, hormonal imbalances, to name just a few. Similarly, most nonprescription remedies are used for minor problems.

If you are small, elderly, sensitive to medications, or prone to side effects, you may find that by starting with a low dosage, you may not need the higher, standard recommended dosage to obtain relief from nonacute problems. Starting with lower doses allows you to determine the lowest effective dose without immediately resorting to higher doses than actually necessary. And by starting with a lower dose, you reduce your risk of side effects.

WHEN A LOW-DOSE APPROACH SHOULD NOT BE USED

Using a low-dose approach sometimes takes time to arrive at the proper dosage, but time is not a luxury in every circumstance. In acute or severe medical situations, rapidly controlling the condition takes precedence. Severe hypertension, sepsis (blood infection), extreme pain, uncontrollable anxiety, serious injuries, deep depression, severe inflammatory disorders, and major cardiac, pulmonary, and renal conditions are among those that require immediate, intensive treatment. In these situations, full doses are usually the surest way to ensure adequate treatment within the shortest period of time, although even here physicians differ over what is enough treatment and what is too much. When the crisis is controlled and the situation stabilized, a reduction in medication dosage to maintenance levels may then be possible. This is often the case, for example, in the treatment of ulcers and sometimes hypertension.

Even in a crisis, however, careful dosaging is still necessary. Overmedication won't help the situation. Your physician must still match the medication not only with the illness but with you, the patient. If you are medication-sensitive or small or elderly or taking other drugs, the standard recommended doses may be too high even for an acute problem. If you are medication-sensitive, selecting the best drug and dosage in an acute situation can be challenging, requiring not only deliberation but also careful follow-up and, often, dosage adjustments. Physicians who have a healthy respect for side effects will rarely overlook them.

The use of antibiotics can also be especially problematic with those who are sensitive to medications. The purpose of antibiotics is not to directly reduce your symptoms or balance your physiology, but to eradicate invasive bacteria or other microorganisms. In this situation, it is the bacteria's sensitivity that is the key to cure. But your tolerance to the drug is also a factor and must also be weighed against the need to get enough antibiotic into your body to ward off the infection. Antibiotic dosages tend to be fairly standard. Yet even here, studies show that the blood levels from a specific dose of some antibiotics may vary from 100% to 200% or more from individual to individual. So, at least with less severe infections, there may be some opportunity to work with the lower ranges of recommended antibiotic doses.

LOW-DOSE TREATMENT UTILIZING NONPRESCRIPTION REMEDIES

Over the last few years, there has been a surge of newly released nonprescription drugs that had previously been available only by prescription—and only at higher doses. These newcomers to the already crowded drugstore shelves include Zantac 75, Tagamet HB, Pepcid AC, Aleve, and Orudis KT. Several older nonprescription remedies, such as Benadryl, Tavist, and the various forms of ibuprofen (Motrin IB, Nuprin, Advil, and others) also have prescription-only origins.

Although some physicians do recommend lower-dose nonprescription remedies in selected situations, from what I've seen, most physicians don't. This is probably because they are unaware of the surprising effectiveness of nonprescription doses, particularly in medication-sensitive people. Another reason may be that the medical literature makes little mention of nonprescription drugs and the valid role they can play in many conditions. For instance, many drug references emphasize the importance of using the very lowest effective doses of anti-inflammatory drugs, but nonprescription doses of these drugs are rarely recommended.

There's also an important transactional aspect to the giving of a prescription. Doctors feel that their patients expect prescriptions, not suggestions for nonprescription remedies patients can easily obtain for themselves. This feeling isn't misguided. I've heard patients complain when doctors have recommended a nonprescription remedy for colds or the flu instead of writing a prescription for an antibiotic.

Yet although some patients expect a prescription from their physician and many physicians sense that expectation, the terms of the doctor-patient interaction aren't written in stone. If you are medication-sensitive, if you are concerned about side effects and prefer to initiate medication treatment at the lowest possible dose, share your views with your physician. Tell your physician that if the type of remedy you require is available in a low-dose nonprescription form, you'd prefer to start there. With his support, it's easy enough to increase the dosage or obtain a prescription if the nonprescription dose is insufficient.

The many medications that are now available in nonprescription sizes offer you and your physician expanded flexibility in the treatment of many conditions. They also allow for dose adjustments in smaller, more gradual gradations. (They are also much cheaper.) Using lower doses and increasing by smaller gradations—these are the keys to reducing the risk of medication side effects.

NEW NONPRESCRIPTION REMEDIES = ADDITIONAL NEED FOR CAUTION

The downside of the increasing array of nonprescription drugs is that their easy accessibility may lull us into a false sense that these drugs are quite safe and free of serious side effects. This isn't the case. For instance, Motrin IB and other forms of ibuprofen, Aleve, and Orudis KT, like aspirin, all can cause gastric irritation and bleeding, or kidney damage, especially with frequent usage. The risk may be reduced at nonprescription doses, but it still exists.

Yet the availability of these drugs without prescription and the extensive advertising extolling their usage for a wide variety of symptoms may give us the impression that these drugs are benign. I've known people who take ibuprofen almost daily for headaches or other symptoms for which ibuprofen offers no advantages over acetaminophen (Tylenol), which most physicians believe to be a much safer drug.

Again, interindividual variation is the determinant. For example, for headaches Tylenol works better for some people, ibuprofen or Aleve or others work better for others. Taken infrequently, all of these medications usually are safe. Taken frequently or daily, ibuprofen and other anti-inflammatory drugs, even at nonprescription doses, may entail considerable risks.

Lately there's been a lot of advertising directed at influencing parents to use ibuprofen or other anti-inflammatory drugs for treating fever in children. Yet acetaminophen is just as effective in reducing fever and much less likely to cause stomach irritation, especially in a child with an upset stomach.

Anti-inflammatory drugs such as Motrin IB, Advil, Nuprin, Aleve, and Orudis KT are clearly superior to Tylenol in the treatment of muscle strains, bursitis, tendinitis, and similar injuries and conditions that involve inflammation. But for simple pain or fever, Tylenol is usually as effective and generally preferred by physicians. Furthermore, the frequent usage of anti-inflammatory drugs is associated with an increased incidence toward gastric irritation, ulcers, internal bleeding, and death. Lower dosages reduce the degree of risk, but with frequent usage, the risk increases. Even Tylenol has its disadvantages. When used in large quantities for long periods, Tylenol has been associated with an increased, although still infrequent, incidence of kidney disease.

Whichever nonprescription drug you select, the surest way to avoid provoking side effects is to avoid overusage. Used infrequently, most of these drugs are fairly safe; used frequently, all of them can cause problems.

A LOW-DOSE APPROACH THAT'S ALREADY WIDELY USED

The low-dose approach advocated in this book isn't entirely new to the medical community. For years, some physicians have started patients with hypertension on lower than standard doses of antihypertensive drugs. This approach, known as the steppedcare program, entails starting people at low, sometimes so-called subtherapeutic dosages, increasing the dosage very gradually and, if necessary, adding additional medications just as carefully in intransigent cases—in other words, the essence of the "start low, go slow" philosophy. As a hypertension specialist explained to me: "My philosophy's real, real simple. I give just enough to make it work. I usually start by underdosing people. If their hypertension isn't horrible, and if you 'crawl up' with the dosage, you can avoid scaring people by overmedicating them and giving them side effects. Very often their blood vessels relax over a period of time and you wind up ultimately needing less medication."

Despite the commonsense wisdom of this approach, its acceptance is far from universal. Its efficacy has been difficult to prove scientifically because:

1. It doesn't work with every patient (not everyone is medication-sensitive).
2. Because of the variability of response, its efficacy is difficult to establish in clinical studies.
3. It requires more time and, sometimes, extra visits to arrive at the ideal dosage.

For these reasons, the use of a stepped-care approach in treating hypertension, as well as low-dose methods in other medical arenas, has remained controversial. Yet one of the leading textbooks on medical therapeutics, *Conn's Current Therapy 1993*, while acknowledging the limited data on the efficacy of the step program, recommends it anyway: "The stepped-care approach does have one important attribute: it has worked." And when it works, it reduces the incidence of side effects, often the most troublesome aspect of antihypertensive treatment.

You see, all medical science, all previous knowledge and experience in medicine, ultimately converge at one point: the meeting of the physician and you, the patient. In that single interaction, do we take all we know and try to fit you into our already preset methods and doses? Or do we try to fit our doses to you?

The respected textbook *Melmon and Morrelli's Clinical Pharmacology: Basic Principles in Therapeutics* makes a point of emphasizing that clinical studies may not be relevant to an individual case, because different people will respond differently to the same drug. Such interindividual variation isn't a rarity—it's the norm. Indeed, in the conclusion of this textbook, this fact is pointedly underscored: "The thrust of this book is to reemphasize that given a particular antianginal, antihypertensive, antiparkinsonian, antiasthmatic (and so on) agent, different patients respond differently."

Perhaps a firm validation of the stepped-care approach to hypertension has been elusive, but this really isn't surprising because the number of people intolerant of the standard doses of a specific medication may be a minority. Scientifically validating a medication or treatment approach that may be effective for 30% to

40% of the population can be difficult, but that doesn't mean the method isn't worthwhile.

Interindividual variation is unquestionably a real phenomenon. And different people with the same condition will respond to different doses of medication. And some people are definitely medication-sensitive. Yet when I asked the hypertension specialist quoted above whether his peers shared his enthusiasm for the step-care approach, he replied: "Most physicians don't use such low doses in treating hypertension. It takes time to explain. It's not very time efficient."

But neither is provoking side effects and then having to deal with them. Or having people drop out of treatment only to return years later in medical crisis, an unfortunately common occurrence with hypertensive individuals. This is the reason that over the last few years, some authorities on hypertension have begun to recommend an alternative approach that reduces the risk of side effects. They are suggesting that the traditional approach of increasing a single antihypertensive drug higher and higher to control the condition causes too many side effects. Instead, they now advocate an approach that utilizes very low doses of two or three medications, thereby obtaining a cumulative antihypertensive effect while provoking far fewer side effects. This approach is discussed at greater length in Chapter 12.

USING SIDE EFFECTS AS A GUIDE

If you know you have a particular sensitivity such as sedation with alcohol or cold remedies, or overstimulation or anxiety with coffee or other stimulants, sharing this knowledge with your physician should allow you to avoid other medications that provoke similar side-effect tendencies. This strategy was discussed in Chapter 1, and the pages 19–22 in that chapter list medications that may cause sedation or anxiety/insomnia.

Advising your physician of your personal tendencies can help avoid unnecessary adverse drug reactions. Many medications are prone to causing constipation, headaches, dizziness, blurred vision, diarrhea, ringing in the ears, stomach upset, or other mild but bothersome effects. If you already have a tendency toward one of these, it's wise to avoid medications that may exacerbate it.

AVOIDING CONFUSION OVER DOSES AND INGREDIENTS

Do you sometimes find yourself standing in front of a row of remedies in the drugstore, unable to choose between 325-mg Tylenol, 200-mg Motrin IB, Advil, Nuprin, generic ibuprofen, and 12.5-mg Orudis KT? Or trying to choose between a cold or allergy remedy that contains the one medication you most need or another that contains four different ingredients that might handle all of your symptoms and then some. Television advertisements don't help. One states that Orudis KT is more powerful because only 12.5 mg of the drug is needed, but another claims that Nuprin or Advil offer more medication for your money because they contain 200 mg in each pill. Of course, Tylenol contains even more—325 mg per regular-strength pill and 500 mg with the extra-strength variety.

These claims are at the very least confusing, and at the worst misleading. Drugs are big business. Objectivity is not the goal of advertising; attracting your dollar is.

The fact is that Orudis KT, Aleve, ibuprofen, and aspirin have fairly similar effects. The differences are more a matter of personal preference, ease of dosage, and cost. Here, too, interindividual variation plays a role, for your response to each of these medications may be different from another's. You may find that one of these drugs is more effective or more prone to causing you side effects than another.

Over the years I've had patients swear that for them Tylenol, ibuprofen, aspirin, or Excedrin (aspirin and caffeine), etc., is the most effective nonprescription pain reliever. I've heard similar testimonials about Contac, Sudafed, Tavist, Comtrex, and many others. The difference in preference is amazing. Whichever medication you select, understand that even though it is available without a prescription, it still can cause side effects, especially if used frequently. That's why selecting the safest, most appropriate drug and utilizing the lowest effective dose is of primary importance.

WHICH IS BETTER: SHORT-ACTING OR LONG-ACTING MEDICATIONS?

Another area of confusion is whether to use short-acting or long-acting prescription and nonprescription remedies. There is no inherent superiority to either approach, but the specific condition and situation may make one preferable.

Long-acting drugs are more convenient to take and easier to remember. Studies have shown that the less often a medication has to be taken, the less often it's forgotten. For serious conditions that require ongoing medication treatment, you may find that taking a long-acting drug once or twice a day is easier to remember and therefore assures consistent treatment.

On the other hand, short-acting drugs allow you to adjust the dose more easily and quickly according to your body's needs. This can be an advantage with conditions that don't require constant treatment and that allow for dose manipulation. Short-acting drugs also exit your system sooner, an advantage if you encounter side effects.

THE BOTTOM LINE ON LOW-DOSE MEDICATION THERAPY

Not every person prescribed low-dose treatment will respond adequately. Some people will ultimately require higher dosages. But some won't. Unless you are given the opportunity to try lower dosages when appropriate, you'll never know whether you might have responded. Medication-sensitive people often respond to lower dosages.

Remember, the key issue here is avoiding side effects. With almost any drug, the risks of side effects increase with the dose— about this there's no debate. And since most conditions are non-acute, there's little to lose and much to gain from first trying lower doses when the situation allows.

Even if you eventually need higher doses, the ''start low, go slow'' approach offers advantages. It takes time for some people's systems to adjust to medications. Initiating treatment with lower doses allows your system to adapt gradually as doses are increased. This in turn reduces the risk of adverse reactions.

In addition, by starting low and, if necessary, adjusting the dose gradually, you will know that you are taking the amount of medication your body needs, and no more. Considering that all medications are foreign chemicals that exert powerful effects on our bodies, and that side effects are a frequent and sometimes serious result of drug therapy, it's reassuring to know that you are using the lowest amount of medication necessary.

PART 2

Medications for the Treatment of
Psychiatric Disorders

SIX

✑

Antidepressants

Treatment should be initiated with very low dosages because patients are often apprehensive about medication and exquisitely sensitive to side effects.

—R. B. Lydiard and J. C. Ballenger,
Journal of Affective Disorders

In-Depth Analyses

SSRI Antidepressants
    Prozac (Fluoxetine)
    Paxil (Paroxetine)
    Serzone (Nefazodone)
    Zoloft (Sertraline)
Others
    Effexor (Venlafaxine)
    Wellbutrin (Bupropion)

Additional Medications

SSRI Antidepressants
    Luvox (Fluvoxamine)
    Desyrel (trazodone)

Tricyclics Antidepressants
    Anafranil (clomipramine)
    Elavil (amitriptyline)

Additional Medications (cont'd)

Norpramin (desipramine)
Pamelor (nortriptyline)
Parnate (tranylcypromine)
Sinequan, Adapin (Doxephin)
Tofranil (imipramine)

Brief Comments

Asendin (amoxapine)
Ludiomil (maprotiline)
Remeron (mirtazapine)
Nardil (phenelzine)
Vivactil (protriptyline)

About Depression and Antidepressant Medications

Over the last decade, one of the most revolutionary advances in medication therapy has occurred in the treatment of depression. Since the introduction of Prozac in 1988, a succession of remarkably effective drugs have been released (see page 83) that have not only improved doctors' ability to treat depressive disorders, but also have shown promise in anxiety/panic/agoraphobia disorders, premenstrual stress syndrome (PMS), social phobias, obsessive-compulsive disorders, pain syndromes, post-traumatic stress syndrome, postpartum depression, bulimia, anorexia, and a continually expanding list of other problems.

Before initiating antidepressant drug therapy, other causes of depression must be ruled out. Infections, central nervous system diseases, thyroid disorders, and heart, liver or kidney ailments can be the cause of depression-like symptoms. Depression can also be a side effect of medications such as Tenormin, Lopressor, Inderal, sedatives, sleep medications, and sedating antihistamines. These possibilities should be considered before antidepressant drugs are prescribed.

HOW ANTIDEPRESSANTS WORK

Antidepressants work by improving nerve transmission within the emotion centers of the brain. These drugs accomplish this by optimizing the amount of specific chemicals, called neurotransmitters, that are required for the normal transmission of impulses between nerves. The brain utilizes many types of neurotransmitters. Antidepressant drugs work by increasing the reservoirs of serotonin and norepinephrine, the two primary neurotransmitters that are thought to be deficient in depressive disorders.

Types of Antidepressant Medications and the Neurotransmitters They Enhance

S = serotonin; N = norepinephrine

New-Generation Antidepressants
Selective serotonin reuptake inhibitors (SSRIs)

Paxil (paroxetine)	S
Prozac (fluoxetine)	S
Luvox (fluvoxamine)	S
Serzone (nefazodone)	S
Zoloft (sertraline)	S

Others

Effexor (venlafaxine)	N and S
Remeron (mirtazapine)	N and S
Wellbutrin (bupropion)	N

First-Generation (Older) Antidepressants: Except for Anafranil, most of these drugs primarily increase norepinephrine in the brain, but some also increase serotonin to a lesser degree.

Tricyclics

Anafranil (clomipramine)	S
Elavil (Endep, amitriptyline)	N
Norpramin (desipramine)	N

Pamelor (Aventyl, nortriptyline)	N
Sinequan (Adapin, doxepin)	N
Surmontil (trimipramine)	N
Tofranil (imipramine)	N
Vivactil (protriptyline)	N
Monamine oxidase inhibitors (MAOIs)	
Nardil (phenelzine)	N
Parnate (tranylcypromine)	N
Others	
Desyrel (trazodone)	S
Asendin (amoxapine)	N
Ludiomil (maprotiline)	N

INTERINDIVIDUAL VARIATION AND ANTIDEPRESSANT MEDICATIONS

As discussed earlier, a wide range of individual variation is seen when people take the same dose of the same drug. With antidepressants, this variability can be enormous, up to 40-fold (that's 4,000%) or greater. People have been known to respond to doses as low as 1 mg a day or as high as 80 mg a day of Prozac.

Unfortunately, the dose ranges recommended for most antidepressants are much narrower. This means, as a 1993 article commented, ''Treating all patients with standard dosing regimens can result in either undermedication or toxicity for many.''

Alert physicians quickly learn to use antidepressant drugs flexibly, selecting doses on a case-by-case basis. They learn not to rely solely on the PDR, which omits much of the low-dose data. As one physician put it: ''In most cases, I start adult patients at 10 mg of Prozac, or 25 mg of Zoloft, or 10 mg of Paxil.'' These doses are all 50% lower than the starting doses recommended in the PDR.

And in some medication-sensitive individuals, even these low doses may be too high. As mentioned, a small percentage of patients respond to 1 or 2 mg a day of Prozac; at even slightly higher doses they develop side effects. The physician quoted above told me of a patient, a hard-working dentist, who couldn't tolerate 2.5 mg a day of Paxil, one-eighth the standard starting dosage. The man did tolerate 10 mg a day of Pamelor (manufacturer-recommended dosage, 75 to 100 mg a day), and his depression responded well when the dose was increased to 15 mg a day.

"Dosage is an art form," stated a psychiatrist quoted in a psychiatry newsletter. "There is really very little scientific basis to making a guess at what dose somebody is going to do well on." Yet, if you have informed your physician that you are medication-sensitive or are concerned about drug side effects, starting antidepressant treatment at lower than recommended doses makes a lot of sense.

DIFFERENT DISORDERS, DIFFERENT DOSES

If you consult the dosage guidelines for most antidepressants in the PDR, you'll find a recommended starting dose and a dose range. For example, the PDR recommends 20 mg of Paxil as the starting dose for most patients, and a dose range of 20 to 50 mg. But most guidelines fail to mention an important fact: these recommended doses are usually specific for one type of depression, a severe condition known as major depressive disorder. They also fail to mention that many of the other disorders for which antidepressants are prescribed may require different, often lower, doses.

The reason for this is that most antidepressants are FDA approved for treating only one or two conditions, so the doses and data are limited to these disorders. Physicians, however, use these same drugs for many other conditions. Over time, a wealth of information has accrued from case reports and studies involving other uses of antidepressants, but little of this data make their way into the PDR—yet it's to the PDR that doctors most often turn for dosage guidelines.

For example, many physicians aren't aware that individuals with a mild type of depression, dysthymic disorder, often respond to lower than standard doses of antidepressants. Dosages such as 25 mg twice a day of Effexor, 10 mg of Paxil, 10 mg of Prozac, or 50 mg of Serzone can be quite effective. Dysthymic disorder is a mild but chronic condition that makes it difficult to enjoy life or fulfill one's potential. It's the most common form of medical depression, yet few if any manufacturers involve dysthymic patients when developing new drugs. Major depression, a more severe disorder, is easier to study—and usually requires higher dosages. The recommended antidepressant dosages in the PDR are for major depression, but this usually isn't made clear in the dosage guidelines. Thus, many physicians prescribe these same dosages to dysthymic individuals (or those with reactive depressions or seasonal affective disorder). The result is that a large proportion of these people get overmedicated. In some cases, the side effects are severe and the individual withdraws from treatment—a shame, considering that a milder dose of the very same medicine may have completely resolved the disorder.

Panic disorder is a condition that frequently requires extremely low initial antidepressant doses. People with this condition seem to be unusually sensitive to the effects and side effects of antidepressants of all types. Panic patients often show a quick response to Prozac 2.5 to 5 mg a day or imipramine 10 mg a day or Effexor 18.75 mg twice a day, or Paxil, Zoloft, Pamelor, or Norpramin in similarly low dosages. Serzone starting at 25 mg twice daily is also effective and usually causes neither the anxiety and insomnia seen with other antidepressants. In time, most panic patients develop some tolerance to these drugs and can take gradually increased dosages, but they rarely require the full dosages recommended in the PDR for depression.

HIGH OR LOW ANTIDEPRESSANT DOSES?

For decades, psychiatrists have debated the efficacy of higher versus lower doses of antidepressant drugs. Some argue that lower doses are inadequate for many patients, while others counter that higher doses cause too many side effects. It's an old debate that has never been resolved because both goals, prescribing adequate doses yet avoiding unnecessary side effects, are important.

The problem was underscored in a 1988 study comparing Zoloft and Elavil. Subjects were started on low doses and gradually increased toward target doses, which with Elavil was 150 mg a day, an amount some consider the minimum for an antidepressant effect, but others consider high. In this study, only 8% of the subjects were able to reach the 150-mg dose of Elavil; some couldn't tolerate even 40 mg a day, a dose well below the manufacturer's recommended initial dose. Yet others did reach 75, 100, 125, and 150 mg a day. In essence, the study found that with Elavil some subjects required very low doses of Elavil, others moderate doses, and others the full 150 mg a day dose.

This diversity of response isn't really surprising considering the known wide range of interindividual variation seen with Elavil and other antidepressants. Thus, the best approach isn't necessarily low-dose or high-dose, but instead one that offers flexibility. One that, as suggested in a 1995 study entitled "Minimizing and Managing Antidepressant Side Effects," uses "the lowest effective antidepressant dose for a given individual. . . . initiating antidepressants at lower rather than higher doses and titrating the dose upward according to tolerability and response."

SIDE EFFECTS WITH ANTIDEPRESSANTS

The popularity of the newer antidepressants is due not only to their greater effectiveness in a wide range of disorders, but also their improved side effect profiles. That's not to say that side effects occur infrequently; in fact, antidepressants still rank as one of the groups of drugs most prone to side effects. For example, in a 1996 study, 58% of patients given antidepressants developed side effects, despite the fact that only newer antidepressants were used.

The list of side effects in the PDR for any antidepressant drug is daunting. Headaches, nausea/vomiting, insomnia, agitation/anxiety, constipation, dizziness, sedation, excessive sweating, dry mouth—each of these occurs in more than 20% of patients taking many of these drugs. A dropout rate of 20% due to side effects is not unusual.

It makes sense that except in severe conditions, antidepressant drugs should be initiated cautiously, starting with low doses in order to avoid unnecessary side effects that often complicate or terminate treatment. A 1997 report from the respected *Medical Letter on Drugs and Therapeutics* concurred: "Jitteriness and insomnia [with Prozac, Paxil, Zoloft, and others] early in treatment can be minimized by beginning with low doses.''

ANTIDEPRESSANTS AND SEXUAL DYSFUNCTION

Sexual dysfunctions are common with several groups of antidepressants, particularly the SSRIs and tricyclics. Dysfunctions include diminished or absent sexual drive, delayed ability or inability to reach orgasm, impaired ability for male erection. There have also been infrequent reports of reduced sensation in the penile or vaginal areas.

When Prozac and subsequent SSRIs were first released, the incidence of sexual dysfunctions was downplayed. Initial estimates of these problems often were listed as far less than 10%. A 1997 study has shown that when based on spontaneous reports, the recorded incidence of sexual dysfunctions with Prozac was 9%, with Paxil 11%, and with Zoloft 19%. But when measured by a specific questionnaire or direct interview, the rates jumped to 50%, 47%, and 39%, respectively. These latter figures match what many practitioners have long insisted—that sexual dysfunctions occur in 50% or more of patients taking SSRIs.

In recent years, antidepressant-related sexual dysfunctions have become more widely recognized because they cause many patients to discontinue treatment. Because these dysfunctions are dose-related, the first approach should be an attempt to lower the antidepressant dosage, if possible. Reducing the amount only a bit, such as from 20 mg to 15 mg of Prozac, may make a big difference.

If dose reduction is impossible or ineffective, the next step is usually to switch to an antidepressant such as Wellbutrin that doesn't cause these problems. Switching often works, but if you are doing well on Prozac, Zoloft, or another SSRI, there's no guarantee you'll do as well on a different type of antidepressant, or that switching will be an easy process. For this reason, the psychiatric community has long sought a treatment that might prevent SSRI-related sexual dysfunctions without altering their antidepressant effects. Unfortunately, no such treatment was readily found.

In 1997, an unexpected potential solution was announced at the annual meeting of the American Psychiatric Association. Dr. Alan J. Cohen reported that in a small open trial, ginkgo biloba, an herbal compound found at most health stores, alleviated erectile failure, anorgasmia, or diminished libido in 30 out of 33 (91%) women and 23 out of 30 (76%) men. The overall effectiveness was 84%.

Purported to improve overall blood flow to various parts of the body, ginkgo is touted for improving memory problems and decreasing mental confusion, dizziness, ringing in the ears (tinnitus), and circulatory problems to the arms or legs.

In Dr. Cohen's trial, patients were typically started at 60 mg twice a day of ginkgo. The dose was increased as necessary to 120 mg twice a day, up to a maximum dose of 420 mg a day. The average dose was slightly above 200 mg a day—apparently most people improved at 90 or 120 mg twice a day.

Ginkgo can cause side effects including gastric upset, gas, diarrhea, and light-headedness. It is said to decrease the clotting ability of blood platelets and therefore should be used carefully with other anticoagulant drugs such as aspirin and Coumadin (warfarin).

More rigorous trials are necessary to confirm Dr. Cohen's findings. Yet this report is encouraging because it follows other reports of using ginkgo biloba successfully to treated impotence. Because ginkgo is readily available and generally considered safe, there's little reason not to try this approach for antidepressant-related sexual dysfunctions.

DIFFERENT SIDE EFFECT TENDENCIES OF DIFFERENT ANTIDEPRESSANTS

The best way to minimize side effects is by choosing the drug and the dose that is least likely to produce problems for you. This can be accomplished by matching the side effect profile of specific antidepressants with your side effect history.

For example, some antidepressants are prone to causing agitation and insomnia, whereas others are more likely to produce sedation (see page 90). The former group is preferable if your depression includes symptoms of sluggishness or low energy, whereas the latter group works better if you are experiencing anxiety or insomnia.

Antidepressant Sedating/ Energizing Tendencies

ANTIDEPRESSANTS THAT MAY (BUT DON'T ALWAYS) CAUSE SEDATION.

These medications should be prescribed cautiously in disorders with symptoms including low energy or increased sleep, but they can be very beneficial in conditions associated with anxiety or insomnia.

Elavil (amitriptyline)
Desyrel (trazodone)
Ludiomil (maprotiline)
Luvox (fluvoxamine): Sedating/energizing effect variable
Pamelor (Aventyl, nortriptyline)
Paxil (paroxetine): Sedating/energizing effect variable
Remeron (mirtazapine)
Serzone (nefazodone)
Sinequan, Adapin (doxepin)
Tofranil (imipramine): Sedating/energizing effect variable; often causes agitation in panic patients

ANTIDEPRESSANTS THAT MAY (BUT DON'T ALWAYS) CAUSE AGITATION, NERVOUSNESS, OR INSOMNIA.

These medications should be prescribed cautiously in conditions with symptoms of anxiety or insomnia, but they can be beneficial in conditions with low energy or excessive sleeping.

Anafranil (clomipramine)
Effexor (venlafaxine)
Luvox (fluvoxamine): Sedating/energizing effect variable
Nardil (phenelzine)
Norpramin (desipramine)
Parnate (tranylcypromine)
Paxil (paroxetine): Sedating/energizing effect variable
Prozac (fluoxetine)
Tofranil (imipramine): Sedating/energizing effect variable; often causes agitation in panic patients
Vivactil (protriptyline)
Wellbutrin (bupropion)
Zoloft (sertraline)

MIXING ANTIDEPRESSANT MEDICATIONS

In the occasional case that doesn't respond to treatment despite attempts with a number of antidepressants, a good result can sometimes be obtained by combining the effects of two different drugs. This is a delicate maneuver that requires the expertise of a highly experienced psychopharmacologist (a psychiatrist or other physician who works extensively with psychiatric medications). Mixing the wrong medications, or even the correct drugs but in too high a dosage, can provoke serious side effects. One such reaction is the serotonin syndrome, due to an excessive accumulation of serotonin in the brain. Symptoms include increased heart rate and blood pressure, nausea, vomiting, agitation, diarrhea, confusion, and in severe cases, delirium, seizures, and coma. This reaction is seen when two serotonergic drugs are combined, or one serotonergic drug and an MAOI antidepressant, or a serotonergic drug and the diet medication Pondimin.

ANTIDEPRESSANTS AND THE ELDERLY

Depression is a common and often serious illness among the elderly. Treatment combining psychological, social, and medication therapies can be highly effective.

Many seniors are extremely sensitive to antidepressant drug effects because they metabolize antidepressant drugs more slowly and therefore develop higher blood levels of the medication than younger persons. For example, in the elderly, Paxil can reach up to three times the maximum blood level as compared with younger adults. Similar increases in blood levels and drug duration of action are seen with other antidepressants. For this reason, many elderly patients do well on very low doses.

ARE ANTIDEPRESSANTS ADDICTIVE?

Questions about addiction, tolerance, and dependence invariably arise when people are told they require antidepressant treatment. Addiction means craving, as seen in the cases of alcohol, cocaine, and heroin—but not antidepressants. Depressed individuals don't crave antidepressant drugs; they just want to feel better. In fact, rather than crave antidepressants, many people taking them dislike having to rely upon a medication to feel "normal." It's just the same as diabetics who dislike relying on insulin and hypertensives who dislike needing their antihypertensive drugs.

Antidepressants aren't mood elevators or uppers. Normal individuals taking an antidepressant obtain no high or feeling of euphoria. Instead, most simply get side effects. Antidepressants work only in those who are deficient in neurotransmitters, just as insulin helps only those deficient in their own production of insulin. And just as with insulin, discontinuation of antidepressants should be done gradually. Abrupt discontinuation may cause withdrawal phenomena in some people, producing symptoms such as low energy or sluggishness, dizziness, numbness or tingling in the limbs, vivid dreams, irritability, lowered mood, nausea, anxiety, or tremors.

Minor degrees of tolerance may occur with antidepressant drugs, as it does with many types of medications. This is usually due to the body's enhanced metabolism of the drug, not to the sudden development of addiction. Minor adjustments of dosage upward or downward are occasionally necessary.

Some types of depression require continuing treatment. This is no different from many cases of heart disease, hypertension, diabetes, arthritis, or seizures. Unfortunately, many people with psychiatric disorders equate the need for medication with a failure to cope. This is no more true than with medical disorders. The need to take antidepressant medication is an issue of neurochemistry, not of character or willpower.

DOING WELL WITH ANTIDEPRESSANTS

Antidepressants are very effective medicines that when used properly produce a high rate of success. Yet antidepressants are also notorious for causing a high incidence of side effects. Therefore, the difference between success and failure depends on how these drugs are utilized. The best approach was articulated to me by the medical director of a psychiatric hospital in North Carolina: "When antidepressant treatment fails, it's usually the doctor's fault, not the patient's. I always explain to my patients that there are six groups of antidepressants, and several members in each group. There are no blood tests to guide treatment, so I'm choosing the one I think will work, but it might not and we may have to try others. I explain that I am starting with the lowest doses in order to test their sensitivity and minimize side effects. I discuss specific doses with my patients and involve them in the decisions. Because they understand the process and are participants in the decisions, most patients are very cooperative and do well."

Antidepressant treatment is a long-term process, lasting at least six to twelve months. Because finding the best medication at the best dose may take time, good communication between patient and physician is required. With a thorough understanding of the medication sensitivities of each individual and the differences between antidepressant drugs, side effects can be minimized or avoided, and antidepressant drug therapy can be exceedingly successful.

In-Depth Analysis: Prozac (Fluoxetine)

VERY EFFECTIVE, BUT NOT ALWAYS BENIGN

Standard doses of fluoxetine [Prozac] may be higher than "optimum."

—J. W. Cain, *Journal of Clinical Psychiatry*

America's and the world's best-selling antidepressant drug, Prozac has received more attention than any medication in recent memory. Much of this attention is deserved, for Prozac is a very effective drug, a giant step forward in the treatment of depression and other disorders. This is why 1 million prescriptions for Prozac are written monthly worldwide, netting $1 billion per year for its manufacturer.

Yet Prozac has also caused problems. From the start it was obvious that Prozac wasn't benign. When it was released for general usage in the United States in 1988, its manufacturer acknowledged an overall 38% rate of side effects—that's more than one in three patients, a high ratio. Since 1988, new side effects have been identified and higher rates of already recognized side effects have been uncovered. Table 6.1 lists the manufacturer-acknowledged incidence of the most common side effects with Prozac, all of which are dose-related. Many of these reactions can be severe, and even when mild they can be distinctly unpleasant. And according to many practicing physicians, the listed incidences may be underestimates.

Table 6.1. Prozac's Most Common Side Effects
(Percent of subjects reporting the following adverse reactions to Prozac; adapted from the 1996 PDR)

	DEPRESSION STUDIES	OBSESSIVE-COMPULSIVE DISORDER STUDIES
Headache	20.3%	33%
Nervousness/anxiety	24.3%	16%
Insomnia	13.8%	30%
Drowsiness	11.6%	Not Listed
Asthenia/low energy	4.4%	15%
Tremor	7.9%	9%
Decreased libido	1.6%	11%
Sexual impotence	1.7%	Not Listed
Abnormal ejaculation	Not Listed	7%
Sexual dysfunction	1.9%	Not Listed
Nausea	21.1%	27%
Diarrhea	12.3%	18%
Loss of appetite	8.7%	17%
Excessive sweating	8.4%	7%

If we consider just the known rate of side effects, it's not surprising that studies have revealed a high dropout rate with Prozac. One study reported: "Of the 27 patients with both depression and panic disorder, [only] 13 tolerated the full 20 mg dose of fluoxetine [Prozac] without any problems."

TOO MUCH OF A GOOD THING?

When Prozac was first released, 20 mg a day was the manufacturer-recommended starting dose for everyone. Indeed, the smallest pill was a 20-mg capsule, so lower doses were rarely considered by most physicians.

Today, 20 mg a day remains the manufacturer-recommended

initial Prozac dose for everyone except patients with liver or kidney impairments. Nor do the manufacturer's dosage guidelines take into consideration the 7% of the population that the PDR itself states have deficiencies in one of the enzymes (cytochrome P450 2D6) necessary to metabolize the drug, making them slow metabolizers. Because Prozac will accrue in the blood and tissues and higher levels, these people will be highly vulnerable to side effects with standard dosages.

The experience of myself and others suggests that far more than 7% are sensitive to Prozac. In the study quoted above, less than half of the subjects, who other than their psychiatric disorders were healthy, tolerated the recommended dose. In fact, the authors noted: ''When adverse reactions developed, they were considered so unacceptable that the patients abruptly stopped fluoxetine [Prozac] and refused to try a lower dose.''

With lower doses, these and other side effects are less likely to occur, and if they do, they are usually less severe. But most doctors start their patients on the standard recommended 20-mg Prozac dose, regardless of their size, age, or history of medication sensitivities.

UNUSUAL REACTIONS RAISE
DISTURBING QUESTIONS
ABOUT PROZAC

The issue of dosage becomes even more important when one considers not only the high incidence of side effects, but also the *kinds* of side effects Prozac provokes in some patients. Most controversial is Prozac's association with violent behavior. Bizarre and impulsive attempts at suicide by patients receiving Prozac, although rare, have occurred often enough to raise concerns, including a federal hearing in 1991.

The issue has not been resolved, but some researchers seem convinced that Prozac can cause sudden and acute mental disorganization in certain patients. Many physicians, including me, believe that this reaction is real and related to Prozac's tendency to cause agitation, which in severe instances can cause sufferers to feel they're losing control and to become suicidal.

Recently I was introduced to a man who spent most of the year in Alaska. The reduced sunlight and gloomy weather produced a form of depression known as seasonal affective disorder (SAD). He told me, "I tried Prozac. In a week I was so wired, I became suicidal. I stopped the medication immediately and have never felt that way before or since."

Even in mild cases, Prozac-induced acute agitation can be extremely disruptive. As one therapist related to me: "A mildly depressed patient of mine became acutely agitated on Prozac. Her first thought was to jump in her car and crash it into a wall. She'd never had suicidal thoughts before. She knew it was crazy, but it really shook her up."

Most of Prozac's side effects are mild, but whether mild or severe, nearly all of them are directly related to dosage.

PROZAC AND SEXUAL DYSFUNCTION

One of the least publicized yet greatest problems with Prozac is its tendency to cause sexual dysfunction such as diminished libido (decreased or absent sexual urge), the inhibition of or total inability to achieve orgasm, and male impotence. From 1988 through 1995, while tens of millions were prescribed Prozac, the manufacturer listed the incidence of each of these problems at less than 2%. Meanwhile, studies began to reveal rates as high as 34%, and after considerable experience with Prozac many clinical physicians estimate the rate at 50% or higher.

Finally, in the 1996 PDR, seven years after Prozac's release, the manufacturer added a new side effect chart based on its studies with obsessive-compulsive disorders, in which the rate of Prozac-related sexual dysfunctions is listed at 18%. So now the PDR offers two charts, one based on its studies with depression, listing sexual dysfunctions at a combined rate of less than 6%, and another listing them at 18%. So which rate is to be believed? Or are both numbers gross underestimates based on independent studies and physicians' estimates?

Sexual dysfunctions with antidepressants are dose-related. Reducing the dose even a small amount, such as from 20 to 15 or 10 mg a day of Prozac, may make a difference. Also, as discussed previously, a recent report has suggested that ginkgo biloba, an

herbal preparation, may be highly effective in negating the sexual
dysfunction caused by Prozac and some other antidepressants.

IMPRESSIVE RESULTS WITH LOW-DOSE PROZAC

When Prozac was released in 1988, it came in only one size,
20 mg. Worse, the Prozac pill was a capsule, making dose adjustments virtually impossible. Yet many patients, about 50% of
my caseload, couldn't tolerate 20 mg. They clearly required less
Prozac, a reduction in dose that could be accomplished only by
twisting open the capsules and emptying out some of the contents.
"I feel like I'm using some illicit drug when I have to mess
around with these capsules and dump out half of the powder,"
one patient told me. Yet these hand-fashioned reduced doses of
5, 10, and 15 mg worked for her and many others.

Some patients were able to attain lower doses of Prozac by
taking the medication every other day. Because Prozac is a long-
acting drug, the blood level of Prozac remains high enough to
remain effective on a schedule of every other day. This approach
worked for some, but others simply couldn't tolerate 20 mg of
Prozac taken at one time, even if the medication was skipped the
next day. These patients did much better with 5 or 10 mg on a
daily basis.

Outside the office, several friends of mine, many of them the
spouses of psychiatrists, confided that they were taking Prozac,
and each was taking less than 20 mg a day. Another friend had a
less satisfactory experience. Given the recommended 20 mg by
her physician, within days she developed unbearable side effects
and quit the medication. I suggested that she might have a more
positive result at a lower dose of Prozac, but she wouldn't hear
of it; her experience with Prozac had been that unnerving.

Low-dose Prozac is effective and safer for many people. Yet,
as pointed out earlier, even today none of the data supporting
lower doses of Prozac is offered in the package insert or PDR, so
doctors, over 90% of whom rely on the PDR as their primary
source of medication information, aren't aware of and therefore
don't make use of this alternative. This is the reason that although
Prozac's manufacturer now produces a 10-mg capsule and a Pro-

zac liquid, they aren't prescribed nearly as often as the standard 20-mg dose.

LOW-DOSE PROZAC FOR MILD CONDITIONS AND MEDICATION-SENSITIVE INDIVIDUALS

There is a considerable and growing literature regarding the effectiveness of low-dose Prozac. Typical is a case study in the renowned British journal *The Lancet*. Upon receiving 20 mg a day of Prozac for severe depression, the patient developed restlessness, agitation, nausea, and headaches, as well as a worsening of his depression, suicidal thinking, cognitive impairments, and a sleep disorder. Rather than discontinuing the Prozac, the doctors decreased it to 10 mg a day. The side effects abated, and the patient's condition stabilized.

Noteworthy about this case is that the condition was a very severe depressive disorder, the treatment for which Prozac is officially approved. The manufacturer-recommended dose for this condition is 20 to 80 mg a day. Yet for this individual, the so-called minimum 20-mg Prozac dose was excessive.

This explains why other conditions such as mild depressions (e.g., dysthymic disorders), anxiety/panic disorders, premenstrual stress syndrome, and others often respond to even lower doses. A 1992 journal article recommended starting Prozac at doses as low as 2.5 mg a day for patients with histories of mild depressions or panic disorders. Prozac isn't FDA approved for usage in these conditions, yet doctors often prescribe it anyway because of its high rate of success—often at very low doses.

Year after year, more and more articles and letters appear in the literature supporting the effectiveness and safety of low-dose Prozac. For example, an article in a 1994 issue of the *New England Journal of Medicine* stated, "the results of three dose-effect studies . . . [demonstrated that] a dose of 5 mg per day was as effective as any of the higher doses." Unfortunately, most comments about low-dose Prozac appear in psychiatry journals that aren't read by the majority of physicians.

The diverse uses of Prozac have added to the already considerable confusion regarding the proper doses for physicians to prescribe. Because no pre-release research was done with Prozac in dysthymic or anxiety/panic disorders, the PDR offers no information whatsoever about prescribing Prozac to these patients, many of whom are highly sensitive to antidepressant drugs. Yet because Prozac's PDR dosage guidelines don't say a word about this, many physicians assume that the recommended 20 mg a day applies to all usages, and they initiate treatment with all disorders with that dose. This can be disastrous with milder conditions or medication-sensitive individuals.

EVIDENCE ON THE EFFECTIVENESS OF LOW-DOSE PROZAC BEFORE ITS RELEASE

About the same time that Prozac was released, a study appeared in *Psychopharmacology Bulletin* (J. Wernicke et al.) entitled "Low-Dose Fluoxetine [Prozac] Therapy for Depression." Published in early 1988, this study was likely completed in 1987, before or during the time that the manufacturer sought FDA approval for Prozac at the one-size-fits-all initial 20 mg a day dosage.

The study compared Prozac doses of 5, 20, and 40 mg a day, and a placebo. The results were revealing: 54% of subjects improved on 5 mg a day; 64% on 20 mg a day; 65% on 40 mg a day. These results are close, but they were even closer when you consider that fewer side effects allowed more subjects to complete the study on the 5 mg dose, and because of this the overall number of positive responses (43, 45, and 44 subjects, respectively) was virtually identical (Table 6.2). Thus the authors acknowledged that the differences between 5 mg and the 400% higher dose of 20 mg and the 800% higher 40 mg were minimal.

Moreover, the 5-mg study was brief, just six weeks, a time frame that may have skewed the results in favor of the higher doses. With more time, the 5-mg dose may have performed even better, and 20- and 40-mg doses, as the subjects' blood levels of long-acting Prozac rose, may have caused more side effects.

Furthermore this study was performed on subjects with major depression, a severe type of depressive disorder. The 5-mg dose would likely have performed even better in outpatients with milder conditions, as the authors themselves commented: "No lower limit for an effective dose of [Prozac] has been demonstrated in moderately depressed outpatients.''

Another article addressing lower, safer dosages was published the year of Prozac's release. It reviewed the response rates to various Prozac doses in several studies. The results: 54% rate of response with 5 mg, and 64% and 53% (separate studies) with 20 mg. Equally important, the 5-mg dose caused fewer side effects. Thus, the authors acknowledged: ''The 5 mg dose appears to have been effective in the treatment of depression,'' but then added: ''While this observation of efficacy for the 5 mg dose was made in a large, powerful study, it requires to be confirmed before this dose is generally accepted as effective.''

Table 6.2. Results from the Manufacturer-Sponsored "5 mg Study"
(Adapted from J. Wernicke, et al.,
Psychopharmacology Bulletin, 1988)

PROZAC DOSAGE	NUMBER OF SUBJECTS	RESPONSE RATE
Placebo	78	33%
5 mg/day	96	54%
20 mg/day	96	64%
40 mg/day	93	65%

This study was completed before Prozac was approved by the FDA and released for public usage at an initial recommended dose of 20 mg/day (for everyone!). In this study, the 5 mg/day dose attained a response rate nearly equal to doses 400% and 800% higher. In addition, the 5 mg group had the fewest dropouts, with the highest percentage of subjects successfully completing the study. Nevertheless, Prozac was released in only one size, a 20-mg capsule, making the use of lower doses and gradual dose titration extremely difficult.

Such confirmatory studies do not appear to have been undertaken by the manufacturer. Thus, initiating treatment at a one-size-fits-all dose of 20 mg a day became the recommended approach, and even today none of the impressive low-dose Prozac data is contained in the PDR.

It should be noted that FDA regulations require a new drug to be proven "safe and effective." The regulations don't require that it be the safest. They don't require that it be shown whether lower doses might be safer or equally effective.

So, in the United States, Prozac was approved with its one-size-fits-all 20-mg initial dose. Not all countries agreed. According to Public Citizen's *Health Letter*: "Having noticed that patients responded in a wide range, 5 mg/day–80 mg/day, the Swedish and Norwegian authorities in 1991 refused to give Prozac a license—because it was supplied [only] in a 20 mg size."

NEW POSSIBILITIES, NEW PROBLEMS WITH PROZAC

Although officially approved only for treating major depressive and obsessive-compulsive disorders, Prozac has shown effectiveness in a remarkable range of other conditions. These many new uses have further embellished Prozac's record as one of the breakthrough drugs of this era. At the same time, new problems and side effects have also been identified. Some of these new uses and dangers are listed below.

New Possibilities, New Problems with Prozac

POSSIBILITIES
Premenstrual Disorders (PMS)
Multiple studies have now shown Prozac and other SSRI antidepressants to be effective in treating depressive symptoms related to premenstrual physiologic changes. The most recent data suggest that women should start on the medication at the fourteenth day of the menstrual cycle and con-

tinue until menstruation first begins, but some doctors claim that merely starting Prozac at the first sign of premenstrual depression is sufficient. The ideal dose of Prozac for PMS may vary from woman to woman depending on age, size, and history of medication sensitivities, but many have done well at doses as low as 5 or 10 mg a day. Women interested in trying Prozac for PMS should be aware that Prozac's package insert and PDR write-up offer no guidelines for treating this condition, and that many gynecologists are unaware of the effectiveness of low-dose Prozac. Women concerned about Prozac's side effects and wanting to start with lower doses should request either the 10-mg Prozac pills or the more flexible Prozac liquid. If lower doses prove insufficient, they can easily be adjusted upward under a physician's guidance.

OBSESSIVE-COMPULSIVE DISORDERS

Prozac is also approved for treating obsessive-compulsive disorders. The recommended initial dose is 20 mg a day, but clinicians have found that lower doses work for some individuals.

OTHER CONDITIONS

Studies with Prozac have shown promise in treating: anxiety/panic/agoraphobic disorders, dysthymic and other depressive disorders, post-traumatic stress syndromes, bulimia, anorexia nervosa, narcolepsy, pathological jealousy, and overly aggressive and overly sexual behavior in people with brain damage. In a small study of patients with repetitive deviant sexual fantasies/behaviors (paraphilias), Prozac was effective in doses ranging from 10 to 80 mg a day. And according to a 1997 report, Prozac, when combined with the appetite suppressant Ionamin, may be as effective for weight loss as "fen-phen" without the risks of the serious, sometimes fatal side effects of pulmonary hypertension and heart valve disfigurement seen with fen-phen.

PROBLEMS

PROZAC/DILANTIN TOXICITY

The May 1994 *FDA Medical Bulletin* contained an alert about Prozac's interference with Dilantin's elimination, causing the blood levels of Dilantin to soar an average of 161%. Dilantin toxicity can be dangerous, and several of the patients required hospitalization. Lower Prozac doses would likely cause less interference with Dilantin elimination.

PROZAC WITHDRAWAL PHENOMENA

Evidence is mounting that withdrawal symptoms such as low energy, malaise, headaches, and weakness may occur when Prozac (and other antidepressants) is discontinued abruptly. Lower Prozac doses would likely reduce or eliminate withdrawal tendencies, but it may be wise to taper the dose gradually downward over several weeks.

PROZAC RISKS DURING PREGNANCY

A 1996 study suggests that taking Prozac during pregnancy poses increased risks of birth defects. Also, women taking Prozac during their third trimester appeared to have more premature births than those taking Prozac early or not at all.

And, if Prozac isn't already popular enough, in June 1997, Dr. Michael Anchors reported in a letter to the *Archives of Internal Medicine* of successfully treating of over 550 obese patients with a combination of Prozac and the weight-loss drug Ionamin. Ionamin, when used with Pondimin, became the fleeting weight-loss fad "fen-phen." Fen-phen is no longer approved because of serious pulmonary and heart valve side effects that are attributed to Pondimin, not Ionamin. Pondimin's chemical cousin, Redux, has been withdrawn from the market for similar problems. If Dr.

Anchors's report proves accurate, your local weight-loss clinic many soon be combining Prozac, which doesn't appear to cause the side effects of Pondimin or Redux, with Ionamin. The new combination, as described in Dr. Anchors's report, will be Ionamin (phentermine)–Prozac (fluoxetine), sometimes referred to as "phen-pro." By the way, Dr. Anchors utilized low doses of Prozac—10 mg a day.

LOW-DOSE PROZAC AND THE ELDERLY

For elderly individuals, the manufacturer-recommended initial dose of Prozac is 20 mg a day, the same as for younger adults, except for those with other illnesses or taking other medications. For the latter, the manufacturer recommends a lower dosage, but doesn't offer a specific amount. Nevertheless, this is an improvement—when Prozac was released in 1988, the lowest dosage possible was 20 mg for *everyone*.

Soon after Prozac's release, a 1988 study with older subjects given the 20-mg dose produced a daunting array of side effects: nervousness/anxiety, 34.5%; nausea, 23.5%; dry mouth, 20.6%; tremor 14%; insomnia 14%; excessive sweating 13.2%; drowsiness, 11.8%; dizziness 11%; visual disturbance, 10.3%; upset stomach, 10.3%; and so on. The overall dropout rate in this study was 23.5%, nearly one in four.

Clearly, the 20 mg a day dose is excessive for many healthy elderly persons. That's why 10 mg a day is the initial dose preferred by many physicians when treating the elderly, and even lower doses such as 5 mg for those with histories of medication sensitivities, liver impairment or other illnesses, or taking other medications. Some drug references recommend starting all elderly individuals as low as 5 mg a day.

Even when Prozac was available only as a 20-mg capsule, some doctors were recommending lower doses for the elderly. A 1990 article summarized what many of us were telling our older patients:

> At present, fluoxetine [Prozac] is available in the United States only as a 20-mg capsule. A single daily dose of 20 mg may overmedicate some older depressed patients. Ex-

*perienced geriatric clinicians sometimes advise older pa-
tients to open the capsule and sprinkle small amounts of
fluoxetine in a flavored beverage such as orange juice. Al-
ternatively, the contents of an entire capsule may be dis-
solved in a beverage, but only a portion (such as one
quarter or one half) is consumed each day.*

Reports of Prozac-related slowing of the heart rate have
prompted physicians to be even more cautious with Prozac in the
elderly. Some physicians start with doses as low as 2.5 or 5 mg,
which can now be more easily attained using Prozac liquid.

APPLYING GRADUAL, LOW-DOSE
METHODS WITH INDIVIDUALS
REQUIRING HIGHER PROZAC DOSES

Prozac's inflexible dosing recommendations also handicap physicians when adjusting patients' doses upward. One despondent
patient told me of how Prozac had worked for him at 40 mg, but
over time the effect had waned. His doctor increased the Prozac
to 60 mg, but intolerable side effects developed. The Prozac had
to be discontinued, and the patient lapsed back into depression.

I explained to the patient that over time an individual's blood
level of a drug and his rate of metabolizing it may vary. A slight
adjustment in dose may be required—this is common procedure
with drugs such as digoxin, insulin, and antidepressants. This man
simply needed a bit more than 40 mg of Prozac, not a leap of
50% to 60 mg. But physicians are taught to prescribe Prozac at
20–40–60 mg intervals, jumps of 100% and 50% respectively, and
most physicians follow these recommended guidelines without
considering safer alternatives.

Indeed, the February 1995 *Journal of Clinical Psychiatry* contained an article about depressive patients who initially derived
benefit from 20 mg of Prozac but relapsed while remaining on
that dose. The subjects were then increased to 40 mg of Prozac
with good results—67% improved fully. The study was considered a success, but what about the 33% who didn't improve? What
about the 17% who dropped out because of intolerable side effects? The article said nothing further about these "failures," but

when you think about it, it seems obvious that if 20 mg of Prozac was insufficient and 40 mg too much, an intermediate dose such as 25, 30, or 35 mg may have been ideal.

The 20–40–60 mg Prozac dosing method is the accepted approach within the medical community, but a medication expert told me, "Except in an extremely acute case, I never increase patients directly from 20 to 40 mg of Prozac. I always increase more gradually. It just works better that way for many of them."

He's not alone. As Dr. Sidney Wolfe wrote in his highly successful book, *Worst Pills, Best Pills II,* "Many consultants to *The Medical Letter* think that the manufacturer's dosage recommendations are too high."

PROZAC'S LONG DURATION OF ACTION REQUIRES CAREFUL DOSING

Another reason to start low and increase gradually with Prozac is its long duration of action. Prozac and its active breakdown product, norfluoxetine, linger in the bloodstream for weeks, far longer than any other new-generation antidepressant now available. Consequently the full effect of a daily 20-mg dose of Prozac may not be fully realized for weeks or months, during which time the blood level continues to rise. This tendency is further magnified in the elderly.

The dangers of Prozac accumulation were underscored in an 1992 article that described two patients in whom an initially effective 20 mg a day dose of Prozac began to cause severe side effects over a period of two to seven weeks. Uncertain as to the cause of his patients' regressions, the physician increased the Prozac, but this worsened the problems. Improvement occurred when he realized that long-acting Prozac's level had increased to toxic proportions and he discontinued the drug. After allowing the patients' systems to clear, the Prozac was restarted at a lower dose, with both patients responding favorably at 10 mg a day.

RECOMMENDATIONS FOR MEDICATION-SENSITIVE INDIVIDUALS AND OTHERS INTERESTED IN LOW-DOSE PROZAC

Prozac is a very effective medication with an extraordinary range of uses, which explains its rank of No. 7 on the list of outpatient prescriptions in the United States in 1996. But like all antidepressants, Prozac causes a high incidence of side effects. The key with Prozac is a flexible approach that identifies the very lowest dose needed for a given individual.

People with histories of medication sensitivities, or tendencies toward anxiety or insomnia, or edginess with a cup of coffee, should be started at very low doses, such as 2.5 or 5 mg. Even with patients lacking histories of medication sensitivities, some doctors nevertheless recommend starting no higher than 10 mg, half the PDR-recommended dose, for all but the most severe cases.

The range of individual sensitivity to Prozac is very broad, yet the standard dosing approach remains 20–40–60–80 mg. Replacing this with a more flexible approach encompassing doses and increases as low as 2.5, 5, and 10 mg permits greater flexibility and reduces the risks of side effects.

In-Depth Analysis: Paxil (Paroxetine)

Paxil is a highly effective, top-selling antidepressant belonging to the same family, the SSRIs, as Prozac and Zoloft. Paxil is also used for conditions such as anxiety/panic disorders, social phobias, obsessive-compulsive disorders, PMS, and others, which explains its 1996 ranking of No. 24 in U.S. outpatient prescriptions among all drugs.

Like Prozac, Paxil causes a substantial amount of side effects, but it is still a major improvement over earlier antidepressants such as Elavil and Tofranil. Most of Paxil's side effects are dose related; as Table 6.3 demonstrates, 10 mg of Paxil produces considerably fewer side effects than 20 mg. The overall dropout rate in pre-release studies with Paxil at standard dosages was 23%.

What distinguishes Paxil from other popular antidepressants is that Paxil may cause more sedation but less anxiety, agitation, or insomnia than Prozac or Zoloft, although these latter side effects can also occur with Paxil. Paxil can also cause sexual dysfunction.

The manufacturer-recommended initial dose of Paxil is 20 mg a day; maximum dose, 50 mg a day; 10 mg a day initially is recommended for the elderly, for all seriously ill individuals, and those with severe liver or kidney impairments.

Table 6.3. Paxil Doses and Side Effects
Paxil 10 mg caused significantly fewer side effects than 20 mg, as shown in the manufacturer's own studies.

SIDE EFFECTS	10 MG/DAY	20 MG/DAY
Somnolence	12.7%	18.3%
Asthenia (weakness)	2.9%	10.6%
Excessive sweating	1.0%	6.7%
Dry mouth	10.8%	18.3%
Nausea	14.7%	26.9%
Diarrhea	9.8%	19.2%
Constipation	4.7%	7.7%
Anxiety	2.0%	5.8%
Impotence	1.9%	4.3%
Male genital disorders	3.8%	8.7%

According to the manufacturer (1995 PDR), adverse drug effects caused 21% of all Paxil patients in worldwide clinical trials to discontinue treatment. How many of these people would have obtained a good response at a lower Paxil dosage? This has never been determined.

LOW-DOSE PAXIL

A 45-year-old Ph.D. with dysthymic disorder was switched from Prozac to Paxil because Prozac suppressed her libido. Begun at a low, 10 mg a day dose of Paxil, she gradually was upped to 15 mg, still 25% below the recommended initial dose. Out to dinner with her husband, she became dizzy and nauseated after one and a half glasses of wine. ''I ended up unconscious on the ladies' room floor. I spent the evening in an emergency room.''

Although studies with Paxil and alcohol showed no unusual problems compared to other antidepressants, this woman's experience reminds us that different individuals can respond very differently to even low doses of the same drug. When this woman stopped the Paxil, she experienced withdrawal symptoms of nausea, malaise, and insomnia. Withdrawal symptoms may be dose related—clearly 15 mg a day of Paxil was too much for this person. Tried on several other antidepressants, she finally obtained a good response with a very low dose of Serzone.

According to one of my colleagues, just 5 mg of Paxil was too much for one medication-sensitive patient who became oversedated at that extremely low dose. Ultimately, he did fine on Pamelor at 15 mg a day (the PDR suggests 75 mg a day initially), with 20 mg causing side effects and 10 mg being ineffective.

Why is it that these people had difficulty even at lower doses of Paxil while others do fine at the recommended 20-mg dose or higher? In a study involving people with highly differing rates of drug metabolism, a 25-fold variation in Paxil blood levels was found. In other words, at an identical dose of Paxil, medication-sensitive subjects developed blood levels up to 25 times higher than other subjects. This is why some physicians initiate Paxil treatment at 10 mg, and even lower doses with medication-sensitive individuals.

THE ELDERLY AND PAXIL

The elderly exhibit a wide range of individual variation with Paxil. A 1994 study found that ''in the elderly group, maximum plasma paroxetine [Paxil] concentrations after a single dose were, on average, about three times higher than those in the younger group.'' The elderly also experience a high rate of side effects—partly because older individuals metabolize antidepressants more slowly and develop higher drug blood levels than younger persons.

Unlike Prozac, Paxil is recommended at a reduced initial dosing for *all* elderly patients. The dosage is 10 mg a day and it works satisfactorily for some older individuals. However, with medication-sensitive elderly patients or those at higher risk of side effects, a 5-mg initial dose of Paxil may be considered. ''I start elderly patients at either 5 or 10 mg,'' one physician says. ''It depends on the situation.''

TREATING OTHER CONDITIONS WITH PAXIL

The dose recommendations in the PDR are specific for major depression, a severe depressive disorder. No information is offered about the use of Paxil for mild depressive disorders such as dysthymic disorders, or for other conditions such as panic disorders/agoraphobia or PMS. Experience with other antidepressants in these conditions has shown that many individuals respond to much lower doses. This is particularly true with panic/agoraphobia patients, who may not tolerate initial doses of Paxil above 5 or 10 mg a day.

COST FACTORS

Although cost savings should never be the reason for using a lower dose of any drug, when low-dose Paxil is effective, it can also save money. For example, based on local pharmacy prices in 1997, using 10 mg (half a 20-mg tablet) instead of the manufacturer-recommended initial 20 mg a day saved approximately $360 a year.

RECOMMENDATIONS

Unusually wide variations in dose response are common with antidepressant drugs. Because most Paxil side effects are directly related to dosage, starting low and going slow should be the standard approach with all individuals except in severe cases. If the lower dose proves ineffective, it can be easily and gradually increased per your doctor's instructions. This is exactly what many informed physicians already do, starting with 10 mg a day with most adults and 5 mg a day with high-risk individuals.

In-Depth Analysis: Serzone (Nefazodone)

Unlike other members of the SSRI group, Serzone usually doesn't cause the agitation or insomnia seen with Prozac and Zoloft. And unlike these two drugs and Paxil, Serzone is less prone to causing sexual dysfunctions.

In addition to its antidepressant effect, Serzone, like some other antidepressants, is effective in treating panic disorders and premenstrual stress syndrome (PMS). For panic disorders, Serzone is a good choice because it isn't as likely to cause anxiety or agitation, sometimes a problem with Prozac or Zoloft in panic cases, especially when they are prescribed at the usual recommended doses. On the other hand, Serzone may cause sedation, a side effect that may be of some benefit in people who are anxious or can't sleep. Similarly, Serzone may be useful in weaning people dependent on high doses of Xanax or Valium.

MANUFACTURER-RECOMMENDED DOSES OF SERZONE

The manufacturer-recommended initial dose of Serzone is 100 mg twice a day. Interestingly, the manufacturer notes that for treating major depression, doses of 300 to 600 mg a day are usually needed, but recommends starting at the lower dosage to allow patients' systems to adjust to the medication. A good idea, but according to reports and practicing physicians, even 100 mg twice a day is too much for many patients, often causing sedation or nausea.

MOST FREQUENT SIDE EFFECTS

Serzone's most common side effects are: headache, 36%; dry mouth, 25%; somnolence, 25%; nausea, 22%; dizziness, 17%; constipation, 14%; weakness, 11%; insomnia, 11%. Many of these side effects occur at the beginning of treatment and may disappear over a number of weeks. Serzone is contraindicated with the antihistamines Seldane (terfenadine) and Hismanal (astemizole); problematic interactions may occur with Halcion (triazolam), Xanax (alprazolam), and other benzodiazepines.

LOW-DOSE SERZONE

"Serzone offers a nice alternative to Prozac, Paxil, or Zoloft because it doesn't cause agitation or insomnia," one psychiatrist told me. "But it's not selling well. A lot of doctors have quit prescribing it because half of their patients get sedated at [the manufacturer-recommended initial dose of] 100 mg twice a day. As with a lot of the newer antidepressants, Serzone's manufacturer underestimated the sensitivity of many people to the drug's side effects, especially initially." This explains a dropout rate of 16% in pre-release studies with Serzone.

Indeed, in one study, the subjects were started at 100 mg a day, half the manufacturer-recommended dosage. After three days, those not experiencing side effects were increased to 200 mg a day; the majority stayed at 100 mg. Nevertheless, as the authors stated, "Nearly all patients experienced some side effects": nausea, 23%, headache, 21%, fatigue, 17%; chills or flushing, 15%; dry mouth, 13%; gastrointestinal problems, 13%; insomnia, 11%; agitation, dizziness, or increased appetite, 9%.

Two studies have shown that Serzone is effective at low doses. In contrast to the manufacturer-recommended effective dosage range of 300 to 600 mg a day, these studies demonstrated that as little as 50 mg once or twice daily is effective for some patients.

Although Serzone will be used long-term with many people,

the 1996 PDR notes that the "effectiveness of Serzone in long-term use, that is, for more than 6 to 8 weeks, has not been systematically evaluated in controlled trials." In other words, before Serzone's release it wasn't extensively studied for long-term usage, despite the fact that most patients will take it for many months or years. This lack of long-term experience is another reason to start with the very lowest effective dosage.

THE ELDERLY AND SERZONE

For elderly or debilitated persons, the manufacturer does recommend a lower initial dose of 50 mg twice a day. Based on the frequency of side effects in young adults at this dosage, 25 or 50 mg once daily may be a safer and more tolerable initial dose for older individuals.

RECOMMENDATIONS

The reports discussed above amply demonstrate that the manufacturer-recommended initial dose of 100 mg twice a day of Serzone is too high for many people, even those who aren't medication-sensitive or otherwise at risk for side effects. Even at an initial dose of 100 mg a day, half the manufacturer-recommended amount, a very high proportion of people develop side effects. Therefore, a dose of 50 or even 25 mg once daily may be considered an appropriate initial dose for those who are small, elderly, medication-sensitive or prone to side effects, or those who just want to start with the lowest possible effective dose.

Also, because the manufacturer-recommended dosages for Serzone are gauged for treating major depression, people with milder disorders such as dysthymic disorder, panic/anxiety disorders, or PMS may respond well to lower doses of Serzone. For example, it has been shown that Serzone may have specific pain-reducing effects when used alone or in combination with pain medications. For this purpose, recent reports suggest initiating treatment with doses beginning at 25 mg twice a day.

Many people may need to gradually increase their dose of Serzone to obtain maximum benefit. To minimize the risk of side effects, you may increase by 25 mg or 50 mg at a time. This also will ensure that you are taking only as much medication as necessary for your specific condition. Fortunately, Serzone is made in multiple sizes that allow for flexible dosing: 100- and 150-mg scored tablets, and 200- and 250-mg unscored tablets.

In-Depth Analysis: Zoloft
(Sertraline)

Zoloft is a top-selling antidepressant of the SSRI (selective serotonin reuptake inhibitor) group, the same family as Prozac. Like Prozac, Zoloft is a highly effective antidepressant with a favorable side effect profile compared with older antidepressants such as Elavil and Tofranil; nonetheless Zoloft, like all antidepressants, has a substantial capacity for causing side effects. In addition to its effectiveness for depressive disorders, Zoloft is also prescribed for other conditions such as social phobias, obsessive-compulsive disorders, post-traumatic syndrome, and premenstrual syndrome (PMS).

Zoloft has become the first-choice antidepressant of many physicians because Zoloft doesn't linger in the system nearly as long as Prozac, making treatment and dose adjustment easier and less prone to error. In addition, Zoloft appears to have fewer effects on liver enzymes than Prozac or Paxil, especially at higher dosages. Also, Zoloft doesn't appear to reduce patients' heart rates as seen with Prozac in elderly individuals. For these reasons, Zoloft has quickly risen in U.S. outpatient prescriptions, ranking No. 11 in 1996, just four spots behind Prozac.

According to practitioners, Zoloft's most common troublesome side effects are jitteriness and insomnia, although some individuals develop somnolence or fatigue. The latter side effects can be minimized by taking Zoloft before bedtime. For those developing insomnia, taking Zoloft in the morning may cause less of a problem. Like most of Zoloft's side effects, these problems are dose related and can be reduced or eliminated by using the very lowest effective dose of this medication.

A problem for about 15% of Zoloft users is persistent diarrhea, a side effect that often develops after days or weeks on the medication. Before decreasing an otherwise effective dosage of Zoloft, one journal report suggests that the problem may be simply solved with lactobacillus, the bacteria found in yogurt; lactobacillus capsules or powder can also be purchased at health food stores.

The initial manufacturer-recommended dosage of Zoloft is 50 mg once daily; its usual dose range is 50 to 200 mg a day. Dose increases should not be made more rapidly than once per week. The dosages for the elderly are the same as those for younger adults; however, because of reduced metabolism of sertraline, dose increases should not be made more frequently than two to three weeks. Zoloft is manufactured in 50- and 100-mg scored tablets. It is not available as a generic.

MOST FREQUENT SIDE EFFECTS

The most frequently reported side effects with Zoloft are nausea, 26%; diarrhea, 18%; somnolence, 13%; fatigue, 11%; insomnia, 16%; agitation/anxiety/nervousness, 12%; headache, 20%; male sexual dysfunction 16%; dry mouth, 16%; tremor, 11%; dizziness, 12%. Zoloft must be used with caution with Tagamet, hypoglycemic drugs, other antidepressants. It must be used with caution in individuals with seizure disorders, schizophrenia, and manic-depressive illness. (Please consult the package insert for a full listing of side effects, precautions, contraindications, and drug interactions.)

LOW-DOSE ZOLOFT

Like all antidepressants, Zoloft can cause a high rate of side effects. At lower doses, such as 25 to 50 mg a day, the side effect rate is much lower. In a study in which subjects were started at the recommended initial dose of 50 mg a day, the side effect rate was low, but when subjects were increased to higher doses, 89% complained of side effects. When subjects were started at 200 mg a day, 36% dropped out because of intolerable side effects.

Even the lowest recommended dose, 50 mg a day, may be too much for some individuals, according to journal reports:

> *A 62-year-old man with severe depression began stuttering within 24 hours of his first dose of 50 mg of Zoloft. The doctor reported, ''The stuttering was severe and involved virtually every word spoken.'' Other side effects included somnolence and increased appetite. All side effects disappeared quickly after the Zoloft was discontinued.*

> *A 28-year-old patient developed panic attacks after 6 days on 50 mg/day of Zoloft. He'd been started at 25 mg/day without any reactions, then increased to 50 mg/day after one week.*

In the first case, one wonders whether starting at 25 mg a day, or reducing to that level after side effects occurred, would have been sufficient. In the second case, waiting longer before increasing the dosage may have precluded the need to do so. Reports and studies have suggested that in nonacute situations, waiting two to four weeks before increasing the dosage may be preferable.

In one study of severe depression, 76% required no increase from an initial 50 mg a day. If severe depression often requires no more than 50 mg a day, milder conditions may require even less. Indeed, articles and anecdotal reports suggest that lower doses are indeed effective. For example, a woman with a 25-year history of dysthymic disorder responded well to 25 mg a day of Zoloft. ''I always begin with 25 mg of Zoloft unless circumstances dictate otherwise,'' one psychiatrist told me.

A man with obsessive-compulsive tendencies, a type of anxiety disorder, was given 25 mg of Zoloft and developed agitation and insomnia, common side effects with Zoloft. Unfortunately, it didn't occur to the physician that an even lower dose—e.g., 12.5 mg—might be appropriate for this patient. Individuals with anxiety/panic disorders often require extremely low doses of antidepressant drugs; 12.5 mg of Zoloft may indeed be sufficient for some anxiety-prone individuals.

THE ELDERLY AND ZOLOFT

For elderly patients, the manufacturer-recommended initial dose of Zoloft is 50 mg a day, the same as for younger adults. However, older individuals metabolize Zoloft more slowly than younger adults and quickly develop higher blood levels of the drug. Because of this, some physicians start elderly patients at lower doses, 12.5 to 25 mg a day.

RECOMMENDATIONS

Extensive clinical experience with Zoloft has shown that doses lower than those recommended by the manufacturer are effective in many people. If you are small, elderly, medication-sensitive, or prone to side effects, or you simply want to start at the lowest possible effective dose, you might consider starting with a low dose of Zoloft—25 to 50 mg a day. The manufacturer-recommended dosages of Zoloft are based on treating major depression, a severe disorder. If you are treating a milder depressive disorder such as dysthymic disorder, or an anxiety or panic disorder, doses as low as 12.5 to 25 mg a day are effective.

The standard dosing schedule with Zoloft is 50–100–150–200 mg—i.e., jumps of 100%, 50%, and 33%. More gradual increases—increments of 12.5 to 25 mg—may work better for some people.

In-Depth Analysis: Effexor (Venlafaxine)

In 1996, Effexor ranked No. 143 in U.S. outpatient prescriptions among all drugs. Effexor is chemically different than the SSRIs (Prozac, Zoloft, Serzone) and tricyclics (Elavil, Tofranil), but possesses some properties of each of these two groups. Effexor can cause a high incidence of side effects, especially when used in higher doses, but as is the case with the other new antidepressants, the frequency and severity of Effexor's side effects are less than those of the older groups. Because of its unique chemical structure, Effexor may sometimes be effective when other antidepressants have failed. It has been suggested that Effexor should be reserved for this role because it can elevate blood pressure, heart rate, and cholesterol levels.

MANUFACTURER-RECOMMENDED DOSES OF EFFEXOR

Initially, 75 mg a day (either 25 mg three times a day or 37.5 mg twice a day) with food. Maximum dose in outpatients: 225 mg a day; hospitalized patients, 375 mg a day. Elderly doses: same. Dose increases should be made at intervals of four days or more. Reduced doses for individuals with liver and/or kidney impairment. Effexor is produced in 25-, 37.5-, 50-, 75-, and 100-mg scored tablets, easily split or cut. Not available as generic.

MOST FREQUENT SIDE EFFECTS

The most reported side effects with Effexor are nausea (37%), somnolence (23%), dry mouth (22%), dizziness (19%), insomnia (18%), constipation (15%), nervousness and anxiety (13% and 6%, respectively), sweating (12%), asthenia (12%), abnormal ejaculation/orgasm in males (12%), diminished appetite (11%), impotence (6%), orgasm disturbance in females (2%). Effexor can cause elevations in blood pressure, especially at higher doses (7% of subjects at 200 to 300 mg a day). Must be used with caution in pregnancy and nursing mothers, as well as in individuals with liver and/or kidney impairment, seizures, schizophrenia, manicdepressive illness. Must be used with caution with Tagamet (cimetidine), as well as other antidepressants. In pre-release studies, 19% of subjects discontinued Effexor treatment because of side effects. (Please consult the package insert for a full listing of side effects, precautions, contraindications, and drug interactions.)

LOW-DOSE EFFEXOR

A physical therapist I know is prone to chronic depression, a condition that runs in his father's side of the family. His father takes a low dose of Elavil, 40 mg a day; the physical therapist has done very well on low-dose Effexor, 50 mg (25 mg twice a day).

The manufacturer-recommended starting dose of Effexor is 75 mg a day. Articles and anecdotal reports suggest that lower doses are useful with some individuals. One psychiatrist starts all Effexor patients at 37.5 mg a day (18.75 mg, or half a 37.5 mg tablet twice a day), 50% lower than the manufacturer-recommended dose. Some patients, he says, respond at this low level. Those who don't are then increased gradually to higher doses.

According to my discussions with the manufacturer and a review of the literature, only one pre-release study was conducted involving a dose lower than that which the manufacturer recommends. The 312 subjects in this study, all outpatients with major depressive disorders, received either placebo or Effexor 50 mg a day (25 mg twice a day), 100 to 150 mg a day (50 to 75 mg twice a day), or 300 to 400 mg a day (150 to 200 mg twice a day). When the study ended after six weeks, all three Effexor groups demonstrated greater improvement than the placebo group. Interestingly, the performance of the 50-mg dose very nearly equaled that of the highest dose group and outperformed the intermediate Effexor dose on all three depression scales. Not surprisingly, more subjects in the higher Effexor groups dropped out because of side effects. This study involved people with severe depression, which suggests that people with milder disorders may do even better with low-dose Effexor.

As with most antidepressants, people with histories of panic disorders or sensitivities to stimulant drugs may be unusually sensitive to Effexor. A 1995 article described the complete cessation of panic episodes in three patients as soon as Effexor was started at 18.75 mg twice a day. A fourth person could not tolerate even this low dosage and was given 9.375 mg (one-fourth a 37.5-mg tablet) twice a day. Ultimately, these people were able to gradually reach dosages of 50 to 75 mg a day, with continued total control of their panic episodes after nearly a year.

THE ELDERLY AND EFFEXOR

Elderly patients are often highly sensitive to the side effects of antidepressant medication. Somnolence in particular can be dangerous in older patients because of the risks of automobile accidents or falls. Starting with lower doses should be considered with all elderly patients, particularly those with other illnesses and/or taking other medications.

RECOMMENDATIONS

Most side effects caused by antidepressant drugs are dose-related. For example, in one study, 58% of subjects developed nausea at an Effexor dose of 375 mg a day, 38.2% at 225 mg a day, and 32.6% at 75 mg a day. Effexor may cause either sedation or agitation in different individuals; the incidence of somnolence, nervousness, and insomnia are high. This makes it difficult to anticipate how Effexor may affect a given individual, so again starting with lower doses makes sense. This is especially true because in pre-release studies, 19% of subjects discontinued Effexor treatment because of side effects. This is a very high rate. Lower doses are less likely to cause discontinuance due to side effects.

Neither Effexor's package insert nor the PDR write-up provides specific guidelines in adjusting Effexor doses upward, except to list the maximum dosages. Doctors aren't told whether to increase doses by 12.5, 18.75, 25, 37.5, or 50 mg at a time. As with other antidepressants, increasing Effexor doses by small gradations may provoke fewer side effects and allow the individual's system to adjust to the effects of increases in medication.

In-Depth Analysis: Wellbutrin (Bupropion)

The story of Wellbutrin underscores one of the themes of this book—that despite pre-release research, new problems are often discovered after drugs are approved and released for general use. When Wellbutrin was first released in the early 1990s, it was quickly withdrawn because of spontaneous seizures in some patients. Subsequently, it was re-released at lower recommended doses at which seizure episodes are now infrequent (4 out of 1,000 patients) and usually occur with higher doses or when Wellbutrin is mixed with other medications that may also increase seizure susceptibility.

Still, Wellbutrin's manufacturer continues to urge caution in dosing because the risk of seizures increases with the dosage. In addition, the total daily dosage of Wellbutrin should be divided in three or four doses spread over the day. Lower doses and multiple daily doses reduce the seizure risk.

Wellbutrin is a new antidepressant unrelated to either the SSRIs or the tricyclics. Overall, Wellbutrin's effectiveness and tendency toward side effects is comparable with other new antidepressants. Wellbutrin energizes many individuals, and it is often prescribed for depressive disorders characterized by low energy and increased sleep. Wellbutrin causes fewer sexual dysfunctions than the SSRIs (Prozac, Paxil, Zoloft, Serzone)—a point that the manufacturer has advertised excessively—and it often is the drug of choice for people who develop sexual dysfunctions with SSRIs.

MANUFACTURER-RECOMMENDED DOSES OF WELLBUTRIN

Initially, 100 mg twice a day; on the fourth day, increase if necessary to 100 mg three times a day. Maximum dose of 450 mg should be attempted only after several weeks at 300 mg a day; maximum dose should be given in four divided doses at least four hours apart. Elderly doses: same. Wellbutrin is produced in 75- and 100-mg unscored tablets. A sustained-release form, Wellbutrin SR, has recently been introduced.

MOST FREQUENT SIDE EFFECTS

The most frequently reported side effects include excessive sweating, 22%; anxiety/agitation, 35%; insomnia, 19%; tremor,

21%; dizziness, 22%; nausea/vomiting, 23%; constipation, 26%; anorexia, 18%; weight loss, 23%; weight gain, 14%; dry mouth, 28%; headache, 26%; sedation, 20%; blurred vision, 15%; increased heart rate, 11%. Must be used with caution in pregnancy or by nursing mothers and in seizure disorders, schizophrenia, or manic-depressive illness.

LOW-DOSE WELLBUTRIN

The manufacturer-recommended initial dose of 100 mg twice a day (200 mg a day), which is to be increased to 300 mg a day if no response is seen within three days, may be excessive for some people. Sometimes it takes a few weeks for antidepressant drugs to work, so jumping the dose 50% on the fourth day may be premature. Also, studies before and after Wellbutrin's release, as well as anecdotal reports, indicate that doses of 50 to 150 mg a day are sometimes effective. Some physicians start Wellbutrin at 25 to 50 mg a day in medication-sensitive or elderly individuals.

The range of manufacturer-recommended Wellbutrin dosages, 200 to 450 mg a day, is narrow considering, per the PDR, "the wide variability among individuals and their capacity to metabolize and eliminate drugs." The PDR states that the variation between individuals in blood concentrations of Wellbutrin is as much as 5-fold. A 1983 study found a 10-fold range of variation in blood levels. In addition, the time required for different individuals to metabolize and excrete Wellbutrin (elimination half-life) ranges from eight to twenty-four hours, again suggesting wide variability in individual requirements of this drug.

Although approved for the treatment of major depressive disorders, reports suggest that Wellbutrin is effective for dysthymic disorder, chronic fatigue syndrome, chronic pain, and attention deficit syndromes in adolescents and adults. However, unlike other antidepressants that are helpful for anxiety/panic disorders, Wellbutrin should be used cautiously because it may cause agitation.

An additional attribute of Wellbutrin may soon make it as well known as Prozac. For years, anecdotal reports and a small study have suggested that Wellbutrin may be uniquely effective in reducing the extreme drug craving seen in crack-cocaine addicts.

Now it seems that Wellbutrin also may curb the craving and withdrawal phenomena associated with smoking cessation. The FDA agrees. In 1997 it approved bupropion, which is Wellbutrin, for the treatment of nicotine addiction. Although it is the same drug, the manufacturer is marketing it under a different name: Zyban (see Chapter 9).

THE ELDERLY AND WELLBUTRIN

The recommended doses for elderly individuals are the same as for younger adults, yet the PDR acknowledges that prior to its release, "Wellbutrin [had] not been systematically evaluated in older patients." Caution would suggest that with the elderly, especially those with other illnesses and/or taking other medications, starting with lower doses and increasing the dosage only gradually would be prudent.

RECOMMENDATIONS

Depending on the severity and nature of your disorder, you may want to consider starting with low doses of Wellbutrin. The high incidence of side effects at the manufacturer-recommended dosages, the occasional occurrence of seizures, and the studies and anecdotal reports of effectiveness at lower doses support the use of initial low doses of Wellbutrin, especially if you are small, medication-sensitive, elderly, or just want to start at the lowest possible effective dose. Starting with lower doses may be especially useful for conditions other than major depression, the disorder upon which the manufacturer-recommended Wellbutrin doses are based. Milder depressive disorders such as dysthymic disorder, as well as anxiety and panic disorders, usually require lower doses. Some physicians start medication-sensitive individuals at dosages as low as 25 or 50 mg a day. If these are insufficient, your dosage can be gradually increased by gradations of 25 to 50 mg.

Other Antidepressants

This section offers information on one new SSRI antidepressant, Luvox, as well as Desyrel, an older antidepressant that primarily enhances serotonin in the brain. The tricyclic antidepressants are discussed next. Like all antidepressants, these drugs can cause high rates of side effects, and the older preparations are particularly prone to producing problems. Most side effects are dose-related. Lower doses reduce the frequency and severity of many side effects.

SEROTONIN-ENHANCING ANTIDEPRESSANTS

LUVOX (FLUVOXAMINE)

A member of the SSRI group, Luvox exhibits typical SSRI side effect tendencies: nausea, 40%; headache, 22%; somnolence, 22%; insomnia, 21%; anxiety/nervousness, 17%; gastric irritation, sexual dysfunctions. In pre-release trials, 22% of patients quit treatment because of side effects.

Like Prozac and other antidepressants, Luvox has been shown to be effective in treating obsessive-compulsive disorders, for which it is officially marketed. However, it is also prescribed for depression. Luvox was released after Prozac, Paxil, and Zoloft, and its manufacturer appears to have recognized that many individuals are very sensitive to these drugs and has suggested starting all patients at a low dose. Thus, although the manufacturer lists Luvox's effective dosage as 100 to 300 mg a day, the recommended initial dose is 50 mg a day. However, one journal article suggests starting at 25 mg a day with some patients.

Luvox is produced in 50- and 100-mg scored tablets, so doses of 25 mg (half a 50-mg pill) or even lower can be used for initial dosing or subsequent dose increases in medication-sensitive individuals. Luvox affects liver enzymes of the cytochrome P450 group and should be used carefully in patients taking theophylline,

Coumadin (warfarin), Seldane, Hismanal, other antidepressants, methadone, and other drugs.

DESYREL (TRAZODONE)

Released in the mid-1980s as the first new-generation antidepressant, Desyrel could have preempted Prozac if it had demonstrated superior effectiveness or markedly reduced side effects compared with other available drugs. Desyrel never accomplished this, although with its highly sedating properties, Desyrel did compete with Elavil in the treatment of depressive disorders characterized by insomnia or agitation. Desyrel remains useful in this capacity. It is also frequently prescribed as a nonaddictive sleep remedy. These uses helped generic trazodone to be ranked No. 21 among generic drugs in U.S. outpatient prescriptions in 1995.

Though the manufacturer recommends an initial dose of 150 mg a day, including the elderly, many people cannot tolerate anywhere near this dose. Nor are such high doses necessary, according to the medical literature: "Data from studies on trazodone . . . suggest that lower dosages may prove as effective (if not more effective) than very high dosages." For these reasons, initial doses of 50 to 75 mg are often prescribed. Most frequent side effects with Desyrel included drowsiness, headache, nausea, dizziness, light-headedness, fatigue, dry mouth, blurred vision; the infrequent side effect of penile engorgement requires discontinuance of the drug. Because of its side effects, particularly oversedation, the use of Desyrel with elderly patients has been questioned.

Others have questioned the common usage of Desyrel, which increases serotonin levels in the brain, to offset the insomnia caused by serotonergic antidepressants such as Prozac. Mixing serotonin-enhancing drugs can cause a sometimes serious condition called serotonin syndrome. At the low Desyrel doses used for insomnia, clinicians tell me they've rarely encountered this problem.

TRICYCLIC ANTIDEPRESSANTS

From their introduction in the 1950s to the arrival of Prozac in the late 1980s, the tricyclic antidepressants were the most prescribed antidepressants in the world, including top sellers Elavil, Tofranil, Sinequan, Pamelor, and Norpramin. Although supplanted by newer antidepressants, the tricyclics remain useful in treating depression in people unresponsive to or encountering problems with other drugs. The tricyclic antidepressants are also used for anxiety/panic disorders, pain syndromes, insomnia, and other conditions.

The tricyclic antidepressants characteristically display very wide ranges of interindividual variation in dose response. Individual differences in blood levels of a specific dose of drug may vary as much as 30- to 40-fold—that's 3,000% to 4,000%. Not surprising, initial doses recommended in the PDR and many medical textbooks are too high for medication-sensitive individuals. Routine methods of increasing tricyclic doses are often too aggressive, making large jumps too rapidly for medication-sensitive persons.

Tricyclic antidepressants frequently produce side effects. The PDR does not list specific percentages for the incidence of side effects with Elavil or Tofranil, but the more newly approved Anafranil does provide a glimpse of the potential for side effects in drugs of this group (1996 PDR): somnolence, 54%; dry mouth, 84%; constipation, 47%; dizziness, 54%; tremor, 54%; headache, 52%; insomnia, 25%; fatigue, 39%; problems with ejaculation, 42%, and impotence, 20%; and many, many more. Most of these side effects are dose related.

Interestingly, my patients seemed to develop more side effects with Elavil (amitriptyline) and Tofranil (imipramine), the best-known and best-selling members of this group. Over time I stopped using these drugs, and instead found Pamelor (also Adapin, nortriptyline) and Norpramin (desipramine) more palatable for my patients when tricyclic antidepressants were required. Many psychiatrists have told me that they too have come to prefer Norpramin and Pamelor among the tricyclic group. Several journal articles have recommended that Elavil, Tofranil, and Sinequan be avoided with elderly individuals because of the frequency of side effects.

ANAFRANIL (CLOMIPRAMINE)

Like Luvox, this member of the antidepressant family is actually marketed for the treatment of obsessive-compulsive disorders.

Nevertheless, it is also prescribed for depression, PMS, pain syndromes, panic disorders, and other conditions. Like other members of the tricyclic group, Anafranil causes a high incidence of side effects.

The manufacturer-recommended initial dose of Anafranil is 25 mg, increasing to 100 mg over the first two weeks. Because Anafranil is produced only in 25-, 50-, and 75-mg capsules, starting with doses lower than the manufacturer recommends is difficult. Increasing from 25 to 100 mg over fourteen days, as the manufacturer recommends, is too aggressive for many patients. Indeed, studies utilizing Anafranil for pain syndromes, anxiety/panic disorders, and PMS have shown that doses of 10 to 40 mg were effective (the researchers apparently fashioned 10-mg pills). In one study with panic and agoraphobic subjects, eight of thirteen subjects responded at doses of 25 mg or less.

ELAVIL (AMITRIPTYLINE)

The manufacturer-recommended initial dose for outpatients is 75 mg a day in divided doses (e.g., 25 mg three times a day); this can be increased to 150 mg a day. Most frequent side effects include severely dry mouth, blurred vision, sedation, and constipation; also weight gain, menstrual irregularity, sexual dysfunction, cardiac abnormality, and memory impairment.

Variability in individual response to Elavil can be striking. As one journal article stated: "The literature contains a number of case reports of patients developing very high, and in some cases toxic, concentrations of amitriptyline [Elavil] following relatively small doses."

Indeed, many people cannot tolerate doses of Elavil above 10 to 25 mg a day; starting at these doses minimizes risks with medication-sensitive individuals. Over time, some people become more tolerant of this drug and are able to increase their dosage; others don't. And still others tolerate doses of 100 or 200 or 300 mg a day with little difficulty.

Despite its tendency toward side effects, Elavil in the form of its generic, amitriptyline, remains a widely prescribed medication. In 1996, just one of the many preparations of amitriptyline ranked No. 65 in U.S. outpatient prescriptions and No. 29 among generic drugs.

When a patient is using Elavil, dose adjustments should be very gradual; the effective dose is often signaled by the first signs of sedation, dry mouth, blurred vision, constipation, or other early side effects. Further dose increases should be performed carefully. Elavil and generic amitriptyline are usually available in many pill sizes, enabling flexible dosing.

NORPRAMIN (DESIPRAMINE)

Norpramin is often preferred over Elavil and Tofranil when tricyclic antidepressant treatment is necessary. Norpramin rarely causes sedation, and produces blurred vision, dry mouth, constipation, and other typical tricyclic side effects less often. Cardiac irregularities, palpitations, agitation, and weight gain do occasionally occur. Norpramin can cause anxiety or insomnia in anxiety-prone individuals.

The PDR recommends a usual adult dose of 100 to 200 mg a day of Norpramin, then suggests starting at a lower level without actually defining it. To many doctors, this means starting at 50 to 75 mg a day, which is often too much for medication-sensitive individuals. I started most of my patients at 10 to 25 mg a day. Many never reached 50 mg, and fewer still needed 100 mg. For some, especially anxiety-prone folks, 10 mg is sufficient.

PAMELOR (NORTRIPTYLINE)

Pamelor, like Norpramin, is the preferred tricyclic antidepressant of many medication experts. In 1995, generic nortriptyline ranked No. 47 among generic drugs in U.S. outpatient prescriptions.

Although Pamelor can cause many of the side effects seen with other tricyclics—dry mouth, constipation, blurred vision, light-headedness, cardiac irregularities, weight gain—it seems to do so less often and less severely than Elavil or Tofranil. Also, Pamelor causes neither the severe sedation of Elavil and Sinequan nor the palpitations seen with Tofranil. Because of these advantages, in 1995 Pamelor's generic, nortriptyline, ranked among the top 200 prescribed outpatient drugs in the U.S.

The manufacturer-recommended starting dose of Pamelor is 75 to 100 mg a day. I started most patients at 10 to 25 mg a day, depending on their history. With those having histories of medication sensitivities, starting at 10 mg worked best.

The manufacturer does recommend lower doses for the elderly, 30 to 50 mg a day. However, doses of 10 to 20 mg a day may be sufficient in some cases.

SINEQUAN (ADAPIN, DOXEPIN)

Some years ago an old medical school friend called to ask my advice about an agitated and depressed patient of his. The patient was very wary of taking medication but had finally agreed to try something. I suggested Sinequan at 10 mg a day. My friend was skeptical, suggesting that perhaps the manufacturer-recommended starting dose, 75 mg a day, might be more effective. "Possibly, but you may overwhelm him with side effects," I replied. This issue was key because the patient was likely to quit treatment if side effects developed. I told my friend how to adjust the dose steadily upward, if necessary. The patient responded beautifully at 20 mg. Afterward my friend mused, "If I'd given him 75 mg, I'd have blown him out of the water. I'd have lost his trust forever."

The manufacturer-recommended dose of Sinequan is 75 mg a day for mild to moderate depression, up to 300 mg a day for severe cases. The PDR notes that some cases with "very mild symptomatology" have been controlled at 25 to 50 mg a day. There are no specific geriatric doses. Sinequan, like Elavil, can be very sedating; other common side effects include dry mouth, constipation, blurred vision, light-headedness, difficulty urinating. It may cause cardiac irregularities or weight gain.

Many people are easily sedated by Sinequan. This can occur whether the case is mild or severe; my friend's patient had symptoms that were in fact fairly severe. For people who usually aren't sensitive to sedating medicines, starting at 25 mg a day may be reasonable; otherwise, 10 mg a day is a safer dose for initiating treatment. Because of its sedating properties, Sinequan is most useful in depressions characterized by agitation or insomnia. It also has been useful in treating anxiety disorders and pain syndromes. Its multiple uses are the reason that doxepin ranked No. 38 among generic drugs in 1995 U.S. outpatient prescriptions.

TOFRANIL (IMIPRAMINE)

For decades, Tofranil was one of the top-selling antidepressants in the world. Although it is now displaced by Prozac and other newer drugs, Tofranil and its generic, imipramine, continue to be widely used for treating depression, pain disorders, and anxiety/panic syndromes. In 1995, imipramine ranked No. 29 among generic drugs in U.S. outpatient prescriptions.

Imipramine was the first antidepressant discovered to have antipanic properties. Although it is now known that many other antidepressants exert similar antipanic effects with fewer side effects than Tofranil, the latter still retains its (undeserved) reputation as a superior antipanic drug.

For major depression, the manufacturer recommended starting dose for outpatients is 75 mg a day; the geriatric dose, 30 to 40 mg a day; the dose range is 50 to 150 mg a day. For hospitalized patients, 100 mg a day initially, increased to 200 to 300 mg a day as necessary. Most frequent side effects include blurred vision, dry mouth, constipation, agitation, tremor, memory loss, difficulty urinating, palpitations, light-headedness; Tofranil may cause cardiac irregularities or weight gain.

As with Elavil and other tricyclic antidepressants, many people are highly sensitive to side effects with imipramine. Starting at doses of 10 or 25 mg a day reduces the risks of an adverse reaction. Many people respond at doses of 10 to 50 mg a day without ever requiring the higher doses recommended in the PDR and some textbooks.

Anxiety/panic patients are often particularly sensitive to this and other tricyclic antidepressant drugs. In 1978 I prescribed imipramine for the first time to a woman with a severe panic disorder. Ten mg of imipramine was ineffective; 20 mg caused her severe difficulty in urinating. We settled with a dose of 15 mg, which nearly completely halted her panic episodes.

Brief Comments on Other Antidepressants

The following antidepressants should also be used with care with medication-sensitive individuals. Starting with low doses and increasing gradually, when necessary, will lessen the likelihood of side effects and side-effect-related treatment failures.

Asendin is generally well tolerated at lower doses, the most frequent side effects being drowsiness, dry mouth, constipation, and blurred vision—all of which are dose-related. The manufacturer-recommended initial dose is 50 mg twice or three times a day; some patients require gradual increases to 200 to 300 mg a day. For the elderly, the manufacturer-recommended dose is 25 mg twice or three times a day; 100 to 150 mg a day is usually adequate for elderly patients not responding to lower doses. If you are small, medication-sensitive, or only mildly depressed, consider starting with 25 mg once or twice daily. If this dosage isn't adequate, increase it gradually by 25 mg.

Ludiomil is often sedating. Other side effects include dry mouth, constipation, dizziness, and nervousness. The manufacturer-recommended initial dose is 75 mg a day, but 25 mg a day is recommended for the elderly and "some patients." If you are small, medication-sensitive, or only mildly depressed, consider starting with 25 mg a day of Ludiomil at bedtime.

Nardil (phenelzine) and Parnate (tranylcypromine) belong to the family of monamine oxidation inhibitors, or MAOIs. These drugs produce high incidences of side effects, require special changes in diet, and must be used very carefully with other medications— but they can be effective when all other drugs fail. The manufacturer-recommended initial dose of Nardil is 15 mg three times a day; maximum dose, 90 mg a day. If you are small, medication-sensitive, or only mildly depressed, 15 mg once or twice daily may be an adequate initial dose.

Remeron (mirtazapine) is a newer antidepressant with a recommended initial dose of 15 mg a day; the dose range is 15 to 45 mg a day. Remeron is said to be as effective as the other new antidepressants. However, side effects such as increased appetite and weight gain may pose difficulties for some patients. Other side effects include sedation, dizziness, dry mouth, constipation, and an additive effect with alcohol. Remeron has a long half-life of twenty to forty hours, meaning that with each daily dose, the blood level rises until reaching a plateau after one to two weeks. This makes dosing difficult; shorter-acting antidepressants such as Zoloft and Wellbutrin are much easier to work with.

Vivactil (protriptyline) is a tricyclic antidepressant that is similar to Norpramin in that it tends to produce energizing effects. Vivactil can provoke agitation or insomnia in some people. The manufacturer recommends that the "dosage should be initiated at a low level and increased gradually." The manufacturer-suggested usual dosage is 15 to 40 mg a day; maximum dosage, 60 mg a day; elderly dosage, 15 mg initially. Vivactil may be useful in depressions that are characterized by low energy and excessive sleep. However, for these conditions, newer drugs such as Prozac, Zoloft, and Wellbutrin are usually tried first. If you are medication-sensitive, small, or only mildly depressed, consider starting at 5 mg once or twice daily.

SEVEN

Anti-Anxiety and Anti-Panic Medications

In-Depth Analyses

Xanax (alprazolam)
Valium (diazepam)

Other Medications

Ativan (lorazepam)
Klonopin (clonazepam)
Librium (chlordiazepoxide)
Serax (oxazepam)
Tranxene (chlorazepate)

Brief Comments

Atarax and Vistaril (hydroxyzine)
BuSpar (buspirone)

About Anxiety Disorders and Anti-Anxiety Medications

Anxiety disorders come in many forms (see below). About 15% of Americans will develop an anxiety disorder sometime during their lifetime, and this number excludes simple phobias, which affect 30% to 40% of the population.

The treatment of anxiety disorders varies with the type and severity of the anxiety condition and the individual characteristics of each person. If you have an anxiety disorder, you should receive a thorough evaluation, including a search for possible physical causes such as thyroid disease, adrenal tumors, cardiac arrhythmias (e.g., mitral valve prolapse syndrome, which is sometimes associated with panic attacks), respiratory problems, subtle seizure disorders, and, especially, medication side effects.

This latter cause is often overlooked. For example, people have told me of having anxiety reactions to anti-inflammatory drugs such as Relafen, Voltaren, and Clinoril; any drug of this group, including nonprescription preparations (ibuprofen, Aleve, Orudis KT, and others) can provoke an anxiety reaction. So, too, can many antidepressants: Prozac, Zoloft, Wellbutrin, Paxil, Serzone, Effexor, Tofranil, Norpramin, and others. Even drugs that aren't normally associated with anxiety reactions may cause them in a rare case. If you notice that you suddenly have become more and more anxious, or have developed insomnia, and there are no stresses in your personal or emotional life to explain it, you should look carefully at any medication or other health supplement that you've recently started.

Types and Characteristics of Anxiety Disorders

In the past, anxiety disorders were considered entirely mental conditions. For decades, the term *neurosis* was used to indicate the psychological origins of these problems. However, recent advances in medical technology have revealed that many, if not all, anxiety disorders may have a neuro-chemical component—an imbalance of brain chemistry. *Neurosis* was dropped as a diagnostic term more than decade ago.

SITUATIONAL ANXIETY DISORDER

A short-term condition resulting from a severe stress such as loss of a job, the development of a major illness, or the death of a loved one. The degree of anxiety may be mild or severe, and it may involve physical symptoms such as shaking, dizziness, palpitations, nausea, or shortness of breath. It may also impede mental functioning such as concentration, memory, or sleep.

Medication: Benzodiazepines, as needed, on a short-term basis.

GENERALIZED ANXIETY DISORDER

A general tendency toward frequent or constant anxiety, nervousness, or unnecessary or excessive worry, and a tendency to react excessively to common daily stresses. Like chronic depressive disorders, many general anxiety disorders are chronic conditions that may appear to be part of the individual's personality, when in fact the disorder may have more to do with altered brain functioning.

Medication: Benzodiazepines, buspirone (Buspar), sedatives (Atarax, Vistaril), antidepressants, or a combination of drugs (such as benzodiazepines and antidepressants).

PANIC DISORDER

Panic attacks are sudden, unexpected episodes of over-powering anxiety. They are associated with several of the following symptoms: shortness of breath, smothering sensation, dizziness, unsteadiness, faintness, palpitations, rapid heartbeat, trembling, sweating, hot flashes or chills, tightness in the chest, nausea, intense feelings of losing control or fears of dying, going crazy, or acting impulsively or inappropriately. Panic episodes leave the sufferer feeling defenseless and needing to retreat to a safe environment. Without treatment, panic episodes can increase in frequency and severity, ultimately leading in some individuals to agoraphobia. Because the symptoms are mostly physical, panic disorders are often misdiagnosed.

Medication: Benzodiazepines, antidepressants (many have anti-panic effects), beta blockers.

AGORAPHOBIA

Agoraphobia is the fear or avoidance of situations from which escape may be difficult or help unavailable. The fear is usually associated with concerns about physical or psychological well-being, such as fears of fainting, cardiac problems, or loss of control. As a result, the person avoids specific, anxiety-provoking situations that, in severe cases, may limit the individual to their home. Agoraphobia sometimes but not always develops as the end result of progressive panic disorders.

Medication: Same treatment as panic disorder.

SOCIAL PHOBIA

A social phobia is the fear or avoidance of anxiety-provoking situations occurring in social contexts. The person usually fears being scrutinized or ignored by others, or drawing the attention of others in a humiliating or embarrassing manner. Social phobias include difficulty urinating in public facilities, stumbling over words in conversation, difficulty chewing or swallowing when eating with others, and the inability to converse normally with others.

Medication: Usually doesn't require medication; benzodiazepines as needed can be helpful.

SIMPLE PHOBIA

Phobias are recurrent, panic-like reactions to a specific situation such as heights, crowded elevators, airplanes, or seeing a spider or snake. Because of the severity of phobic reaction, phobic individuals avoid the triggering situation whenever possible. Phobic persons usually recognize that their fears are excessive and irrational, but neither this insight nor willpower are enough to overcome the phobic reaction.

Medication: Same treatment as social phobia.

OBSESSIVE-COMPULSIVE DISORDER

Obsessions are intrusive and persistent thoughts, impulses, or images that seem extreme or bizarre to the individual. Compulsions are repetitive behaviors that the person recognizes as extreme or irrational, but feels he must perform because of obsessive thoughts.

Medication: Antidepressants, particularly serotonergic drugs such as Prozac, Zoloft, Paxil, Anafranil.

POST-TRAUMATIC STRESS DISORDER

A trauma is an event that is beyond the range of typical human experience and would cause severe, lingering distress in anyone. Traumatic experiences may include sudden destruction of a person's home, being the victim of violence, the loss of a loved one (especially a child), or the terror of a catastrophe or war experience. Post-traumatic stress syndrome (PTSS) is marked by recurrent, unpleasant memories and dreams, flashbacks in which the traumatic event appears to be reoccurring, and severe anxiety when exposed to situations that symbolize the traumatic event.

Medication: May require treatment with benzodiazepines or antidepressants.

OTHER DISORDERS OFTEN CAUSED BY AN UNDERLYING ANXIETY STATE

Hypochondriasis: Our culture tends to mock and minimize the severity and psychological pain of hypochondriasis. We also usually fail to recognize that this is an anxiety disorder. Hypochondriasis is a severe anxiety or panic disorder that is focused on body sensations and that cause the sufferer to have exaggerated fears and reactions regarding illness and death. Medication treatment usually involves anti-anxiety and/or antidepressant medication.

Hysteria: Emotional dyscontrol, may be caused by anxiety, depression, manic-depressive illness, or other conditions. Medication treatment is directed at the underlying condition. ·

Somatic Conditions: Examples are headaches, stomach or bowel problems, increased heart rate or blood pressure, weight gain or loss, back pain—somatic conditions can involve any system of the body. Medication treatment may involve drugs specific for the system involved (gastrointestinal, cardiovascular, obesity); anti-anxiety and/or antidepressant treatment may be helpful.

Insomnia: In addition to the sleep medications discussed in Chapter 8, Valium and generic diazepam and Ativan and generic lorazepam are frequently prescribed for sleep disorders.

Once it is determined that you do in fact have an anxiety disorder, initial treatment should incorporate nondrug methods such as avoidance of caffeine and other stimulants, exercise, stress reduction, or psychotherapy/counseling. These methods alone may be sufficient, but if your anxiety problem is acute or severe, medication treatment may be both necessary and very helpful.

EVERYDAY ANXIETY VERSUS ANXIETY DISORDERS

Anxiety is an emotion we all experience. It is a natural part of everyday life. Anxiety is similar to fear in the way it causes us to feel and affects our bodies physiologically. Although anxiety and fear are often defined as separate emotions, anxiety may be just another word for a vague type of fear. Certainly when anxiety reaches panic proportions, anxiety and fear become indistinguishable.

Everyday anxiety has both good and bad aspects. Anxiety is unpleasant. It may make you feel nervous, unsettled, uncertain, insecure, or indecisive and may affect your sleep. It may cause you to lose concentration, be forgetful, or make mistakes. You may lose your appetite or eat compulsively to blot out your tension.

But anxiety also can serve as a motivation. It may sharpen your focus, drive you to perform better, or motivate you to aspire to greater things.

Increased levels of anxiety are normal when you are under pressure, such as a job interview, a school test, dealing with illness, getting promoted or fired, getting married or divorced. Some people perform better under these pressures. Others don't. Interindividual variation is a factor with emotions as well as medications.

The difference between everyday anxiety and a medically defined anxiety disorder is one of proportion. It's normal to be anxious under certain circumstances, such as when you are late. It's not normal to be excessively anxious most of the time, to the exclusion of positive feelings such as joy or satisfaction when the situation warrants. It's normal to be fearful when threatened by a mugger or undergoing surgery. It's not normal to have sudden episodes of full panic when everything seems fine.

By definition, the diagnosis of an anxiety disorder indicates a degree of anxiety that exceeds normal emotion and can dominate a person's inner life and outer experience. The anxiety generated by these conditions can also impair normal functioning and in severe cases cause severe disability.

Dysfunction is a hallmark of an anxiety disorder. Although often not apparent to others, people with anxiety disorders are usually compelled to find alternate ways of functioning in order to control their anxiety. Claustrophobics avoid closed-in spaces. Social phobics avoid parties and crowds. Severe agoraphobics avoid everything, preferring the unhappy limitations of their homes to the panic that occurs when they step outside.

People unfamiliar with these disorders aren't usually aware of the degree of suffering they can cause. Severe anxiety disorders are serious conditions. Secondary depression is common. So, too, are thoughts of suicide. Indeed, in the June 24, 1996, issue of *Newsweek*, there was a moving article about a successful television anchorman who was suddenly overcome by a panic disorder and contemplated crashing into a freeway abutment. Treatment halted his terrible panic episodes.

NOT A CASE OF WILLPOWER

Anxiety disorders have nothing to do with willpower or strength of character. Some of the bravest people I've known are those who battle anxiety disorders. I've treated career military officers, successful businesswomen and businessmen, teachers, attorneys, mothers, and other highly accomplished souls who have tried their best to suppress their anxiety problems. As in the case of depression, a person can't always will away a powerful psychological disorder. Indeed, many patients have told me that the most frustrating aspect of their anxiety disorder is that they realize their anxiety makes no sense—indeed, is irrational, excessive, and unnecessary—yet are not able to control it.

The reason may be that anxiety disorders are more than simply psychological, or "mental," conditions. As we learn more and more about how the brain functions, it has become apparent that many anxiety and depressive disorders have physical—i.e., biochemical—underpinnings. We know that chemical imbalances in the brain play a role in many, if not all, anxiety disorders.

An example is a simple phobia, a disorder in which people are morbidly fearful of normally nonthreatening situations such as heights, cramped elevators, harmless spiders, or nonpoisonous snakes. In a simple phobia, the individual is fully aware that his phobic reaction is not only irrational and excessive but embarrassing. Once, an intern told me how he learned that his fiancée also an intern, had a severe phobia to snakes. One night, while they were watching television, she suddenly left the room. When she didn't return, he asked her what was wrong. She called from the other room: "Is the snake gone?" The movie contained a scene with a snake. She was terribly afraid of snakes, so phobic that just the image of a snake on the TV screen was too nerve-racking to bear. She knew her reaction was absurd, but despite her embarrassment, she had to leave the room.

RECOGNIZING AN ANXIETY DISORDER

The symptoms of anxiety are fairly consistent: feelings of fear, doom, dread; uncertainty, forgetfulness, impaired mental functioning. Depression may develop as a result of anxiety problems. Physical symptoms may include palpitations, sweating, tight muscles, jitteriness, a feeling of tightness or a lump in the throat, stomach upset, decreased or increased appetite, impaired sleep. Anxiety can affect virtually any system of the body, thereby creating symptoms that may mimic many illnesses. Anxiety sufferers often think they have heart or stomach or memory problems. Back pain, headaches, and impaired sexual performance are often associated with anxiety problems. Children who underperform in school may be beset with anxiety.

If your anxiety is severe, you are probably well aware of it. It's not normal to feel constantly nervous, or to have panic attacks while doing nothing unusual, or to feel compelled to check the lock on the front door or wash your hands a dozen times before going to bed, or to be so incapacitated by anxiety that you are unable to talk to others at a party.

On the other hand, physicians often miss the diagnosis of an anxiety disorder. Unless you are having a panic attack right before the doctor's eyes, he may tend to minimize or dismiss the importance of what you're trying to tell him. Part of the problem is that he's human; unless he's experienced the crippling power of severe anxiety or a panic attack, it's impossible to appreciate.

Your anxiety disorder is also difficult for doctors to identify because you are likely educated, presentable, and productive. To physicians, you look just like everyone else. You appear okay. If you suffer panic attacks, you were probably amazed the first time you suffered through a panic episode at a restaurant or in line at the supermarket and no one noticed. Inside, you were dying, but to everyone else nothing seemed unusual. For these reasons, as well as the fact that most physicians aren't well trained about the importance and severity of anxiety disorders, the diagnosis is frequently missed.

The impact of a missed diagnosis can be great. You may leave your doctor's office feeling confused, unsure of yourself, misunderstood, or angry. It took a lot of effort to try to tell your physician about your anxiety problem. Your succumbing to uncontrollable emotions of anxiety or panic feels like a failure. Failing to get the doctor's attention adds to your sense of futility. Most of all, your physician's failure to understand means that treatment is postponed—a shame, because anxiety disorders are very treatable.

ANTI-ANXIETY MEDICATIONS:
THE BENZODIAZEPINES

Many groups of medications can be employed in the treatment of anxiety disorders (see below). By far the most utilized and best-known anti-anxiety medications belong to a group known as the benzodiazepines. Members include household names such as Xanax and Valium. Several well-known sleep medications—for example, Halcion, Restoril, and Dalmane—are also benzodiazepines.

Medications Used for Anxiety Disorders

BENZODIAZEPINES
Ativan (lorazepam)
Klonopin (clonazepam)
Librium (chlordiazepoxide)
Serax (oxazepam)
Tranxene (chlorazepate)
Valium (diazepam)
Xanax (alprazolam)

BUSPAR (BUSPIRONE)

SEDATIVES

Atarax, Vistaril (hydroxyzine)
Other antihistamines: Benadryl (diphenhydramine),
others

ANTIDEPRESSANTS

Many people with anxiety disorders, especially panic disorders, are highly sensitive to antidepressant drugs. Treatment should be started at very low doses.
For agitation or to provide sedation
Sinequan, Adapin (doxepin)
Elavil (amitriptyline)
For anti-panic effects
Tricyclic antidepressants: Pamelor (nortriptyline),
Sinequan or Adapin (doxepin), Norpramin (desipramine), Tofranil (imipramine)

Serotonin enhancers: Prozac (fluoxetine), Zoloft
(sertraline), Paxil (paroxetine)

Monoamine oxidase inhibitors: Nardil (phenelzine)

BETA BLOCKERS

Useful for the physical manifestations of anxiety (tremor,
quivering, palpitations) or mitral valve prolapse syndrome
(sometimes associated with panic attacks)

Inderal (propranolol), Tenormin (atenolol), others

Great popularity and great controversy has surrounded the benzodiazepines for decades and continues to do so today. Once America's top-selling medication, Valium (diazepam) has been controversial for over fifteen years, yet it is still widely used. Xanax has been the center of contention for at least a decade. The sleep remedy Halcion, closely related chemically to Xanax and made by the same manufacturer, continues to be embroiled in a twenty-year controversy of its own (Chapter 8).

Why are such controversial drugs so popular? Why do doctors prescribe them? Why aren't benzodiazepines simply banned, as a handful of physicians have demanded? Because *when they are used properly*, benzodiazepines are very effective, useful, and safe medications. When prescribed in safe amounts, benzodiazepines control anxiety with a minimum of side effects. That's why the American Medical Association states: ''The benzodiazepines are often the drugs of choice when an anti-anxiety, sedative, or hypnotic [sleep-inducing] action is needed.''

On the other hand, when the benzodiazepines are used in excess, side effects abound. The 1997 PDR includes the following among the list of Xanax's side effects when used for generalized anxiety disorders: drowsiness, 41%; light-headedness, 21%; depression, 14%; dry mouth, 14%; headache, 13%; confusion, 10%. These rates were obtained in studies with Xanax dosages as high as 4 mg a day. With the even higher doses of Xanax used for panic disorder, side effects were even more pronounced: drowsiness, 77%; fatigue and tiredness, 49%; impaired coordination, 40%; irritability, 33%; memory impairment, 33%; light-headedness or dizziness, 29%; headache 29%—the list goes on and on.

⁓

Benzodiazepine Adverse Reactions

Most benzodiazepine adverse reactions are dose-related. Benzodiazepines are usually well tolerated at low and moderate dosages, but individual response can vary considerably. Some benzodiazepines are more prone to causing sedation than others. If you are medication-sensitive, or if you are easily affected by alcohol or sedating medications such as antihistamines or muscle relaxants, you will likely be sensitive to benzodiazepines and should start with a low dose of a less sedating preparation. This list of adverse reactions is not comprehensive; less frequent adverse reactions can be found in the PDR and other medication references.

Side Effects: Drowsiness, light-headedness, fatigue or tiredness, depression, impaired coordination, dry mouth, irritability, confusion, memory impairment, dizziness, headache, constipation, diarrhea, nausea/vomiting, appetite changes, joint pain, cognitive (thinking) disorder. Benzodiazepines should be used cautiously in people with tendencies toward depression or psychosis, respiratory problems, or impaired liver functioning. These drugs are usually contraindicated in people with histories of drug addiction or addictive tendencies. They are avoided whenever possible in pregnancy because of evidence of fetal malformations. These drugs pass into breast milk and are therefore avoided in nursing mothers. Benzodiazepines can impair the mental alertness or physical coordination necessary for driving, operating machinery, or similar activities.

Paradoxical Reactions: Occasionally, these drugs can cause a paradoxical reaction, also known as an idiosyncratic effect. This reaction occurs more commonly in elderly individuals or in those taking other drugs affecting the brain or nervous system. Reactions may be mild or severe, including some or all of the following: increased stimulation, excitability, irritability, muscle tightness or spasticity, sleep disturbances, agitation, hostility, rage, aggressive behavior, confusion, hallucinations.

Withdrawal Symptoms: Withdrawal problems can be prevented by avoiding long-term, high-dose benzodiazepine treatment. People using these drugs for prolonged periods must be tapered very gradually off of their medication. Withdrawal reactions usually become evident within one to four days, may be mild or severe, and may include anxiety, sweating, insomnia, diarrhea, irritability, headache, tremors, muscle twitching, abdominal cramps, blurred vision, appetite loss, tingling sensations, feelings of unreality, sensory hypersensitivity to sound or light, confusion, incoordination, hallucinations, psychosis, or seizures.

Drug Interactions: Benzodiazepines can cause heightened or unexpected effects when given with other drugs that effect the brain or nervous system: antidepressants, antihistamines, antipsychotic drugs, seizure medications, codeine and other narcotic pain relievers, barbiturates, some nonprescription sleep and cold remedies, alcohol, and illicit drugs. Benzodiazepines also can interact with other drugs including Tagamet (cimetidine) and Prilosec (omeprazole) oral contraceptives, lithium, and possibly erythromycin antibiotics (erythromycins, Biaxin, Zithromax). A report in the *Psychiatric Annals* (Ayd, 1994) stated that grapefruit juice enhances the effects of Xanax, causing increased sedation in study subjects.

I have always taken issue with the prescribing of high doses of Xanax and other benzodiazepines, for these are the doses that produce many adverse reactions and high rates of dependency. My experience has been that used in moderation and only when necessary, benzodiazepines work well and pose few problems.

CONTROVERSIAL BUT POPULAR

Prior to the release of the first benzodiazepine, Librium, in 1960, the drugs most prescribed for treating anxiety were phenobarbital and meprobamate—both sedating and highly prone to cause drug dependency. Hailed as nonaddictive when they were first marketed, the benzodiazepines, particularly Valium and Librium, quickly dominated the market—a market so large that a 1979 survey found that 11% of Americans were taking antianxiety drugs. Studies show that although the specific type of benzodiazepine has changed, overall usage remains about 11%

(not including benzodiazepines used for sleep; see Chapter 8). Six different preparations of benzodiazepines ranked among the top 200 drugs filled by pharmacists in 1995: brand-name Xanax, Valium, and Klonopin; generic alprazolam, diazepam, and lorazepam.

As a group, for thirty-five years the benzodiazepines have ranked among the most prescribed drugs in the world.

Why have such controversial drugs remained so popular? Because anxiety is pervasive. Because anxiety is painful. Anxiety is psychological pain, and benzodiazepines are very effective at stopping it. These drugs work fast and work well. When prescribed properly, they cause few problems. Compared with alternative medications such as sedatives or antidepressants, side effects with benzodiazepines are generally less frequent and less severe.

As Dr. David Sheehan, an expert on benzodiazepines, has written: "These drugs are safer to use, quicker in onset of action, easier for the physician to prescribe, and more pleasant for the patient to take than the alternatives." The continuing popularity of the benzodiazepines, despite the notoriety surrounding them, underscores their effectiveness and general tolerability. That's why even people without anxiety disorders use an occasional Xanax or Valium when their stress gets beyond control.

HOW BENZODIAZEPINES WORK

Benzodiazepines work by inhibiting brain activity via GABA, an amino acid that is found in many areas of the brain. GABA inhibits brain activity. The benzodiazepines enhance the effect of GABA, thereby decreasing anxiety, excitability, and muscle tension; in high dosages, they produce drowsiness, sleep, and impaired coordination. Anecdotal reports state that relaxation or sedation can be obtained by taking GABA, which can be purchased in health food stores. Whether GABA actually works, in whom, and at what dosages is presently not clear.

THE PROBLEM OF BENZODIAZEPINE DEPENDENCY

So why are benzodiazepines controversial? Mainly because, despite the early pronouncements, they can cause dependency, though not as often as their predecessors. When these drugs are used in high dosages and/or for prolonged periods, dependency—the need to continue taking a drug to avoid withdrawal reactions—is common. In 1994, the *Clinical Psychiatry News* reported: "An estimated 1.6% of Americans are on long-term benzodiazepine therapy—an enormous population of physically dependent patients."

It took about fifteen years after Valium's release for its potential for dependency to become widely known, after which this bestseller plummeted in sales. More recently, it's been determined that about half of the people taking high doses of Xanax, including dose regimens recommended in the PDR, will have difficulty stopping the medication because of withdrawal reactions. Indeed, studies have shown that some people continue taking these medications to avoid rebound or withdrawal reactions, even though the original cause of their anxiety is gone.

Withdrawal is particularly difficult with short-acting drugs such as Xanax and Ativan, but dependency is a problem involving the entire group. This potential for dependency has made benzodiazepines controversial.

But physicians prescribe other drugs that are dangerous or addictive all of the time, and the benzodiazepines aren't nearly as dangerous as some of these. So why have benzodiazepines such as Valium, Xanax, and Halcion attracted such scrutiny? Perhaps because dependency with benzodiazepines is unnecessary and avoidable. People don't seek treatment for their anxiety disorders just to become dependent on the drug that's supposed to be helping them. Especially if they haven't been warned by their physicians of the potential problem.

The PDR provides ample warnings about the dangers of dependency and actually cautions about using benzodiazepines beyond two to three weeks. Yet the disorders for which these drugs are suggested—generalized anxiety disorders, panic disorders—are long-term, sometimes lifelong conditions. Manufacturers know that a panic patient cannot be placed on 6 mg a day of Xanax and then stopped after three weeks.

My belief has long been that the benzodiazepines themselves aren't usually the problem, but rather the doses that are recommended and prescribed. I'm not alone. In an article in *Consumer Reports*, a physician stated: "For anxiety, in general, these medications [benzodiazepines] tend to be used much too long and in too high doses."

WHEN TO USE ANTI-ANXIETY MEDICATIONS

The decision to prescribe anti-anxiety medications is based on the cause, nature, and severity of the condition. Not every instance of intense anxiety requires drug therapy. Many athletes experience intense anxiety before a big game—some of them vomit (an excellent example of anxiety causing a physical, or somatic, reaction)—but we don't medicate them. Most people can get through brief periods of intense anxiety without medication, especially if they utilize other resources such as support from family or friends, physical exercise, keeping themselves mentally occupied, meditation or other types of stress reduction, or counseling/psychotherapy.

Anti-anxiety medication is best used when anxiety becomes so severe or lasts so long that it affects functioning. When the distress is extreme or chronic or causes dysfunction, anti-anxiety medication can be very useful by stabilizing the emotions and permitting improved functioning. Many people take a small dose of Xanax or Valium before flying—it's little different from having an alcoholic drink—and it changes flying from an intense, anxiety-provoking experience into a very tolerable one.

CAREFUL DOSAGING WITH BENZODIAZEPINES

Many physicians prescribe Valium or Xanax or Librium or Ativan to be taken three or four times a day every day. This practice follows the recommendations generally found in the PDR and other drug references. I've always considered this approach a recipe for dependency.

Granted, there are circumstances in which people experience incapacitating anxiety, and it may be necessary to briefly prescribe doses four times a day—in essence round-the-clock treatment. Such instances may include the death of a spouse or child, a rapid succession of panic episodes, or unbearable anxiety that renders the sufferer acutely dysfunctional. Even so, within a few days the medication should greatly decrease the suffering, and further evaluation will determine whether the medication can be reduced, or if other, non-dependency-causing drugs should be added to avoid benzodiazepine dependency.

Most cases, however, are less acute. Even severe conditions such as panic disorders and agoraphobia don't develop overnight. Although the sufferer may feel the need for acute, intense treatment—and he may be right—medication therapy is a stepwise approach that may indeed utilize Xanax or Valium or Klonopin, but also other dependency-free medications to control the condition.

For instance, when prescribing for someone with severe anxiety, I've often used Sinequan, an antidepressant with anti-anxiety properties, at doses of 10 or 25 mg three times a day. In addition, I've often prescribed a benzodiazepine to be used for brief anxiety flare-ups. Working with this combination and, if necessary, adjusting the dosage on a daily basis, I've found that relief can often can be attained within days. With this approach, the benzodiazepine is used as it should be—as an immediate, only when necessary, quick-acting agent.

Unfortunately, starting in the 1980s doctors began prescribing high-dose Xanax as the main medication treatment of anxiety disorders—a rationale I never understood or endorsed. From the day of its release in 1981, it was apparent to me that Xanax would be as prone to cause dependency—indeed, more so—as Valium. Yet Xanax has been prescribed in dosages as high as 4 to 10 mg a day—despite the obvious risk of drug dependency. The result was that patients came to me seeking help in getting off their high doses of Xanax. They were addicted and they knew it. They had tried to stop the medication themselves, but each time they were forced back on it by withdrawal reactions.

Such dependency isn't surprising. Whatever the drug, dependency can occur when the brain is exposed to a continuous flow of high doses of a benzodiazepine for months or years. In some people it can occur within a period of days or weeks. Valium or Xanax given three or four times a day provides this continuous flow to the brain. Remarkably, some people given high dosages don't develop dependency, but others do, and it's often impossible to determine who will become dependent until it has already happened. Fortunately, the pendulum of medical practice has finally begun to swing away from high doses of Xanax, just as it did with Valium twenty years earlier.

My first rule in preventing benzodiazepine dependency is to avoid dosing a patient three or four times a day for many successive days. With people plagued by chronic anxiety, I usually set this rule: on a bad day, you may use the medication up to four times a day, but on other days you must compensate by using less or none. Through a full week, the average amount taken should be no more than two, or on occasion two and a half doses per day.

If you use these drugs variably and intermittently, the brain isn't as likely to become accustomed to the drug. Most people I've worked with are afraid of medications and particularly concerned about dependency. They've heard the stories about Valium and Xanax. They're quite relieved to be put in control of their medication as opposed to being told to take it three or four times a day without fail. Given the necessary information and guidelines, they usually do very well.

Most people are highly motivated to use as little medication as possible, and they use the medication very responsibly. In fact, you may be so motivated to limit your benzodiazepine usage that you sometimes deprive yourself of the drug when you truly need it. In such instances I have to clarify that although minimizing drug usage is important, controlling the symptom is paramount. Allow yourself a bit more flexibility. Besides, the goal is for you to feel or function better, and one pill more or less over a period of weeks or months won't make much difference.

If this approach doesn't control the anxiety disorder, or if the individual simply isn't able to comply with the guidelines, the individual's anxiety may be more severe than recognized and a more intensive approach, using alternative medications, is required. People with addictive personalities or a history of drug addiction often run into dependency problems with benzodiazepines, so these drugs usually are not prescribed for this population. Some children of alcoholic parents may also be more vulnerable to benzodiazepine dependency.

ADDITIONAL BENEFITS OF FLEXIBLE DOSAGING

Besides preventing dependency, flexible dosing with benzodiazepines has other important benefits. Rather than popping a pill because it's noon or 4 P.M., if you are on a flexible dosing schedule, you have to observe yourself. The source of your anxiety may not be readily apparent. The anxiety or panic episodes may seem to come out of nowhere. Yet most anxiety has an origin. If you must decide when to take your medication, you have to be in touch with how you're feeling and, by association, with what immediate events may have prompted these feelings. Thus you can gain information about the source of your anxiety and take steps to deal directly with it.

On the other hand, if the origin of your anxiety isn't recognized, it can't be dealt with. If you are placed on a rigid regimen of Xanax or Valium, the medication may mask the symptoms but not solve the underlying problem. Indeed, the problem may continue to worsen, so that the underlying anxiety increases and with it the need for medication. The risk of dependency mounts.

Because many anxiety disorders are long-term conditions that require ongoing medication treatment, the long-term usage of benzodiazepine drugs requires a strategy. Flexible, intermittent, variable, only-when-needed dosing allows for the safe, prolonged usage of these drugs while you work through your problems.

Even if your anxiety disorder has a significant biochemical basis, as is frequently the case in panic disorders, phobias, and obsessive-compulsive syndromes, the flexible, intermittent use of benzodiazepines allows you to rely on your medication indefinitely with minimal risk. For instance, if you are phobic, an occasional benzodiazepine may allow you to get on an airplane, go to a theater, feel comfortable at a social function, or undergo an MRI. (Indeed, most people, including many with no phobias or anxiety problems, have great difficulty with MRIs, which provoke acute claustrophobia and sensory deprivation.)

TREATING SEVERE ANXIETY DISORDERS

Anxiety disorders can be quite severe and require continuous, intensive medication therapy. In these cases, benzodiazepines shouldn't be expected to do the job alone. Other medications, such as antidepressants, can be employed. Because they don't cause dependency, antidepressants can be used as regularly and intensively as the condition warrants.

Antidepressant medications often become the mainstays of the treatment of panic disorders and agoraphobia, with Xanax, Valium, or other benzodiazepines reserved for acute episodes of increased stress or anxiety. The television anchorman mentioned in the *Newsweek* article overcame his panic disorder with Prozac. After ten days on the drug, he never had another panic episode.

Tofranil (imipramine) was the first antidepressant discovered to have anti-panic effects, and it remains a favorite of some physicians. In my patients, it often caused jitteriness, palpitations, insomnia, or other problems, and I had better results with other antidepressants such as Pamelor.

You should also be aware that people with anxiety disorders, particularly panic disorders, are often highly sensitive to antidepressant drugs. These medications should be started at very low doses. For example, although the recommended initial dosage of Prozac in the PDR is 20 mg a day, numerous studies have shown that as little as 2.5 or 5 mg a day is all that's needed to control panic attacks. In a 1990 study, 5 mg a day of Prozac provided moderate to marked improvement in 76% of panic subjects. Interestingly, 16% developed intolerable side effects, indicating that they would probably have done fine at 2.5 mg or even lower dosages. The authors rightly concluded: "Initiating treatment of panic disorder with low doses of fluoxetine [Prozac] may increase its acceptability and permit more patients to benefit from fluoxetine."

With other antidepressants such as Zoloft or Paxil, similar low-dose strategies have been successful in panic disorder and agoraphobia. If you have a panic or other anxiety disorder, this information is important because you won't find a word about it in the PDR descriptions or package inserts of these drugs.

Several physicians whom I respect tell me that they use high-dose benzodiazepines alone for severe anxiety and panic disorders. They say that despite employing this approach for months or years, they've had few problems. Once the necessary level of medication is reached, they find that there's little need to increase further, and withdrawal is avoided by decreasing the medication gradually. Again, they don't use this approach in people with histories of drug addiction.

These are careful, conscientious physicians—experts in treating anxiety disorders. I attribute their success to a careful selection of patients and frequent monitoring of the treatment. Clearly this approach is not ideal for every person with an anxiety or a panic disorder. As in just about every other area of medicine, good physicians may embrace entirely different, sometimes conflicting, approaches. I've seen too many Xanax dependency and withdrawal problems to agree with the usage of ongoing high-dosage Xanax. Indeed, a small percentage of people experience withdrawal from Xanax after only one or a few pills. My feeling is that if other, nonaddictive drugs can do the heavy work, and benzodiazepines can cover the intermittent exacerbations, why risk using high-dose Xanax?

My colleagues argue that not everyone can tolerate antidepressant drugs and that other benzodiazepines, particularly long-acting types such as Librium, Tranxene, Valium, and especially Klonopin are less prone to causing dependency and withdrawal problems than Xanax. This is true, but the risk of dependency always exists with these drugs.

One thing is certain: high-dose, long-term benzodiazepine treatment is an approach that you should consider undertaking only with an expert, a specialist who has broad experience in treating anxiety disorders and an extensive knowledge of the uses and difficulties of benzodiazepine drugs.

The good news is that most anxiety disorders are treatable. But to obtain the best results, you should find a knowledgeable physician and involve yourself in all decisions about medications and doses.

INTERINDIVIDUAL VARIATION WITH BENZODIAZEPINES

The wife of a doctor friend of mine is afraid of flying, so her husband gave her the smallest dose of Xanax, 0.25 mg, a usually safe amount, before they left for the airport. "She was so sedated," he told me, "I had to physically hold her up while we walked onto the airplane."

The range of individual variation in response to benzodiazepine drugs is extremely wide. Medication-sensitive individuals such as the doctor's wife require small doses. Anything greater will produce sedation, impaired coordination, or other side effects. Although according to the PDR and most textbooks the lowest dosage of Xanax is 0.25 mg, I've had many patients who need as little as one-fourth to one-half of this amount.

THE KEY TO CHOOSING THE RIGHT BENZODIAZEPINE

Not all benzodiazepines are alike. We speak of Xanax, Valium, Librium, and Ativan as if they are interchangeable, when in fact each is quite different, and each has different effects on different individuals. Selecting the proper benzodiazepine not only ensures the best result, but allows for the usage of the lowest dosage.

Benzodiazepines differ in their potency and in their tendency to produce sedation (see page 157). Although all benzodiazepines can produce sedation, some are more likely to do so than others. Valium, Ativan, Serax, and Klonopin are generally more sedating than Xanax, Librium, and Tranxene. If you are sensitive to the depressant effects of alcohol, antihistamines, or codeine, you will likely have difficulty with sedating benzodiazepines like Valium. If you are very sensitive, no matter how small a piece of the Valium pill you try, you may not be able to reduce anxiety without getting drowsy. Xanax or Librium will likely work much better for you.

Conversely, if you are not sensitive to sedating drugs, you may find Xanax, Librium, and Tranxene too mild unless taken in very high doses. You'll probably get better results and require relatively lower doses with Valium, Ativan, Serax, or Klonopin. If even these drugs are ineffective or only work at exceedingly high doses, you should then try Buspar, sedatives (Vistaril or Phenergan), or antidepressants with anti-anxiety effects (e.g., Sinequan).

Characteristics of Benzodiazepines Used for Anxiety

There are great differences in how various benzodiazepines affect people. These differences are, however, relative and vary with the sensitivity of the individual.

	SHORT-ACTING	LONG-ACTING	ULTRA LONG-ACTING
Less Sedating	Xanax (alprazolam)	Librium (chlordiazepoxide)	
		Tranxene (chlorazepate)	
More Sedating	Ativan (lorazepam)	Valium (diazepam)	
	Serax (oxazepam)		Klonopin (clonazepam)

Another difference between benzodiazepines is in their effect on mental anxiety: worrying, or repeatedly going over the same issue in your head. For this symptom, Xanax usually works, but when it doesn't, Librium often does. If you aren't sedation sensitive, Valium may be even more effective.

These fine distinctions between benzodiazepine drugs aren't widely recognized. They're not mentioned in the PDR or many drug references, or taught at medical schools. In my experience, physicians tend to use these drugs interchangeably, as if they are identical. But they're not, and the distinctions often mean the difference between high dosages and low dosages, between a good response and side effects.

Whichever medication is selected, if you are medication-sensitive, start with the lowest dose and titrate upward according to your sensitivity. Because benzodiazepines are generally fast-acting drugs, it's easy to increase the dosage if necessary. If you take half a Xanax an hour before flying and you are still panicking after takeoff, then another half a Xanax is in order.

SHORT-ACTING VERSUS LONG-ACTING BENZODIAZEPINES

Another key distinction between different benzodiazepines is whether they are short-, long-, or ultra long-acting (see page 157). In the late 1970s and early 1980s, as a result of the Valium controversy, physicians became leery of long-acting benzodiazepines because with frequent usage, the levels of these drugs tend to accumulate in the body. This may cause cumulative side effects such as sluggishness, drowsiness, impaired thinking or memory, or depression, or it may promote dependency. It was Valium's tendency to collect in body tissues when prescribed in high dosages for prolonged periods that led to its fall from grace. This provided the opportunity for manufacturers of short-acting drugs such as Xanax to quickly gain dominance in the huge anti-anxiety drug market.

In fact, short-acting benzodiazepines can create as many if not more problems than longer-acting types. That's why Xanax causes a higher incidence of drug dependency than Valium. Unfortunately, the preference for short-acting benzodiazepines remains strong among physicians, when in fact longer-acting benzodiazepines often may be preferable. I've seen far more dependency with short-acting Xanax than I ever saw with longer-acting Valium or Librium.

The reality is that both short-acting and longer-acting benzodiazepines have their place in the treatment of anxiety disorders. The choice should depend on the situation and the individual. If you are experiencing a panic attack, fast-acting Xanax may be the best choice. Indeed, for an almost instantaneous effect, patients have told me that they chew the Xanax tablet or let it dissolve in their mouths. I equate Xanax in anxiety disorders to nitroglycerin in angina—a great medicine for fast, short-term relief.

CHOOSING THE BEST BENZODIAZEPINE FOR YOU

In the discussion of short-acting and long-acting benzodiazepines, it must be understood that these terms are relative. The duration of action of a specific benzodiazepine varies from person to person. For some, the effect of Xanax wears off very quickly, in three hours or less. But if you are medication-sensitive, Xanax's effect may last five to six hours.

Like Xanax, Ativan is a short-acting drug. More sedating than Xanax, it may be useful with individuals who don't get much relief from moderate doses of Xanax. Conversely, individuals sedated by Ativan may find Xanax a better fit. I prefer Ativan to Serax because Ativan, like Xanax, is available as a tablet, allowing individuals to adjust their doses by splitting or cutting the pill, whereas Serax is a capsule.

For continual, ongoing anxiety, short-acting benzodiazepines make less sense. They wear off too quickly and require too many repeated doses. In some people, Xanax wears off so swiftly that it causes a rebound effect—a strong resurgence of anxiety as the drug rapidly leaves the system. In contrast, long-acting Valium, Tranxene, and Librium provide a more gradual, longer-lasting effect, thereby requiring fewer doses and rare rebound problems. If you are sedation sensitive, or if Valium or Ativan have made you too drowsy, Librium or Tranxene may be preferable. If you aren't sedation sensitive, or if Librium or Tranxene are too mild, Valium may provide better results.

Klonopin, the longest-acting benzodiazepine, is in a class of its own. Klonopin is too slow acting to provide immediate relief for panic attacks, but because of its prolonged activity, its dependency potential is low. In fact, Klonopin was developed as an anti-seizure drug. You won't find a word about its usage for anxiety disorders in the PDR. People using Klonopin for seizure problems take it daily, yet dependency problems with Klonopin have been minimal. For this reason, Klonopin may be the exception to the rule—the one benzodiazepine that may reasonably be considered for use as the primary, daily medication for the control of generalized anxiety disorders, panic disorders, and agoraphobia.

ANTI-ANXIETY MEDICATIONS AND THE ELDERLY

In a small number of people, benzodiazepines cause a paradoxical effect, meaning that rather than becoming calmer, they become agitated, hostile, or confused. In younger adults this reaction is rare, but in the elderly it's common. Also, typical side effects of benzodiazepines such as depression, weakness, disorientation, or impaired memory also occur more frequently in the elderly. When these side effects develop gradually, they can be misdiagnosed as Alzheimer's disease and other disorders. For this reason, some physicians don't prescribe benzodiazepines to older individuals. Unfortunately, alternate drugs cause other, sometimes worse side effects in this population.

Anxiety disorders occur more often in older people than in younger populations, and severe anxiety can be more incapacitating. Most important, a thorough physical evaluation should be done to rule out a medical cause. Second, the person's medications must be carefully reviewed because they are frequently a source of anxiety and other emotional changes.

In treating an anxiety disorder, the best approach with the elderly is to avoid all drugs that affect mental functioning. Stress reduction, activities, exercise, and increased social participation can be helpful, but sometimes anxiety-reducing medication is necessary. Benzodiazepines may be used, but cautiously.

Studies show that these drugs can be very effective in the elderly, but responses to these medications can be even more variable than in younger adults. Older people metabolize benzodiazepines more slowly, producing higher blood levels. Also, nervous system sensitivity to these drugs is increased. Therefore, treatment must be initiated at very low dosages with careful monitoring by the physician and family.

The less sedating benzodiazepines—Xanax, Librium, Tranxene—are probably preferable initially. Because Librium and Tranxene are longer acting, their effects may tend to linger in some elderly persons, but these drugs won't cause the rebound anxiety sometimes seen with Xanax. The choice should depend upon the individual's condition and side effect history, and the initial response should be monitored closely.

USING BENZODIAZEPINES SAFELY

For the immediate treatment of anxiety, no medications surpass the benzodiazepines. When used conservatively, this group of drugs has a long record of effectiveness with minimal side effects. The catch, of course, is proper usage: selecting the right benzodiazepine, taking the lowest effective dosage, using it flexibly, and avoiding dosages that may cause dependency.

Selecting between Xanax, Valium, Ativan, Librium, Serax, Tranxene, and Klonopin merely requires knowing the type of anxiety problem you have and whether you are sensitive to sedating medications. Starting low and adjusting upward is easy and allows you to determine your specific sensitivity to the medication with fewer risks. And although physicians may differ regarding the benzodiazepine they prefer, there is little disagreement about the importance of using the very lowest, effective doses of these drugs.

In-Depth Analysis: Xanax (Alprazolam)

QUICK AND EFFECTIVE—BUT SAFE?

America's favorite anti-anxiety medication, Xanax is a very effective medication. For the relief of anxiety, panic, and general nervousness, Xanax works fast and doesn't linger. In most people, Xanax works within twenty minutes and lasts about four hours. For a quicker effect, patients with panic disorders have told me of chewing or placing a Xanax tablet under their tongue to obtain an almost instant result. This method should be used only with your physician's guidance because of the possible risk of greater side effects.

Another Xanax attribute is that it is less prone to causing sedation or drowsiness than Valium or Ativan. If you are medication-sensitive or if you are sensitive to alcohol or the sedating effects of some antihistamines (e.g., Benadryl, Dramamine) or muscle relaxants, then Xanax is a good choice for quick, short-acting relief of intermittent anxiety.

When used properly, Xanax is a generally safe medication. The problem with Xanax is that when it hit the market in 1981, it was oversold and its dangers vastly underestimated.

XANAX—REPEATING THE MISTAKES OF VALIUM

Because of the way Xanax was marketed in the early 1980s, I knew there would be problems, big ones. Valium, after over a decade of tremendous popularity, was falling into disfavor because of publicity about the physical and emotional dependency it caused in some people. The huge anti-anxiety market that Valium had dominated was suddenly wide open, and manufacturers of other anti-anxiety drugs rushed to fill the void.

Assured that Xanax did not accumulate in the body like Valium, physicians began substituting it for Valium, prescribing Xanax as often, perhaps more so, than they ever prescribed Valium. Xanax rapidly became a top-selling drug, ranking among the top ten medications in outpatient prescriptions for many years. It even outsold Prozac in the early 1990s.

The problem was that Xanax was readily employed not just for occasional anxiety, but for the ongoing, long-term treatment of severe anxiety—just as Valium had been. This often required high dosages—dosages that I have always considered too prone to result in dependency to be used safely.

For panic disorders, even higher dosages of Xanax were recommended and prescribed—dosages of 4 to 10 mg a day. I considered this unwise not only because these dosages risked dependency, but also because other medications were available to help handle panic tendencies. My feeling was that Xanax should be used intermittently for intense surges of anxiety. In contrast to the flood of journal articles extolling the virtues of high-dosage Xanax and the apparent popularity of Xanax among physicians and patients, my views obviously were in the minority.

The result of Xanax overusage was not surprising. Just as the previous overuse of Valium caused many cases of dependency, so too did Xanax—with a vengeance. In fact, more people developed a dependency on Xanax than on Valium. This didn't surprise me either. Because Xanax exits the human body so quickly, withdrawal reactions are likely to be swifter and more severe.

Indeed, Xanax leaves the body so quickly that some people experience a rebound reaction, a feeling of increased anxiety as the dose of Xanax wears off. To avoid the rebound reaction, people with ongoing problems such as panic disorders were often placed on four-times-a-day dosing. This had two effects: it provided better immediate anxiety control, and it also made dependency and withdrawal reactions ultimately more likely.

Because of the frequency and severity of Xanax dependency and withdrawal, reducing or stopping Xanax proved to be very difficult after long-term or high-dose usage. The manufacturer of Xanax acknowledges this in the PDR: "When used at high doses for long intervals . . . Xanax has the potential to cause severe emotional and physical dependence in some patients and these patients may find it exceedingly difficult to terminate treatment."

Indeed, dependency problems have been reported even at modest dosages. Again, per the PDR: "Even after relatively short-term use at the doses recommended for treatment of transient anxiety and anxiety disorder (i.e., 0.75 to 4.0 mg per day), there is some risk of dependence." Not infrequently, I saw this in my own patients. This reinforced my belief that at any dosage, Xanax must be used carefully.

One of the ironies about Xanax is that in treating Xanax dependency, some people have to be switched to Librium or Valium—the drugs Xanax was supposed to replace—because gradually reducing the dosages of these drugs is usually less difficult or dangerous than doing so with Xanax.

After watching my profession repeat the same errors with Xanax that we'd committed with Valium, and after having to slowly withdraw many people from high-dose Xanax given to them by other physicians, in 1988 I finally registered my concerns in a letter to the *Journal of Clinical Psychiatry* (see below). Fortunately, over recent years many physicians have gradually turned away from high-dose Xanax for severe, long-term anxiety disorders.

XANAX USAGES

Despite the excesses, Xanax has a place in medical treatment. Xanax remains perhaps the best anti-anxiety medication for the intermittent, quick treatment of high stress, anxiety, or panic attacks. Xanax also can be very useful in the episodic treatment of social and other phobias (flying, public speaking, etc.), premenstrual stress disorder, unnerving medical procedures such as MRIs, and other conditions characterized by anxiety, agitation, nervousness, or jitteriness.

This is why Xanax and three different types of its generic, alprazolam, continue to rank among the 200 top-selling drugs in outpatient prescriptions.

An Early Warning About High-Dose Xanax

A letter to the editor of the August 1988 issue of the *Journal of Clinical Psychiatry*:

Sir: I am writing in response to an article (February 1988 issue) comparing a variety of medications in the treatment of panic disorder. I wonder, do any physicians besides me get nervous when they read about alprazolam (Xanax) being used in doses as high as 4 mg or more?

Over the last few years, several studies compared alprazolam with a variety of other psychopharmacological approaches, such as antidepressants or beta blockers. In all of these, alprazolam is used at dosage levels that I, for one, consider extremely high. Personally, I am very reluctant to prescribe dosages of alprazolam above 1 mg/day for any prolonged period, because at higher dosages I have frequently run into problems with spontaneous withdrawal and/or acute rebound phenomena. From a pharmacological perspective, it seems obvious to me that, because of the extremely short duration of its clinical effect, alprazolam is potentially more addictive than any of the other benzodiazepine preparations. In practice, I have seen many more problems with alprazolam than I ever did with diazepam [Valium]. Consequently, both science and experience have made me extremely cautious in prescribing alprazolam. Therefore, if a patient does not respond quickly and thoroughly to daily dosages of alprazolam of 1 mg or less, I immediately add antidepressants or beta blockers to the regimen, rather than increase the alprazolam dosage.

There is no doubt that in some patients alprazolam works exceedingly well for panic attacks, especially in those who need a quick-acting anti-anxiety drug on an intermittent basis. On the other hand, the daily use of alprazolam in high doses for the patient who has continually high anxiety or frequent panic attacks has been, in my experience, fraught with difficulty and danger. I wonder if any other physicians out there share this perspective?

—Jay S. Cohen, M.D.

MANUFACTURER-RECOMMENDED DOSAGES OF XANAX

In the PDR, the manufacturer makes multiple statements about the importance of using the lowest effective Xanax dosages and the risks of long-term usage and dependency. For treating generalized anxiety, the manufacturer suggests an initial dosage of 0.25 or 0.5 mg three times a day, increasing if necessary up to a maximum dose of 4 mg a day. For panic disorders, doses range from 1 to 10 mg a day, with the average being 5 to 6 mg a day.

LOW-DOSE XANAX

The PDR and drug references all emphasize the problem of dependency with Xanax, yet they then recommend some dosages that in my opinion are highly likely to cause dependency. Starting Xanax at 0.25 or 0.5 mg a day, as the manufacturer recommends, is generally safe. However, if you take Xanax three times a day every day, you may very well become tolerant to Xanax's effects and soon need higher dosages to accomplish the same result. This is how Xanax dependency often begins.

Dependency is of course a function of usage. It is very difficult to become dependent on Xanax if you use it intermittently, once or twice a day, even three times a day on an occasional bad day, especially if you skip using Xanax perhaps one or two days per week. This variable approach, using an average of about two doses or less of Xanax per day, is usually quite safe and can be utilized for prolonged periods.

If you are medication-sensitive, the lowest Xanax dose, 0.25 mg, may be ideal, or it may be too strong for you. Half or one-fourth a tablet may be enough. One woman, after giving birth to her first child, developed postpartum panic attacks. Her doctor, who hadn't yet accepted the fact of postpartum anxiety and depressive syndromes, also discounted the fact that one-fourth of a 0.25 mg Xanax controlled this woman's anxiety. Nevertheless, using one or two doses a day, in several weeks her anxiety waned, and she easily discontinued the drug. (She wasn't breast-feeding her child; Xanax and other benzodiazepines are excreted in breast milk.)

A wide range of interindividual variation is seen with Xanax. If you are medication-sensitive, start at a very low dose of Xanax and adjust according to your response. Lower doses work for many people, but others require higher doses to obtain the same result. People who are not sedation sensitive may find Xanax too mild for their needs, and they may respond better to Valium, Serax, or Ativan.

ALTERNATIVES TO HIGH-DOSE, LONG-TERM XANAX

High-dose Xanax doesn't always cause dependency, but the risk is not small. If the flexible approach described above isn't sufficient to control your anxiety symptoms, you should instead be treated with alternative medications as discussed earlier in this chapter. Xanax is often used in combination with other medications, thereby negating the need for high dosages of Xanax to control all of your symptoms. For example, Xanax combined with antidepressant drugs is an effective way of controlling panic disorders.

The PDR states that Xanax should be used for no more than two to three weeks, but this warning is impractical with chronic anxiety disorders. People with generalized anxiety disorders, panic episodes, agoraphobia, or other phobias don't get over these conditions quickly. For some, these problems are the result of chemical imbalances in the brain and require lifelong treatment. This is no different than the continuous treatment necessary for disorders such as hypertension or diabetes.

Xanax can be used indefinitely in the treatment of anxiety disorders if it's used cautiously, intermittently, and in the very lowest, effective doses.

XANAX AND THE ELDERLY

Xanax, like Valium and Halcion and all other benzodiazepines, must be used with particular care in elderly persons. Side effects and paradoxical reactions occur more frequently in the older population than the younger. Yet so do many anxiety disorders and insomnia.

Although it's preferable to avoid all medications that affect the nervous system in older people, severe anxiety can cause emotional havoc and impair functioning. In many cases, Xanax or other benzodiazepines may be the safest and fastest-acting choice.

Obtaining a medication history is very important. People who have responded well to Xanax previously are more likely to do well on it again; those who had problems with Xanax will likely have problems again.

Overall, the less sedating benzodiazepines such as Xanax, Librium, and Tranxene are preferable for daytime anxiety. Xanax is the least likely of these to accumulate in the system of older individuals, who metabolize medications more slowly. Librium and Tranxene are less likely than Xanax to cause rebound anxiety, but if overused they can accumulate and cause depression of physical or mental functioning.

RECOMMENDATIONS

Xanax is a very effective, useful drug—*if* it is used properly. My approach has always been to utilize Xanax for the quick relief of acute anxiety, for brief episodes of anxiety such as dealing with a social phobia or undergoing an MRI, or for intermittent usage in controlling the symptoms of long-term anxiety disorders.

I have never subscribed to the use of high-dose Xanax for treating generalized anxiety disorders, agoraphobia, or panic syndromes; other, nonaddictive drugs can be used for this purpose. Xanax can be used in conjunction with other medications, a much safer approach in long-term conditions.

Flexible dosaging with Xanax is easy because both Xanax and generic alprazolam are produced in 0.25-, 0.5-, 1-, and 2-mg scored tablets. If you are medication-sensitive, or are sensitive to alcohol or to the sedating effects of antihistamines or muscle relaxants, start with the very lowest Xanax tablet, 0.25 mg. This pill is breakable and I've had many patients who've responded to a fourth or a half of this amount. Start low and increase gradually if necessary to obtain the desired anxiety control without drowsiness.

Patients with panic episodes have told me that when in a crisis, they've obtained an almost immediate effect by chewing on a Xanax tablet or letting it dissolve under their tongue. You should obtain your physician's advice before using this method because of a possible increased risk of side effects.

The effect of Xanax lasts about four hours in most people. For those with ongoing anxiety, I usually prefer Librium or Tranxene because they last about six hours, providing broader coverage with fewer doses. If Xanax, even at 0.5 or 1.0 mg, isn't potent enough to control your anxiety, you may obtain a better response with relatively lower doses of Ativan or Valium. This is often the case in people who aren't sensitive to sedating drugs.

In-Depth Analysis: Valium (Diazepam)

A DESERVED REPUTATION?

Not long ago, I got into a conversation with a woman at the library. When she learned I was a physician, she asked what I thought about Valium. She said, "My father's doctor keeps prescribing it for him. It scares me."

Her father, age 75, had become more irritable and difficult to deal with. A low dose of Valium seemed to be helping him a lot, but its reputation worried her. I could tell by her tone that she considered Valium to be something like heroin.

She continued, "Isn't there something else his doctor could prescribe? Maybe lithium?"

I chuckled to myself. If Valium is a bullet, lithium is a bazooka. I replied, "Lithium is a potentially toxic drug with long-term side effects. It can be hard to handle and requires repeated blood levels. Valium is a lot easier and more benign."

"But won't he get addicted to it?"

Her father was taking about 2 mg twice a day, hardly a dosage likely to cause dependency. The only real problem was Valium's reputation, which understandably disturbed this woman. I tried to reassure her. "Personally, I'd much rather be taking Valium than lithium or an antidepressant. When used properly, it's a much safer drug and causes few problems. It sounds like your father is being treated properly."

THE TROUBLE WITH VALIUM

As with Xanax and Halcion, Valium itself has never been the problem; the problem is how it has been promoted and prescribed.

Indeed, when Valium and Librium were first marketed in the early 1960s, it was believed that these drugs caused no dependency. They were considered major advancements over the sedatives then available, phenobarbital and meprobamate, both sedating and highly addictive drugs that often were the cause of intended and unintended suicides.

In fact, Valium and Librium *were* significant improvements on meprobamate and phenobarbital. Valium and Librium provided a better anti-anxiety effect and caused less sedation. Overdoses rarely caused death. If prescribed cautiously, Valium would probably still possess the lofty reputation it originally had. Unfortunately, it was frequently prescribed in high dosages and doled out in large quantities for prolonged periods—a perfect recipe for dependency.

By 1980, Valium dependency had become the stuff of newspaper and magazine exposés, best-selling books, and at least one movie. Valium's popularity and sales plummeted—and medical history began repeating itself again with Xanax.

STILL A USEFUL MEDICATION

Despite its mixed record, and despite the fact that Valium is a medication that has been around over thirty years, its usefulness continues. This is demonstrated by the fact that both brand-name Valium and generic diazepam ranked among the 200 top-selling drugs in 1995 as measured by U.S. outpatient prescriptions.

Valium's uses are many. It is prescribed for anxiety disorders, muscular spasms, insomnia, and alcohol withdrawal. Valium is also used intravenously for acute seizures and for the light sedation required for minor medical procedures, such as endoscopy. In this latter usage, Valium sometimes causes anterograde amnesia—incomplete memory of the procedure, which many people prefer. (Versed, a frequently used benzodiazepine anesthetic, often causes this amnesia.) This is the same anterograde amnesia that has made Halcion controversial in the treatment of insomnia. Temporary amnesia is fine when it's medically induced and controlled as with intravenous Valium, but not when it's caused by a sleeping pill that wipes out a person's memory of his or her activities the following morning.

VALIUM AND ANXIETY DISORDERS

No one has ever argued the fact that Valium is an effective anti-anxiety medication. Its effectiveness is what led to Valium's main problem—overusage.

Valium is a longer-acting benzodiazepine. It doesn't cause the rebound reactions seen with short-acting Xanax, but when used in high dosages for a long period, Valium can accumulate in the body and cause sluggishness, fatigue, depression, or loss of mental acuity. Such usage also can promote physical dependency and withdrawal reactions.

Valium is generally more sedating than Xanax or Librium. If you are medication-sensitive, or sensitive to alcohol or the sedating effects some antihistamines (e.g., Benadryl, Dramamine) or muscle relaxants, Valium may make you drowsy or sleepy. Librium, Tranxene, or Xanax may be better initial choices for you. If these medications are too mild or you require very high doses of them to obtain anxiety control, Valium may work better at a lower dosage.

If you aren't sensitive to sedating drugs, Valium may work well for you. It also works well for anxiety that's characterized by mental agitation such as obsessive thoughts or going over the same worries again and again. For these symptoms, Librium and Tranxene may work better than Xanax; Valium and Ativan better than Librium and Tranxene.

MANUFACTURER-RECOMMENDED DOSAGES OF VALIUM

The manufacturer-recommended dosage of Valium for anxiety is 2 to 10 mg, two to four times a day; for muscular spasm, 2 to 10 mg three to four times a day; for the elderly, 2 ½ mg once or twice daily. Valium is also produced in an extended-release pill, 15 mg Valrelease, the equivalent to 5 mg of Valium three times a day. Valrelease is recommended once or twice a day for anxiety disorders or muscular spasms.

LOW-DOSE VALIUM—USING VALIUM SAFELY

I never have been comfortable prescribing Valium or any other benzodiazepine three or four times a day for more than a few days. To me, anything longer is a recipe for dependency.

On the other hand, if used flexibly and intermittently, Valium can be used safely for prolonged periods. This is important because many anxiety disorders are chronic conditions requiring ongoing treatment. The PDR states that Valium should be used for only two to three weeks, but this warning is disingenuous because it's well known that many people prescribed Valium are going to need it for longer than that.

The solution is to use Valium in a low-dose, variable manner. First, you need to find the dose of Valium that provides an anti-anxiety effect without causing sedation. If you are medication-sensitive, you should start at the lowest dose, 2 mg, or even half or a fourth of that amount. Fortunately, flexible dosing is easy because both brand-name Valium and generic diazepam are produced in 2-, 5-, and 10-mg scored tablets.

Once the effective dose is established, whether it's 1, 2, 2.5, 5, or 10 mg, the key is to use it flexibly and intermittently. For example, on a highly stressful day, you may need to take the effective dose three or four times, but on other days just once or twice, and if possible no Valium at least one day a week. The average usage should be about two doses or less per day. By using Valium this way, variably and only when necessary, as opposed to three or four times a day every day, you will minimize the risks of physical dependency. Unfortunately, this method of flexible dosaging is not mentioned in the PDR or many other drug references.

If this method of flexible dosaging isn't sufficient to control your anxiety disorder, then alternate medications should be considered. For example, in panic disorders, antidepressants are often effective in controlling the panic tendency, while Valium or another benzodiazepine is employed as needed for episodes of intense anxiety.

VALIUM AND THE ELDERLY

In the elderly, it is usually preferable to use less sedating benzodiazepines such as Librium, Tranxene, or Xanax instead of Valium. These drugs are less likely to cause undesirable sedation or paradoxical reactions. If these medications are too mild, Valium may be tried at a very low initial dose such as 1 mg. It can be gradually adjusted upward, if necessary, according to the individual's response.

For insomnia, shorter-acting drugs such as Ativan or Restoril are usually preferable to long-acting Valium.

RECOMMENDATIONS

Valium is an effective and safe medication when used properly. If you are medication-sensitive or sensitive to sedating drugs, Valium may be too strong for you. Librium, Tranxene, or Xanax may be better initial choices. If they are too mild to control your anxiety, Valium may provide a better effect.

The key to avoiding dependency on Valium or any other benzodiazepine drug is to use it flexibly and intermittently. By taking Valium only when needed, rather than three or four times a day, you minimize the risk of physical dependency. If Valium is used variably and sparingly, it can be taken for prolonged periods for chronic conditions such as generalized anxiety or panic disorders.

For severe anxiety or panic, adding one of the alternate medications in combination with Valium, rather than depending solely on high-dose Valium, often works better while minimizing the risks of Valium dependency.

If you've been taking daily moderate or high-dose Valium for a prolonged period, discontinuing the medication should be done gradually under the guidance of a physician to prevent withdrawal reactions.

Overall, dependency problems are fewer and less severe with Valium than with Xanax, the drug that replaced Valium as America's top-selling anti-anxiety drug. Another irony is that people unable to withdraw from Xanax are often switched to Valium, from which gradual withdrawal is safer and easier. This is because long-acting Valium doesn't exit the body as precipitously as short-acting Xanax.

The public concern about Valium that began two decades ago was warranted because Valium was being overprescribed and overused. Nevertheless, Valium is an effective and generally safe medication when prescribed and used carefully. This means using Valium flexibly, only when needed, and in the very lowest effective dose.

Other Anti-Anxiety Medications

ATIVAN (LORAZEPAM)

Ativan, like Xanax, is a short-acting benzodiazepine that is less prone to accumulate in the body than Valium or Librium. This attribute has made it a popular anti-anxiety drug—two different types of Ativan's generic, lorazepam, ranked No. 31 and No. 32 among all generic drugs in outpatient prescriptions in 1996.

Unlike Xanax, Ativan is one of the more sedating benzodiazepines. If you are medication-sensitive or sensitive to alcohol or sedating drugs such as some antihistamines (e.g., Benadryl, Dramamine) or muscle relaxants, Ativan may be too sedating for you. You should first consider Librium, Tranxene, or Xanax. If you aren't sensitive to sedation, or if you usually tolerate standard doses of sedating antihistamines or sleep medications well, Ativan may be a good first choice for controlling anxiety.

Because Ativan works quickly and is sedating, it's often used as a sleep medication. Ativan metabolism may be less affected by aging than other benzodiazepines, and very low doses of Ativan may be useful as a sleep remedy for older individuals.

Ativan shares all of the advantages and disadvantages of short-acting benzodiazepines. It works fast and at standard dosages doesn't build up in the body. Yet because Ativan leaves the body rapidly, withdrawal reactions can be severe in people who've been on high daily doses of Ativan for weeks or longer.

Like all drugs of this group, daily Ativan usage, even at doses recommended by the manufacturer and other drug references, can cause physical and emotional dependency. In the PDR, the manufacturer warns about dependency and withdrawal, and states that the Ativan dosage should be individualized. The PDR recommends a starting dosage of 2 or 3 mg a day (presumably 0.5 mg four times a day or 1 mg three times a day). For the elderly, 1 to 2 mg a day. The "usual range" of dosages is 2 to 6 mg a day, with some patients requiring up to 10 mg a day.

In my opinion, some of these dosages are excessive and dangerous. Even 2 or 3 mg can cause dependency in some people. Furthermore, the PDR does not suggest using variable, as-needed dosaging. Anti-anxiety drugs like Ativan cause much less dependency when used flexibly and intermittently. With this method, Ativan can be used three times a day on high anxiety days, but less often on less stressful days. It's particularly helpful if no medication is taken perhaps one or two days a week. Overall, usage should average about two doses or less per day.

A flexible, intermittent approach allows for the ongoing use of Ativan with minimal risk, an important issue if you have a chronic anxiety disorder. Most generalized anxiety disorders, panic disorders, and agoraphobia are chronic conditions. If the flexible usage of Ativan is insufficient to relieve your anxiety, other medications can be added to attain control. In panic disorders, for example, combination therapy includes antidepressants to halt the panic tendency and Ativan or another benzodiazepine for intermittent episodes of intense anxiety.

If you are medication-sensitive, you may respond to even less than the smallest Ativan pill, 0.5 mg. Half or even a fourth of this amount may be a better initial dose until you determine your specific sensitivity. The brand-name Ativan 0.5 mg tablet is not scored, but some types of generic lorazepam are; ask your pharmacist for a scored 0.5-mg tablet. Ativan and generic lorazepam are also produced in 1- and 2-mg sizes; the brand-name tablets are scored in these sizes, but only some generic brands are scored—check with your pharmacist.

If you require higher doses of Ativan, rather than jumping from

0.5 to 1.0 to 2.0 mg, each a 100% increase, you can adjust more gradually by splitting the 0.5 and 1.0 mg pills to obtain intermediate doses of 0.75, 1.25, 1.5, and 1.75 mg. Remember, keeping the dosage as low as possible is the key to avoiding tolerance and dependency.

For elderly individuals, less sedating anti-anxiety medications than Ativan, such as Librium, Tranxene, or Xanax, are usually preferable. If they aren't effective, Ativan can be used, starting with a very low dosage.

If you've been taking daily moderate or high-dose Ativan for a prolonged period, discontinuing the medication should be done gradually under medical guidance to prevent withdrawal reactions.

KLONOPIN (CLONAZEPAM)

Unlike other benzodiazepines that have been marketed extensively for treating anxiety and panic disorders, Klonopin is not FDA approved for this usage. Klonopin was developed and continues to be prescribed for seizure disorders. All benzodiazepines have anti-seizure properties, but only Klonopin is employed as a primary, day-to-day anti-seizure drug. Because Klonopin is an ultra long-acting medication, it's possible to maintain stable blood levels of Klonopin, thereby providing continuous anti-seizure protection.

It's for this very same reason that Klonopin has gradually been adopted for treating anxiety disorders, especially panic disorders. In contrast to quick-acting and -exiting Xanax, Klonopin offers a steady, prolonged effect with little risk of rebound reactions. Because of its multiple uses and relatively safe side effect profile, in 1996 Klonopin ranked No. 52 in outpatient prescriptions in the U.S.

Klonopin works too slowly for the immediate control of extreme anxiety or panic episodes, but when taken on a daily basis, it has proven to be quite effective in controlling the emergence of severe anxiety symptoms. And because Klonopin leaves the body slowly, withdrawal reactions seem to be less frequent or severe.

Nevertheless, dependency can occur with Klonopin and this must be considered when deciding upon medication treatment for an anxiety disorder. As with all benzodiazepines that have been taken in moderate or high daily doses for weeks or months, the Klonopin dosage should be tapered gradually under the guidance of a physician instead of abruptly discontinued.

The PDR contains no information about Klonopin in relation to anxiety disorders, although Klonopin has been extensively used for these conditions for nearly a decade. For the manufacturer to include such information, it would have to reapply to the FDA, an often lengthy and expensive process that often isn't cost-effective. For seizures, the PDR recommends an initial dosage not exceeding 1.5 mg a day with a maximum dosage of 20 mg a day.

Other drug references, which aren't limited by the FDA, do discuss Klonopin in the treatment of anxiety and panic syndromes. The recommended dosages range from 1 to 5 mg a day. In one study Klonopin was effective in about 75% of the subjects with social phobias; the Klonopin dosage range was from 0.5 to 5 mg a day, with an average dose of 2 mg a day. Partial improvement was seen after 2 weeks, with a full response occurring after about 6 weeks on Klonopin. In another study, Klonopin was effective for 78% of the subjects with social phobias versus only 20% of those taking a placebo. Other studies obtained 82% and 84% rates of improvement, respectively.

In a 1997 study of people with panic disorders, Klonopin out-performed Xanax in controlling panic attacks. The average Klonopin dose was 2.5 mg a day, a moderate amount, especially in comparison to the average of 5.3 mg a day of Xanax, a dosage that may be addictive for some people.

Because Klonopin is a sedating drug, if you are medication-sensitive, or sensitive to alcohol or the sedation of some antihistamines (e.g., Benadryl, Dramamine) or muscle relaxants, you should begin with a very low dose of Klonopin, such as 0.25 mg, half a 0.5 tablet. It's preferable to first try the medication at night, so if the Klonopin sedates you, you can go to bed.

Once-a-day Klonopin is sufficient for some people, but others need coverage twice a day or three times a day. When daytime dosages are used, they are usually a fourth to a half the bedtime dosage. Typical Klonopin regimens are 0.25 mg in the morning (or twice a day) and 0.5 mg at bedtime, or 0.5 mg in the morning (or twice a day) and 1.0 mg at bedtime.

In time, you may become tolerant to Klonopin's sedating effects and higher dosages, if necessary, can be used. Or if you aren't sensitive to sedation, you may start at a slightly higher dose such as 0.5 or 1.0 mg, adjusting the dosage according to your response. The usual range of effective Klonopin dosages in anxiety disorders is 0.5 to 5 mg a day.

Before making any changes in your medication or dosing, discuss these issues with your physician. Flexible dosaging is easy because Klonopin and its generic, clonazepam, are produced in 0.5-, 1-, and 2-mg scored tablets.

LIBRIUM (CHLORDIAZEPOXIDE)

Librium was the first benzodiazepine released in America. A drug widely used during the 1960s and 1970s, Librium ranked just behind Valium in popularity. Librium is less sedating than Valium and usually works better for people who are sensitive to the effects of alcohol or the sedation cause by some antihistamines (e.g., Benadryl, Dramamine) or muscle relaxants.

Today, Librium is most often used in treating anxiety disorders, the anxiety preceding surgery, and in alcohol and Xanax withdrawal.

If you are medication-sensitive or if you are sensitive to sedating drugs, Librium is a good choice for anxiety control. Librium doesn't work quite as fast as Xanax, but it lasts longer, about six hours in most people. If Librium is ineffective or effective only at high doses, Valium, Serax, or Ativan may work better at lower doses.

Because Librium is longer acting than Xanax, it rarely causes the rebound anxiety seen with Xanax. On the other hand, because it is long-acting, if Librium is taken frequently for long periods, it may accumulate in the body and cause fatigue, depression, mental sluggishness, or dependency.

For general anxiety, I've found Librium to be an effective, dependable medication, especially in medication-sensitive individuals. When used properly, dependency is rarely a problem. The only time that I prefer Xanax to Librium is in the treatment of acute anxiety or panic attacks. Otherwise, I've found Librium to work more gently and evenly, with far fewer problems, than Xanax.

The manufacturer recommended dosage of Librium for general anxiety is 5 to 10 mg three or four times a day; for severe anxiety, 20 to 25 mg at the same frequency; for the elderly, 5 mg two to four times a day. The manufacturer offers the usual warnings about Librium dependency and the need to individualize dosages. However, I believe that the higher recommended dosages, especially when used three to four times daily, are risky.

Most important, the manufacturer makes no mention of using Librium in a variable, as-needed manner. The key to maintaining the usefulness of this drug and avoiding tolerance and dependency is to utilize it flexibly and intermittently.

In this method, Librium can be used three or even four times a day on bad days, but must be used less often on other days, and preferably not at all once a week. If you use Librium variably, with an average usage of about two doses or less per day, problems are minimized even with prolonged usage. This is particularly important in treating anxiety disorders, which are often long-term conditions.

If this method is insufficient to control your anxiety or panic disorder, alternative medications should be considered. In panic disorders, an effective combination includes an antidepressant to halt the panic tendency and Librium for episodes of intense anxiety.

If you've been taking daily moderate or high dose Librium for a prolonged period, discontinuing the medication should be done gradually under the guidance of a physician to prevent withdrawal reactions.

Dosage flexibility is somewhat limited with Librium because of the way it's manufactured. Brand-name Librium is produced in 5-, 10-, and 25-mg capsules, and also in 5- and 25-mg film-coated tablets that are difficult to split. All generic types of Librium I've seen are capsules. Fortunately, the 5-mg dose is generally well tolerated by medication-sensitive individuals. If greater dose flexibility is required, Tranxene, which is very similar to Librium in its effects, is available as scored tablets in a wide range of doses.

SERAX (OXAZEPAM)

Serax is a short-acting benzodiazepine that is usually more sedating than Xanax or Librium. It is similar to Ativan in its effects and usages. If you are medication-sensitive, or sensitive to alcohol or the sedating effects of some antihistamines (e.g., Dramamine, Librium) or muscle relaxants, Serax may be too sedating for you. Librium, Tranxene, and Xanax are anti-anxiety medications that are less likely to cause drowsiness or sedation.

If you aren't sensitive to sedating drugs, or if Librium or Xanax are too mild, Serax may work well for you. Because Serax works rapidly, it is sometimes used as a sleep remedy. Medication-sensitive or elderly individuals should start with 10 mg, although even this dose may be too strong for some people.

Overall, short-acting benzodiazepines like Serax may be more prone to causing dependency and withdrawal than long-acting types when used in high doses or for long periods. If you've been taking moderate or high-dose Serax for a prolonged time, discontinuing the medication should be done gradually under the guidance of a physician to prevent withdrawal reactions.

The manufacturer recommended dosage of Serax for moderate anxiety is 10 to 15 mg taken three or four times a day; for severe anxiety, 15 to 30 mg taken three to four times daily; for the elderly, 10 mg taken three to four times daily.

I believe that using Serax or other benzodiazepines three or four times a day tends to foster dependency. Although the manufacturer states that Serax should not be used for more than two to three weeks, this is not realistic in treating many types of anxiety disorders, which are chronic conditions requiring long-term, sometimes lifelong treatment.

As with other benzodiazepines, Serax can be used indefinitely if it's used flexibly and intermittently—that is, only when needed. Whereas Serax used three or four times a day may cause dependency, if it is used three or four times a day on high-stress days, once a day on others, and none on others—averaging about two doses or less per day—dependency is unlikely.

If this flexible dosing method is inadequate to relieve your anxiety symptoms, alternative medications can be added to attain control. For example, in panic disorders antidepressants are very helpful in extinguishing the panic tendency, while Serax can be used intermittently for intense, episodic anxiety.

Flexible dosaging is hampered by the fact that Serax and its generic, oxazepam, are usually produced in capsules (10, 15, and 30 mg). Serax also is available as a 15-mg tablet, but overall this drug does not offer the range of dose flexibility of Ativan, which in part may explain the latter drug's wider popularity.

TRANXENE (CHLORAZEPATE)

Tranxene is similar to Librium in its effects and usages. Primarily prescribed for anxiety disorders, Tranxene is also used for its calming effects before surgery and for alcohol and Xanax withdrawal.

Like Librium, Tranxene is less sedating than Valium or Ativan. If you are medication-sensitive or sensitive to alcohol or the sedating effects of some antihistamines (e.g., Benadryl, Dramamine) or muscle relaxants, Tranxene is often a good choice. On the other hand, if Tranxene even at moderate doses is ineffective in curbing your anxiety, Valium, Serax, or Ativan may provide a better effect.

Because Tranxene is a longer-acting medication, it causes fewer rebound effects than Xanax. Tranxene's anti-anxiety effects usually last about six hours, so it doesn't have to be taken as often as shorter-acting Xanax.

The PDR recommended initial dosage of Tranxene is 30 mg a day in divided doses—presumably 15 mg twice a day or 7.5 mg four times a day—with an effective range of 15 to 60 mg a day. For the elderly, lower dosages are recommended but not defined. Tranxene is also produced as extended-release, once-a-day Tranxene-SD, which can be substituted in people already stabilized on a regular regimen of Tranxene.

My view is that Tranxene should not be used three or four times a day on a regular, day-to-day basis because of the risk of dependency. Similarly, I'm not a fan of extended-release benzodiazepines such as Tranxene-SD, which provides an ongoing level of Tranxene in the body. It's this continuous drug exposure that increases the risk of dependency.

Instead, I prefer to have people take Tranxene in a flexible and variable manner. Using Tranxene three or four times a day on high-stress days is acceptable, but must be compensated for by using one Tranxene on others, and no Tranxene if possible one or two days a week. The goal is to use an average of about two Tranxene or less per day. This regimen minimizes the risks of dependency and withdrawal, therefore allowing Tranxene to be used for extended periods. This is important because many anxiety disorders are long-term conditions, requiring treatment for far longer than the two to three weeks of medication usage that manufacturers recommend.

If you are medication-sensitive or sedation-sensitive, the recommended initial dose of 30 mg a day of Tranxene may be excessive. Depending on your degree of sensitivity, you may wish to start with the smallest pill, 3.75 mg, twice or three times a day. Even half of a 3.75-mg pill may be enough for some medication-sensitive or elderly people. As you ascertain your sensitivity to this medication, gradual increases in dosage can be made because Tranxene is produced in scored tablets in three sizes—3.75, 7.5, and 15 mg. Generic chlorazepate is available in similarly sized, scored pills.

If your anxiety is so severe that a flexible approach with Tranxene is inadequate in relieving your anxiety, it is preferable to add alternative medications instead of relying on daily high doses of Tranxene. For example, in panic disorders antidepressant drugs are effective in halting the panic tendency, while Tranxene or another benzodiazepine can be used for intermittent episodes of high anxiety.

If you've been taking daily moderate or high-dose Tranxene for a prolonged period, discontinuing the medication should be done gradually under the guidance of a physician to prevent withdrawal reactions.

Brief Comments

ATARAX AND VISTARIL (HYDROXYZINE)

Atarax and Vistaril are chemically identical medications (hydroxyzine) produced by different divisions of the same pharmaceutical company. Atarax, Vistaril, and generic hydroxyzine are sedating antihistamines that over the decades have been utilized more for anxiety or agitation than for allergy symptoms. Atarax, Vistaril, and generic hydroxyzine are also used for anxiety before surgery.

Like other first-generation antihistamines such as Benadryl, chlorpheniramine, and Dramamine, these drugs cause a high incidence of sedation even in people who aren't medication-sensitive.

The PDR descriptions of Atarax and Vistaril are old and outdated. The recommended dosage of Atarax for treating anxiety is 50 to 100 mg four times a day, a dosage that can be highly sedating. The PDR offers no specific dosages for the elderly.

Because of their sedating tendencies, these medications are rarely employed as first-choice anti-anxiety drugs. However, they can be tried when other anti-anxiety drugs are contraindicated or cause dependency. Atarax, Vistaril, and generic hydroxyzine, which don't usually cause dependency or addiction, can also be used more safely in people with histories of addictive tendencies.

These drugs are usually produced in 25-, 50-, and 100-mg coated, unbreakable tablets. However, even 25 mg is sedating for many people. Atarax is also produced in an unbreakable 10-mg pill, which is the dosage that you should try first if you are medication-sensitive, elderly, or sensitive to sedating drugs. Hydroxyzine is also manufactured as a syrup, which allows maximum dose flexibility but is more expensive.

BUSPAR (BUSPIRONE)

BuSpar is marketed as an anti-anxiety medication, but it is chemically more closely related to the serotonin-enhancing antidepressants (see Chapter 6). Like these drugs, BuSpar does not immediately reduce anxiety in the manner of Xanax, Librium, Klonopin, or other benzodiazepines. Instead, BuSpar must be taken regularly for several days or weeks before its anti-anxiety effect begins. BuSpar is not an addictive medication and can be used in people with drug addictions or addictive tendencies.

The manufacturer-recommended initial dose of BuSpar is 7.5 mg twice a day for everyone, including the elderly. If no response is obtained within a few days, the dose can be increased by 5 mg a day every few days. In pre-release clinical studies, doses of 20 to 30 mg a day were commonly required. Maximum dosage is 60 mg a day. The most common side effects with BuSpar are dizziness, drowsiness, nausea, and headache.

If you are medication-sensitive, 5 mg twice a day may be a sufficient dosage of BuSpar. On the other hand, according to physicians who've used BuSpar frequently, people who aren't medication-sensitive often need 40 to 60 mg a day.

From its description, BuSpar appears to be the ideal anti-anxiety drug because it is nonaddictive. However, in addition to its side effects, BuSpar doesn't work quickly enough for people with severe anxiety or panic disorders. In addition, BuSpar sometimes doesn't work at all, and many weeks can be wasted adjusting dosages without a successful result. For these reasons, BuSpar is often reserved for people with mild to moderate, chronic anxiety disorders—people who would likely require long-term treatment and whose symptoms could be tolerated long enough to see if BuSpar works.

BuSpar is produced in 5-, 10-, and 15-mg scored tablets, making flexible dosing easy.

EIGHT

❧

Sleep Medications

In-Depth Analyses

    Halcion (triazolam)
    Ambien (zolpidem)
    Dalmane (flurazepam)
    Restoril (temazepam)

Other Medications

    Doral (quazepam)
    ProSom (estazolam)

About Insomnia and Sleep Medications

Insomnia is the inability to fall asleep, stay asleep, or otherwise obtain a normal, restorative amount of sleep. Insomnia is a common condition with multiple causes. Brief periods of insomnia are experienced by most people at one time or another. Physical illness, job changes, relationship problems, school exams, antici-

185

pated events, emotional excitement, or jet lag can trigger a few nights of impaired sleep.

Prolonged insomnia is more problematic. Within a given year, more than 15% of adults will experience an episode of insomnia that is serious. Chronic insomnia is often related to emotional or physical conditions: anxiety, depression, chronic stress, mania, drug and alcohol abuse, respiratory difficulties, pain syndromes, muscle cramps, cardiac problems, thyroid and other hormonal diseases, stimulants such as coffee or tea, and many medications (oral steroids, decongestants, some diet pills, antibiotics such as Zithromax and Biaxin, and some antidepressants such as Prozac, Zoloft, Norpramin, and Wellbutrin).

The treatment of insomnia should first address the cause and attempt to ameliorate it. For example, if insomnia is related to stress, worry, anxiety, or depression, treatment of these conditions will usually resolve the sleep problem.

Unfortunately, instead of solving the primary problem with or without their physician's help, people often first turn to drugs, perhaps because of the heavy advertising on television for nonprescription sleep remedies such as Sominex and Nytol. Nonprescription preparations are very widely used, despite the fact that they contain sedating antihistamines that may cause more side effects than prescription remedies. And dependency can occur with nonprescription sleep preparations, just as it can with prescription drugs.

Melatonin has attracted a great deal of recent attention. However, while some people do very well with melatonin, others have complained of side effects, particularly vivid nightmares. Melatonin sometimes wears off by dawn, too early for many people. Also, melatonin plays a complex role in the body's hormonal balance, and the long-term effects of regular melatonin usage are unknown. The dosage range for melatonin varies greatly from individual to individual, ranging from 0.3 to 5 mg taken with dinner or at bedtime. Melatonin is probably a better choice than nonprescription sleep remedies for occasional or regular use for insomnia. Start with a low dose such as .3 mg or .5 mg, increase gradually, if necessary.

Before resorting to any drug therapy, perhaps the best things to try are natural methods such as daytime exercise, avoidance of daytime naps, avoidance of stimulants in the late afternoon and evening, and relaxing pre-sleep activities such as baths, herbal teas, reading, and sex. If these don't work, a thorough evaluation by your physician is in order.

Sometimes, however, despite a thorough medical evaluation and a variety of nonmedicinal approaches, insomnia remains an intractable problem that disrupts not only normal nighttime activity but daytime activity and efficiency as well. In such cases, prescription sleep remedies may work more effectively than anything else. And they cause few problems if used properly.

Because they work well, prescription sleep remedies are popular drugs. In 1989, twenty million outpatient prescriptions were written for sleep medications, and that tally didn't include the millions more written for hospital and nursing home patients.

SLEEP MEDICATIONS AND DEPENDENCY

In recent years, many physicians have become increasingly cautious about prescribing sleep medications, especially for prolonged periods. The reason is drug dependency.

Dependency is always a concern when sleep medications are overused. This applies to both nonprescription and prescription drugs. Dependency usually occurs when dosages are too high or when the drugs are used too often and too long.

People who take high doses of sleep medications every night for months are at the greatest risk of developing drug dependency. When they discontinue the drug, they can't sleep, and many encounter withdrawal phenomena such as nervousness and irritability. In rare cases, especially when the sleep medication is discontinued abruptly, withdrawal reactions occur, causing muscle cramps, vomiting, sweating, tremors, or seizures.

TYPES OF PRESCRIPTION SLEEP MEDICATIONS

Sleep medications are divided into three groups depending on their duration of action (see pages 188–189). The short-acting drugs, Halcion and Ambien, are most effective for people who have difficulty falling asleep. Intermediate and long-acting drugs are more effective for those who awaken early and cannot get back to sleep.

One of the problems with short-acting sleep medications is that they may wear off too soon, causing a "rebound" awakening before the night is over. Long-acting drugs can last well into the following day, causing impaired mental and physical performance.

In actual practice, starting with a short-acting or intermediate-acting medication is usually effective with less likelihood of hangover effects.

Chemically, all of the drugs listed below except Ambien are members of the benzodiazepine family, a group that also includes Valium, Ativan, Xanax, and others. Because they are sedating, Valium and Ativan are sometimes prescribed for insomnia; Ativan is short-acting, Valium long-acting.

SLEEP MEDICATIONS AND THE ELDERLY

Aging brings changes in the sleep cycle, including lighter sleep, more frequent awakenings, and a need for less sleep overall. Almost 90% of people over age 60 experience insomnia at one time or another. Most people adapt to these changes without difficulty, but some cannot. Medical problems can add to the difficulty. Sleep can often be normalized by an active lifestyle, regular daytime exercise, limited napping during the day, regular mealtimes, and limited fluids in the evening.

Duration of Action of Sleep Medications

SHORT-ACTING

Halcion (Triazolam)
Ambien (Zolpidem)

INTERMEDIATE-ACTING

Restoril (Temazapam)
ProSom (Estazolam)

LONG-ACTING

Dalmane (Flurazepam)
Doral (Quazepam)

Many elderly people take sleep medication. In addition to the usual side effects of drugs, the elderly encounter additional risks, especially with everyday usage. Because many of the side effects of sleep medications can be cumulative in this age group, nightly dependence on sleep remedies exposes elderly individuals to insidious side effects such as cognitive and memory impairments that can mimic dementia or Alzheimer's.

When needed, sleep medications should be started at the very lowest dosages and used only when needed. Nightly dependency should be avoided if at all possible.

DO WE USE TOO MUCH SLEEP MEDICATION?

Some health professionals decry our heavy reliance on medications to stabilize sleep. They claim that insomnia shouldn't be treated with drugs. Certainly, they are correct in asserting that we often turn prematurely to medications before identifying the underlying problem and trying other methods first.

On the other hand, studies repeatedly show that untreated insomniacs experience more and greater problems with concentration, memory, fatigue, and other symptoms than do those assisted by sleep medications. The data suggest that medication therapy for insomnia, when used appropriately and in suitable dosages, can be very helpful for most insomniacs.

The debate about the appropriate role of sleep medications remains unresolved because some people, despite all other approaches, just can't sleep without assistance. Until a better solution is found, the regular yet careful use of sleep medications remains the only (if imperfect) treatment. Not everyone who takes regular sleep medication develops dependency—the need for larger and larger doses. Many people take a mild or moderate dose of a sleep medication on a nightly basis without encountering problems. In these cases, people are better off using prescription medications instead of nonprescription drugs. Of course, they should be monitored regularly by their physicians.

Nightly sleep medication is neither necessary nor desirable in most cases of insomnia. In most cases, insomnia is temporary and related to life events. If you are going to use sleep medication, the best approach is to use the very lowest effective dose, use it only when necessary, and try to avoid using it every night. The intermittent use of low-dose sleep medications reduces the likelihood of side effects, drug dependency, and withdrawal reactions when the medication is discontinued.

DOSAGE IS THE KEY

Are sleep medications used appropriately and in suitable—i.e., the lowest and safest—dosages? Studies show that physicians often overprescribe sleep medications, but the problem of side effects with sleep medications extends beyond the overuse of these substances. The dosages of sleep medications that manufacturers select and physicians prescribe may well pose an equally important hazard.

Most of the side effects with sleep medications are directly related to dosage. Yet the recommended dosages of popular sleep remedies such as Ambien (zolpidem) and Dalmane (flurazepam) may be unnecessarily high for many adults, and especially so for medication-sensitive individuals. The recommended doses for Halcion (triazolam) and Restoril (temazepam) were also too high until they were reduced after more than a decade of general usage.

With such deficiencies in the dosage selection and prescribing of sleep medications, it's hardly surprising that the rate of side effects with this group of drugs remains higher than necessary. Side effects can be avoided by using the lowest effective dose. If you are going to take a medication for insomnia, ask your physician to prescribe the lowest dose of whichever medication is chosen. If this dose isn't strong enough, increase the dosage slowly and gradually until the effective amount is determined.

In-Depth Analysis: Halcion (Triazolam)

The most prescribed sleep medication in America from the mid 1980s through the early 1990s, Halcion has prompted one of the longest-running major drug controversies in history. A large part of that controversy has centered around the issue of dosage. Indeed, the story of Halcion is the story of inadequately researched, unnecessarily high dosages.

TROUBLE FROM THE OUTSET

The manufacturer-recommended usual adult dosage of Halcion is 0.25 mg, and some believe it's still too high. Yet when Halcion was first released in Holland in 1979, the recommended dose was 1.0 mg—400% higher than today's recommended U.S. dose. An inundation of reports of side effects led to a quick ban of the drug in that country, and the 1.0-mg recommended dose wasn't marketed elsewhere.

Why did it take the fiasco in Holland for Halcion's manufacturer and governmental agencies to reevaluate Halcion more closely? A good question, because years earlier, one study had already identified Halcion's most troublesome side effect, an unusual type of amnesia. This study didn't mince words: "Because of the finding of amnesia in two of our [7] subjects, and the serious potential of this side effect, specific studies on the effects of triazolam [Halcion] and memory are indicated." In the concluding sentence, the authors added: "Finally, the findings of amnesia associated with triazolam administration need to be more thoroughly evaluated."

The study was published in 1976, three years before Halcion's release in Holland. The dosage tested in the study was 0.5 mg, while in Holland it was 1.0 mg. No wonder immediate problems resulted.

IN SEARCH OF A SAFE HALCION DOSAGE

Following the Holland debacle, Halcion's recommended dosage was slashed to 0.5 mg. When approved in the United States in 1983, it was with a recommended dosage of 0.25 to 0.5 mg. This 0.5-mg dosage was heavily prescribed for five years.

In 1987, the 0.5-mg dosage was banned in France and Italy. A year later West Germany banned it, too, and the manufacturer reduced the recommended dosage in the U.S. The new recommended adult dosage became 0.25 mg, with 0.125 mg suggested for "some patients." Thus it currently remains.

In effect, within a span of nine years, the maximum recommended dosage of the world's most prescribed sleep remedy dropped from 1.0 mg to 0.5 mg to 0.25 mg, a fourth of the original amount. A 400% reduction.

Halcion's Fifteen-Year Saga of Dosage Reduction

1978: Halcion approved in Holland. Dosages recommended up to 1.0 mg—an avalanche of side effect reports follow. Halcion suspended in Holland in 1979.

1983: Halcion's first year on the American market. PDR dosage guidelines state: "The recommended dosage range for adults is 0.25 to 0.5 mg before retiring."

1986: Though the recommended dosage range remains 0.25 to 0.5 mg, additional suggestions appear: "A dose of 0.125 mg may be found to be sufficient for selected [adult] patients, however." And: "As with all medications, the lowest effective dose should be used."

1987: The 0.5-mg dosage is banned in France and Italy.

1988: The 0.5-mg dosage is banned in West Germany. In the U.S., Upjohn drops its recommendation for the 0.5-mg dosage and adds this warning to the PDR: "A dose of 0.5 mg should be reserved for those patients who do not respond adequately to a lower dose since the risk of several adverse reactions increases with the size of the dose administered." Only the 0.25-mg dose remains, with 0.125 mg reserved for "selected patients."

1991: The 0.5-mg pill is no longer offered in the U.S.

1992: By now, Halcion has been banned in Britain, Norway, Finland, Brazil, Holland, and Argentina. The 0.25-mg dosage has been suspended in Spain, France, and New Zealand. Canada and Japan have lowered Halcion's recommended adult dosage to 0.125 mg. Other countries including the U.S. stick with the 0.25-mg dosage recommendation, with 0.125 mg for "selected patients."

THE TROUBLE WITH HALCION

Anterograde amnesia is an after-the-fact inability to remember events in which one participated. It's the failure to create memories while participating in activities with seemingly intact awareness. The person involved, absorbed in the activity, is unaware of his/her lack of memory. To outsiders, there's no evidence of unusual activity. It's only later that the individual, unable to retrieve any memory of a lengthy flow of events, becomes aware that something was amiss.

Many medications affecting the central nervous system can evoke anterograde amnesia. Patients receiving intravenous Valium during medical procedures often incur a loss of memory, but since these circumstances are strictly controlled, the amnesia poses little danger. Indeed, many patients have expressed satisfaction at having little or no memory of their procedures.

In contrast, when anterograde amnesia is triggered unexpectedly in uncontrolled situations in unsuspecting victims, its effects can be dangerous. Most sleep remedies, including nonprescription varieties, have in rare instances caused anterograde amnesia and/or other psychiatric disturbances, but none has elicited a flood of complaints like Halcion. Consider this incident, one of many reported in 1988 in *JAMA*:

> *A 44-year-old woman had to address a meeting of about 200 people. Arriving at the hotel the evening before, she took 0.5 mg of Halcion before bedtime. She "came to" at about noon the next day at lunch with a large group of strangers. Although she didn't remember it, she had given her speech complete with a slide presentation between 8 and 10 earlier that morning.*

THE FIFTEEN-YEAR CONTROVERSY CONTINUES

The reductions in dosage haven't ended the Halcion controversy. A report in the 1993 *British Medical Journal* stated: "In our research we found that triazolam [Halcion] caused anxiety, panics, depression, paranoid reactions, and weight loss in 40 subjects compared with 40 who received placebo and 40 who received [another sleep medication]."

Is Halcion uniquely disposed toward mental disturbances—amnesia, agitation, confusion, anxiety? Is it more dangerous than other sleep remedies? The debate goes on—nearly two decades after the Holland incident, letters and studies continue to argue whether Halcion causes more problems than other prescription sleep remedies.

Studies comparing different sleep remedies have tried to provide an answer. One of the most striking was a 1991 study comparing the frequency of reports to the FDA of behavioral disturbances with Halcion and a top competitor. Its conclusion: "Considering the extent of use, reporting rates for triazolam [Halcion] were 22 to 99 times those for temazepam [Restoril]." Moreover, 43% of the reported complainants had experienced a reaction to Halcion on the first dose. This study summarized its findings as follows: "The data reported herein show a considerably larger number of reports and higher reporting rates with triazolam . . .

for confusion, amnesia, bizarre behavior, agitation, and hallucinations.''

Indeed, a 1993 study reported a rate of 44% of side effects with Halcion. Because Halcion is so short acting, some people experience withdrawal anxiety the following morning. Upon discontinuing Halcion after prolonged usage, withdrawal insomnia, according *Conn's Current Therapy 1994*, ''is prompt and impressive.'' And, as with all medications, new side effects continue to be identified. A 1995 report stated that Halcion's effects were enhanced, and side effects were therefore more likely, by the concomitant use of antifungal agents such as Sporanox (itraconazole) and Nizoral (ketoconazole).

Yet support for Halcion continues as well. A 1993 letter to the *British Medical Journal* captured the pro-Halcion point of view: ''That benzodiazepine hypnotics [Halcion, Dalmane, Restoril, Doral, ProSom] can have side effects is beyond doubt, but many patients who use them for short periods derive remarkable benefit. In our opinion, the weight of evidence does not support the view that triazolam is more prone to produce side effects than other benzodiazepine hypnotics—a conclusion arrived at by both the Collegium Internationale Neuropsychopharmacologium and the World Psychiatric Association in their consensus reports.''

My own experience with Halcion has been mostly favorable. Because it is short-acting, hangover effects with Halcion are infrequent. But I always have started patients at the very lowest dosage, far below the manufacturer's guidelines.

DOCTORS AND HALCION DOSAGES

More than anything, dosage has been the main issue with Halcion. Most of Halcion's side effects, including amnesia and other mental disturbances, are dose related. Many of the incidents that have been reported happened at a dosage of 0.5 mg. Today the recommended dose is 0.25 mg—yet some problems have continued as this report demonstrates:

> *To ensure sleep during an overnight flight to Europe, a traveller ingested 0.25 mg of triazolam. The next night, he had amnesia for how he had gotten from the airport to his*

destination (only train and taxi receipts in his pocket clar-
ified the mystery).

Even at the very lowest recommended Halcion dosage, 0.125 mg, memory problems have occurred. From *Goth's Medical Pharmacology*, 1992: ''Memory impairment and anterograde amnesia have been reported after administration of as little as 0.125 mg of the drug.'' This has led some investigators to conclude that at any dosage, Halcion is dangerous—too dangerous to warrant its continued approval.

Supporters of Halcion respond that individual cases of memory and other psychiatric problems can be found with every sleep medication. Halcion's overall side effect profile is as good as any, and studies show that the rates of patient satisfaction with Halcion are as high as any other sleep remedy.

Furthermore, Halcion's supporters assert, if any blame is warranted, it should be borne by physicians, who as often as not prescribe higher rather than lower dosages of Halcion. This despite Upjohn's recommendation since 1983 in Halcion's package insert: ''It is important to individualize the dosage of Halcion Tablets (triazolam) for maximum beneficial effect and to help avoid significant adverse effects.'' And since 1986: ''As with all medications, the lowest effective dose should be used.''

Unfortunately, doctors don't always heed this advice, as illustrated by an incident described to me by an editor: ''I was having trouble sleeping. My doctor prescribed Halcion. The directions said to take a whole pill, but I took only half and slept fine. I told him about this and asked, 'Why didn't you first prescribe a milder dosage?' He just shrugged, but when it came time for a refill, he prescribed the lower dosage.''

Doctors have also been shown to prescribe Halcion and other sleep medications for unsupportably long periods. A 1992 study in the *American Journal of Medicine* reported: ''We found that 30% of the prescriptions written by internists or surgeons were for inappropriately large quantities of these drugs (180 or more doses).'' In the PDR, Halcion's manufacturer states that Halcion should be used short-term, generally no more than seven to ten days, then adds: ''Use for more than 2–3 weeks requires reevaluation of the patient.'' Unfortunately, this warning is located three columns—a full page—distant from the dosage recommendations where doctors might be more likely to notice it.

WHY WEREN'T LOWER DOSAGES RECOMMENDED INITIALLY?

Why weren't lower Halcion doses recommended in the first place? Why wasn't more effort exerted in determining the lowest effective dose before Halcion's release? Why did it take nearly a decade of usage in the general population to arrive at lower, safer recommended dosages—dosages that some authorities believe are still too high?

One reason may be that for a new drug to compete with already established competitors, it must offer some advantage. Without this, doctors would have little incentive to switch from medications they already know and trust. In other words, a manufacturer must be able to pronounce its new drug superior in some important aspect.

This competitive reality demands that new drugs not only equal but outperform competitors. In the case of Halcion, the 1.0 mg dosage was more successful in controlling insomnia. Yet early studies also indicated that a 0.25 mg Halcion dosage was also effective. In one study, this dosage was preferred by more patients and shown to be equally effective in promoting sleep as the highest dosage of Dalmane, a leading prescription sleep remedy. Still, the higher Halcion dosages, 0.5 mg and 1.0 mg, reduced insomnia more reliably.

But what about the increased side effects with the 1.0-mg Halcion dosage? Weren't the problems obvious?

These problems were missed because many Halcion pre-release dosage studies were performed for very short durations. In some studies, subjects received the drug for only one, two, or three nights. In addition, the findings of many of these studies were based on self-reports, yet subsequent research has shown that many of the memory impairments caused by Halcion weren't apparent to patients or even to their physicians. Self-reporting often misses memory impairments.

Also, in many studies the subjects were young, healthy males. With an average age of around 22, with no illnesses and no other medications, this group would tolerate much higher dosages than the general public. And they would be less likely to manifest side effects. Even so, there was evidence at the time that Halcion caused amnesia, and a call was made for further research on this problem before Halcion was released.

So how was the problem overlooked? Accusations have been hurled back and forth, and the courts may ultimately decide. The purpose here isn't to point fingers, but to emphasize that mistakes and oversights happen, even in the vital arena of prescription drugs.

The balance between efficacy and safety is often a delicate one. The pressure on manufacturers to develop effective yet safe pharmaceuticals, the pressure on the FDA for quick yet cautious action—these dual demands are inevitably in conflict. The demands of a lucrative yet competitive marketplace further complicate the process.

HALCION AND THE ELDERLY

The manufacturer-recommended dosage of Halcion for elderly individuals is 0.125 mg. This may be ideal for some people but too much for others. Memory deficits in adults have been seen with this dosage. Indeed, in some countries 0.125 mg of Halcion is the recommended dose for younger adults. If this is so, surely some elderly persons may require less. The 0.125-mg Halcion pill is scored and easily split.

RECOMMENDATIONS

Is Halcion safe? In 1993, the World Psychiatric Association Task Force on sleep medications offered this opinion: "When treatment is properly supervised and dosage properly chosen, the large majority of patients experience therapeutic benefit [from Halcion and other benzodiazepine sleep medications] with few problems."

The key words here are "properly chosen." With Halcion, the story has been of dosages that have been repeatedly lowered in the face of unexpected, serious side effects. Interestingly, lowering the recommended dosage of Halcion doesn't appear to have dampened the controversy—or Halcion's popularity.

Halcion is produced in 0.125- and 0.25-mg tablets. Halcion tablets are scored, so they can easily be split. If you are medication-sensitive, small, or elderly, or just want to take the very lowest effective dose of Halcion, this can be accomplished by starting very low and, if necessary, increasing very gradually until you reach an effective dosage.

Halcion's manufacturer recommends a dose of 0.125 mg for the elderly and "selected patients," a regular 0.25-mg dose for most adults, and 0.5 for recalcitrant conditions—note that each jump in dosage is 100%. But by starting with half the smallest tablet and increasing by this amount, if necessary, you can fashion doses of 0.0625, 0.125, 0.1875, 0.25, 0.3125, 0.375, 0.4375, and 0.5 mg, a broad and flexible range.

You can even split a tablet in quarters. I've had a few patients for whom a fourth of a 0.125 mg pill has been sufficient.

In-Depth Analysis: Ambien (Zolpidem)

Released in 1993, Ambien is chemically unrelated to Halcion and other benzodiazepine sleep remedies. As such, it was hoped that Ambien would provide effective treatment of insomnia with fewer side effects. With the previous best-seller Halcion beset by negative publicity and lawsuits, Ambien has reaped the greatest benefit, rising to No. 59 in 1995 among the top 200 drugs in U.S. outpatient prescriptions. In 1996, Ambien climbed to No. 45.

Ambien's manufacturer recommends a dose of 10 mg for most adults. A 5-mg dose is recommended for elderly or debilitated patients, those with liver impairments, and those taking other central nervous system depressants (e.g., antidepressant, anti-seizure, or anti-anxiety medications). Other than these groups, Ambien is essentially a one-size-fits-all drug.

Yet the manufacturer also suggests that Ambien's dosage

"should be individualized." A few lines further down it warns that the 10-mg dosage shouldn't be exceeded. In other words, the standard adult dose is 10 mg and the maximum dose is 10 mg. This doesn't leave much room for individualization.

LOW DOSE AMBIEN

The literature reveals considerable research on lower doses of Ambien. One of the earliest and longest low-dose studies was performed in 1989, four years before Ambien's release in 1993. This study compared doses of 2.5, 5.0, 7.5, 10, and 20 mg over a seven-week period. The results: the 5.0-mg dosage demonstrated efficacy on several parameters, and the 7.5-mg dosage was nearly as effective as the 33% higher manufacturer-recommended 10-mg dosage. The authors' summary states it succinctly: "In conclusion, results of this study indicate that zolpidem [Ambien] is hypnotically active at doses as low as 5.0 and 7.5 mg. . . . Also, adverse effects do not occur at these low doses." Indeed, even the lowly 2.5-mg dosage showed some improvement over a placebo. One wonders if some medication-sensitive individuals might respond to this dosage.

Adding emphasis to these impressive findings was the fact that the twelve subjects were males aged 22 to 35 who were healthy and taking no other medications—that is, healthier, younger, and probably bigger than the general patient population. If these subjects responded so well to low-dose Ambien, then the average person would likely respond even better and require even less. It is not surprising, then, that other studies have confirmed the effectiveness of the 5 mg and 7.5 mg doses of Ambien.

Yet not all studies demonstrated the effectiveness of the 5-mg dose. For that matter, not all studies demonstrated the effectiveness of the manufacturer-recommended 10-mg dose. However, the majority of low-dose studies demonstrated that Ambien 5 mg is effective in healthy, young adults.

The 7.5-mg dosage also performed well in most studies. In addition to the 1989 study cited above, a 1988 study stated: "Efficacy, defined as significant difference from placebo, usually occurred at doses of 7.5 mg and above." Ambien's package insert agrees, stating that the 7.5-mg dosage was "superior to placebo on objective measures of sleep latency, sleep duration, and [reduced] number of awakenings.''

Yet Ambien doesn't come in a 7.5-mg pill. Nor does the package insert mention the demonstrated efficacy of the 5-mg dosage in healthy, young adults. Instead, the 10-mg dose is recommended for young or middle-aged, big or small—everyone except the elderly or ill.

IS AMBIEN BETTER?

Is Ambien a newer and better alternative? A 1992 review article examined the results with eight sleep medications including Halcion and Ambien from 38 studies encompassing 5,506 patients. It found ''remarkable similarity . . . among all of these shorter-acting agents in terms of efficacy, side effects, and performance-related effects.'' About Ambien in particular it added, ''Although claims have been made suggesting differences, evaluation of the studies herein showed [Ambien] indistinguishable from triazolam [Halcion] and other benzodiazepine hypnotics in their clinical and pharmacologic activity.''

More recent reports supported these findings. Case studies have appeared describing incidents of tolerance, hallucinatory phenomena, and withdrawal symptoms with Ambien. This isn't entirely surprising because Ambien works upon the same brain receptors as other sleep medications. Indeed, a 1993 article comparing the side effects of Ambien and Halcion found that both similarly impaired psychomotor performance, memory, and balance.

Other Ambien side effects include next-day drowsiness, nausea, dizziness, headache, and vomiting.

AMBIEN AND THE ELDERLY

The manufacturer recommends a lower dose, 5 mg, for elderly individuals than the 10 mg suggested for younger adults. But as we have seen, 5 mg is quite sufficient for many younger adults. Lower doses such as 2.5 mg may therefore be sufficient for some elderly persons. In fact, a 1991 study showed that 2.5 mg of Ambien did significantly affect sleep in elderly subjects. Again, caution and flexibility should be exercised in using any sedating medication with elderly individuals.

RECOMMENDATIONS

A physician's comment in a 1995 journal summarizes it best: "While zolpidem [Ambien] is generally well tolerated, it should not be considered risk free, *even at therapeutic doses* [my italics]. . . . [The] advantages of zolpidem are yet to be determined." Nevertheless, physicians have turned to Ambien, although it's not clear whether this popularity represents Ambien's inherent superiority as a sleep remedy or simply physicians' concerns with Halcion and other benzodiazepines such as Dalmane and Restoril.

In any event, it's clear that any medication that induces sleep is likely to have the potential for side effects, especially those involving coordination and mental clarity. No one medication is going to fit everyone. And no single dosage is going to be ideal for all adults or all elderly persons. One thing is certain: lower doses cause fewer side effects.

The data cited above reveal that many healthy adults will respond to 5 mg of Ambien. Fortunately, Ambien is produced in both 5- and 10-mg tablets that aren't scored but are breakable. If you are medication-sensitive, starting at a low dose such as 5 mg is recommended. Even 2.5 mg of Ambien was found to be active in some studies. Highly sensitive individuals may prefer to start at this very low dose.

When lower doses aren't sufficient, increases should be done gradually. In Chapter 3, I mentioned a case in which a woman developed sensations that her body and bed were moving after taking a standard 10-mg dose of Ambien. Her physician had first tried 5 mg, but although this amount made her mildly sedated, it didn't afford a good night's sleep. When the dosage was increased to 10 mg—a 100% increase—she developed the sensory disturbances. Considering that she had already had a partial response at 5 mg, she apparently required only a little more medication to accomplish the goal. 10 mg was too much, and side effects were the result.

By splitting the 5-mg Ambien tablet, you can fashion doses of 2.5, 5, 7.5, and 10 mg.

In-Depth Analysis: Dalmane (Flurazepam)

Dalmane (flurazepam) and Restoril (temazepam—see page 205) make an interesting contrast. Both are top-selling sleep medications, but Restoril's recommended dosages, which had been similar to Dalmane's, were slashed 50% in 1994. The recommended dosages for Dalmane have remained unchanged for over twenty-five years—dosages that many authorities consider too high.

According to the 1996 PDR, the usual adult dosage for Dalmane is 30 mg. The guidelines then state that "in some patients, 15 mg may suffice." Fifteen mg is also recommended for elderly or debilitated individuals.

Most common side effects include excessive sedation, sedation continuing the following day, incoordination, light-headedness, headache, and apprehension.

Dalmane is produced as 15- and 30-mg capsules.

LOW-DOSE DALMANE

In contrast to the manufacturer's guidelines, for three decades medical journals and textbooks have suggested 15 mg, not 30 mg, as the preferred standard dosage of Dalmane. Indeed, prior to Dalmane's release in 1970, two studies had already indicated that 15 mg might be more than sufficient.

A 1966 article in the *New England Journal of Medicine* reported that 15 mg of Dalmane was significantly superior to a placebo and equal in efficacy to the potent barbiturate sleep remedy, Seconal 100 mg. A 1967 study in *Current Therapeutic Research* compared Dalmane 15 mg and 30 mg head to head. Fourteen of the twenty-two patients did just as well or better on the 15-mg dosage. The authors concluded: "The 30-mg dose could not be shown to be superior to the 15-mg one."

Despite these impressive findings, Dalmane was released with a recommended adult dosage of 30 mg. Subsequent studies have continued to support the 15-mg dosage.

WHY LOW-DOSE DALMANE IS SAFER

Efficacy isn't the only reason for the calls for using lower doses of Dalmane. The manufacturer-recommended dosage of 30 mg of Dalmane causes a significantly higher rate of side effects.

Dalmane's duration of action is longer—i.e., it lingers in patients' systems longer—than that of most other sleep remedies. This means that Dalmane may be superior in keeping patients from awakening too early, but it also may cause hangover symptoms: difficulty in awakening, sluggishness or drowsiness lasting into the day, impaired reflexes, and reduced mental acuity. Dosage is key, as a 1975 study found: "Flurazepam [Dalmane] 30 mg but not 15 mg significantly impaired performance. . . . subjective hangover effects after 30 mg were significantly more frequent than after 15 mg. . . . In all three of the tests, flurazepam 30 mg caused more impairment than 15 mg."

DALMANE AND THE ELDERLY

If 15 mg of Dalmane is more than sufficient for most healthy adults, what can be said about using the same dosage in elderly individuals? Unfortunately, Dalmane isn't produced in a dose lower than 15 mg, so using a lower dosage in the elderly is difficult. Some authorities have recommended that Dalmane be avoided with the elderly.

RECOMMENDATIONS

Because of its prolonged duration of action, Dalmane is most useful in sleep disorders that involve early morning awakening. However, this same property may make it too strong for too long, causing next-day oversedation in some people. Lower Dalmane doses cause fewer side effects.

As the low-dose data indicates, 15 mg of Dalmane is plenty for most people. The manufacturer-recommended 30-mg dosage should be reserved for those who aren't helped by the lower dose. Studies indicate that physicians routinely prescribed the higher, 30-mg dose of Dalmane to hospital patients. The same is likely true of outpatients. If your doctor prescribes Dalmane for you, ask for the 15-mg capsules to afford greater dose flexibility.

In-Depth Analysis: Restoril (Temazepam)

The recommended usual adult dose is 30 mg before retiring. In some patients, 15 mg may be sufficient.

—1993 PDR

While the recommended usual adult dose is 15 mg before retiring, 7.5 mg may be sufficient for some patients, and others may need 30 mg.

—1994 PDR

Halcion isn't the only sleep medication whose dosages have plummeted. The dosage recommendation for Restoril (temazepam) have also been lowered.

Released in 1981, for thirteen years Restoril was available in two sizes, 15 and 30 mg, with the higher dosage being the recommended one for most adults. In 1994, a new 7.5-mg Restoril pill appeared. At the same time Restoril's manufacturer slashed Restoril's recommended dosages by 50%.

In tandem with the arrival of the 7.5 pill, Sandoz mounted a robust advertising campaign. "Effective, low-dose therapy to help patients fall asleep gently" read one of its full-page advertisements, thus underscoring one of the central points of this book—reducing drug dosages can benefit not only patients and physicians but drug companies, too.

Restoril's new dosage guidelines offer an additional advantage—they encourage physicians not only to take the time to individualize dosages but also to diagnose the specific type of insomnia. There are various types of insomnia, yet most doctors treat them all the same. Restoril's manufacturer recommends the 7.5 mg-dosage for transient insomnia, in which the difficulty is falling asleep. In contrast, for people who awaken repeatedly during the night, 15 mg is recommended, or in recalcitrant cases, 30 mg.

Thus, the new dosage recommendations direct doctors to use Restoril flexibly, to identify the type of sleep problem, and to utilize the lower dosages of 7.5 or 15 mg initially rather than the previously recommended 30 mg. These are major improvements, which may explain why Restoril's generic, temazepam, continues to rank among the top-selling drugs in U.S. outpatient prescriptions (No.182 in 1996) at a time when physicians are turning from Halcion and other benzodiazepine sleep remedies.

Restoril is produced as 7.5-, 15-, and 30-mg capsules. The most common side effects include headache, fatigue, nervousness, lethargy, dizziness.

LOW-DOSE RESTORIL

The fact that Restoril's manufacturer produced and the FDA approved a lower 7.5-mg dose of this drug provides sufficient testimony to its effectiveness. Studies have further supported this fact.

RESTORIL AND THE ELDERLY

For thirteen years the recommended Restoril dosage for elderly persons was 15 mg. Now it's 7.5 mg, a reduction of 50%. Some people may need the higher dose, but many will do fine with fewer risks at the lower dosage. Start at 7.5 mg and increase only if necessary.

RECOMMENDATIONS

Restoril is an intermediate-acting sleep remedy that is not as likely to produce next-day sedation as longer-acting Dalmane and

Doral. Available now in a low-dose 7.5-mg size, as well as the traditional 15- and 30-mg sizes, Restoril offers increased flexibility for medication-sensitive and elderly individuals.

While Restoril's manufacturer should be congratulated for voluntarily reevaluating this drug and initiating a lower dose with improved dosage guidelines, we might ask why it took thirteen years to discover that lower doses were effective. The time for intensive dose studies should be *before* a drug is released, not long after.

Other Medications

DORAL (QUAZEPAM)

This long-acting sleep remedy can be best compared to Dalmane. Like Dalmane, it is most useful in treating insomnia characterized by early morning awakenings. Because of its long duration of action, next-day drowsiness is its most common side effect. Next-day impairments in coordination and mental acuity may also occur.

The manufacturer recommends a dose of 15 mg before bedtime; the dosage may be reduced on subsequent nights in elderly, debilitated, or other sensitive patients. Doral is produced in 7.5- and 15-mg unscored caplets.

Recommendations: Although the manufacturer recommends an initial dose of 15 mg for everyone, starting with 7.5 mg of Doral may be preferable in medication-sensitive and elderly individuals. Indeed, those known to be highly sensitive to sedating drugs may want to start with half a 7.5-mg pill, taking the other half an hour or two later if necessary.

Some authorities have questioned the use of long-acting sleep medications in elderly individuals.

PROSOM (ESTAZOLAM)

An intermediate-acting sleep medication similar to Restoril, ProSom can be useful in most types of insomnia. Possible side effects include headache, nausea, light-headedness, next-day sedation or lethargy.

The manufacturer's recommended dosages for ProSom are flexible: 1 mg at bedtime for most adults, including healthy elderly persons; 0.5 mg for small or debilitated elderly; 2 mg for those not helped by 1 mg.

ProSom is produced in 1- and 2-mg scored tablets which are easily broken for flexible dosaging.

Recommendations: A 0.5-mg or even 0.25-mg initial dose may be enough if you are medication-sensitive, sensitive to sedating drugs, small, or elderly. You can increase to 0.75 or 1 mg if necessary. If these doses aren't sufficient, you can increase to 1.25, 1.5, or 1.75 mg before immediately going to the recommended 2 mg.

NINE

〰

Smoking Cessation: Zyban (Bupropion)

In the summer of 1997, a torrent of advertisements began appearing on television and in magazines about a "new" medication to help people stop smoking cigarettes. The name of the new drug: Zyban.

But Zyban isn't a new drug at all. It's Wellbutrin, an antidepressant available for several years (see Chapter 6).

The effect of Wellbutrin on some drug cravings has been recognized for years. In 1995 a psychiatrist treating chemical addictions mentioned to me that Wellbutrin seemed to curb the extremely severe drug cravings of crack cocaine withdrawal. Two years later, Wellbutrin's manufacturer repackaged the same drug, bupropion, and released it as Zyban.

Contrary to the gentle tones of the TV advertisements that make Zyban seem as benign as Tylenol, experience with Wellbutrin indicates that Zyban shouldn't be taken without consideration. In fact, after its original release, Wellbutrin was withdrawn from the market because of an unacceptable incidence of seizures. The risk of seizures was, of course, dose-related, so the manufacturer reduced the recommended dosages, the seizure potential dropped, and the drug was reintroduced and has remained a useful antidepressant. Nevertheless, the seizure potential persists with both Wellbutrin and Zyban, as the manufacturer acknowledges in the Zyban package insert: "There is a chance that approximately 1 out of every 1,000 people taking bupropion hydrochloride, the active ingredient in Zyban, will have a seizure.''

Zyban also causes a substantial incidence of other side effects that are listed below.

MANUFACTURER-RECOMMENDED DOSAGE

The manufacturer recommended dosage of Zyban is 150 mg a day for three days, then 150 mg twice a day (i.e., 300 mg a day) for up to 12 weeks. Elderly dosage is the same. Maximum dosage: 300 mg a day. Zyban doses should be taken at least eight hours apart; avoid taking Zyban late in the day to minimize the likelihood of insomnia.

Counseling and support are important throughout treatment. Smoking cessation should not be attempted immediately, but only after being on Zyban for a week. If Zyban has not helped you stop smoking within seven weeks, it isn't likely to work.

Because of its association with seizures in 0.1% of patients, Zyban is not recommended in people with histories of seizures or head injuries. It also must be used very carefully if you are taking medications that may make seizures easier to trigger—drugs such as antidepressants, oral steroids, theophylline, antipsychotics, and alcohol.

HOW EFFECTIVE IS ZYBAN?

The information sent to physicians upon Zyban's release make Zyban seem very effective, but that's not the full picture. The manufacturer's letter highlights a chart showing a quit rate—patients who quit smoking for four consecutive weeks during treatment—of 49%. When combined with a nicotine patch, the quit rate was 58%. These rates were measured at the seventh week of a ten-week study. But by the tenth week of the study, after the drug had been discontinued for just one week, the quit rates were already dropping to 46% and 51%, respectively. And the most important consideration, Zyban's long-term effectiveness in stopping smoking, wasn't measured in this study.

Another study cited in the Zyban package insert does provide long-term results—and they aren't good. This study compared a placebo with three dosages of Zyban: 100, 150, and 300 mg a day. Treatment lasted seven weeks and included brief counseling sessions. The percentage of people able to quit smoking at 7, 12, and 26 weeks are listed in Table 9.1. The results of this study at 52 weeks were provided to me by the manufacturer; they aren't included in the package insert. Perhaps that's because the difference between the placebo and the highest dose of Zyban, 300 mg a day, is a disappointing 3% and not statistically significant.

If these results aren't discouraging enough, the Zyban package insert adds: "Quit rates in clinical trials are influenced by the population selected. Quit rates in isolated populations may be lower than above rates."

Worse, according to independent studies in the medical literature, Zyban's effectiveness in smoking cessation may be further questioned. According to a 1996 report in the *American Journal of Psychiatry*, "Bupropion [Zyban] itself is not indicated for smoking cessation therapy. Two studies have shown that there is not a dramatic effect between patients who receive bupropion and those who receive placebo.... [As one study demonstrated], there was a significant difference between bupropion and placebo during their study, but 3 months after the discontinuation of therapy, the difference between the two groups was insignificant."

This mirrors the results in Table 9.1. The effectiveness of Zyban, although not particularly impressive, was *statistically* significant compared to a placebo at 7 weeks (Zyban, 300 mg a day, 36%; placebo, 17%), but by 52 weeks the difference was negligible (Zyban, 300 mg a day, 13%; placebo, 10%).

Table 9.1. How Effective Is Zyban?

In this long-term study comparing three doses of Zyban with placebo, the results aren't particularly impressive during the study (7 weeks), and they get progressively worse over time.

(Adapted from the 1997 Zyban package insert and data provided by the manufacturer)

	WEEK 7	WEEK 12	WEEK 26	WEEK 52
Placebo	17%	14%	11%	10%
Zyban 110 mg/day	22%	20%	16%	13%
Zyban 150 mg/day	27%	20%	18%	15%
Zyban 300 mg/day	36%	25%	19%	13%

Initially, the difference between placebo (17% success) and the highest dose of Zyban (36% success) is 19%, statistically significant but not outstanding. Ultimately, the difference between the placebo (10% success) and 300 mg/day of Zyban (13% success) is a mere 3%.

Based on this data, it's difficult to understand how the FDA approved Zyban. Zyban's approval is especially surprising because it was based on very limited data—only two small studies, neither of which were published for independent peer review.

MORE SIDE EFFECTS THAN STATED?

Considering Zyban's limited effectiveness in smoking cessation and its potential for side effects, is Zyban worth taking?

The 1/1,000 risk of seizures has already been mentioned. This risk is dose-related and occurs less frequently at dosages below the manufacturer-recommended 300 mg a day.

Regarding other side effects, the Zyban package insert only lists five that occurred in more than 10% of study subjects, and only one side effect, insomnia, occurring in more than 15%. Seems pretty safe, right? Perhaps not.

Zyban is identical to Wellbutrin. As stated above, both are the same drug, bupropion, made by the same manufacturer. The information below compares the side effects occurring in more than 10% of study subjects with Zyban and Wellbutrin according to the manufacturer's 1997 product information.

Why the discrepancies? Certainly not the dosage, because the recommended dosage of Zyban, 300 mg a day, is actually higher than many psychiatrists often use with Wellbutrin, so we would expect more instead of fewer side effects with Zyban compared to Wellbutrin. Indeed, many people are sensitive to Wellbutrin, just as with other antidepressants, and many physicians start patients at doses as low as 37.5 or 75 mg a day. Increases in dosage, if necessary, are made very gradually. Starting Zyban at 150 mg a day and quickly increasing to 300 mg a day will be too much for many people.

Furthermore, Wellbutrin is generally considered an activating drug: it increases energy in depressed individuals, but may provoke anxiety or agitation in anxiety-prone persons. If Zyban is combined with a nicotine patch, anxiety, insomnia, and other side effects are likely to occur even more frequently and severely.

Different Side Effect Rates with the Same Drug?

SIDE EFFECTS WITH ZYBAN OCCURRING IN MORE THAN 10% OF SUBJECTS

Insomnia, 31–40%
Anxiety or Nervousness, 12%
Runny nose, 12%
Dry mouth, 10–11%
Dizziness, 8–10%

SIDE EFFECTS WITH WELLBUTRIN OCCURRING IN MORE THAN 10% OF SUBJECTS

Anxiety/agitation, 35%
Dry Mouth, 28%
Headache, 26%
Constipation, 26%
Insomnia or impaired sleep, 23%
Nausea/vomiting, 23%
Weight loss, 23%
Excessive sweating, 22%
Dizziness, 22%
Tremor, 21%
Sedation, 20%
Anorexia (loss of appetite), 18%
Blurred vision, 15%
Weight gain, 14%
Confusion or disturbed concentration, 12%
Increased heart rate, 11%
Disturbances of movement or sensation, 11%
Rash or itching, 10%

Perhaps the reason for the short list of frequent Zyban side effects is that the data are based on just two small, short-lasting studies. Yet despite these rosy side effect statistics with Zyban, years of experience with Wellbutrin strongly suggest that people taking this drug, whether it's called Zyban or Wellbutrin, will experience a high incidence of a wide range of side effects. How, in 1997, the FDA could have approved Zyban's not credible side effect statistics while ignoring the wealth of information on Wellbutrin is very troubling.

ZYBAN AND THE ELDERLY

Zyban has a long half-life, meaning that it lingers in the system for more than a day. Repeated dosages lead to increasingly elevated blood levels of the drug. Zyban is metabolized by the liver, a process that the manufacturer acknowledges may be reduced in the elderly. This in turn may lead to even more elevated blood levels and therefore a heightened risk of side effects at the manufacturer-recommended dosage. However, the manufacturer does not suggest lower dosages for elderly individuals.

From experience with Wellbutrin, it is known that the elderly may be particularly sensitive to side effects with this drug. If you are elderly, you and your physician should seriously consider starting at a lower dose and increasing the dose, if necessary, much more gradually than the manufacturer recommends.

RECOMMENDATIONS

The slick TV ads for Zyban make it seem as benign as Tylenol. It isn't. Zyban is bupropion, which is also Wellbutrin, an effective but side-effect-prone antidepressant, especially at higher doses such as the 300 mg a day suggested for Zyban.

Antidepressants, including Wellbutrin, are well known to exhibit a very wide range of interindividual variation. Yet Zyban is recommended at a one-size-fits-all dose of 300 mg a day, a recommendation that defies what we know about bupropion via our experience with Wellbutrin—that different people respond to widely differing doses of this drug.

Indeed, one of the Zyban studies compared doses of 100, 150, and 300 mg a day. Of course, the highest dose produced the best results, and likely the most side effects. However, some people taking the lower doses were successful in quitting smoking, so the highest dose wasn't necessary for everyone. Because this study hasn't been published, we aren't able to analyze it to look at individual responses, but clearly some people did accomplish their goal with lower and less side-effect-prone doses of Zyban. This is important because most side effects with Zyban are dose-related.

With Wellbutrin, doses as low as 50 to 150 mg a day have been effective in treating depression. The same may well prove true for Zyban and smoking cessation. Also, because some people are very sensitive to the effects of Wellbutrin, some physicians start Wellbutrin at doses as low as 25, 37.5, or 50 mg a day.

Even the manufacturer acknowledges the wide range of inter-individual variation with Wellbutrin. The 1997 PDR notes that blood concentrations of this drug varied as much as five-fold between different individuals. A 1983 study demonstrated a ten-fold variation. That's why knowledgeable physicians start low and individualize dosages when prescribing Wellbutrin. Unfortunately, this approach is not suggested by Zyban's manufacturer. And since Zyban is produced in only one size, a 150-mg film-coated, extended-release pill that shouldn't be split, dose flexibility is very limited. For those wanting to start at a lower dose, your physician can prescribe Wellbutrin, which comes in smaller and breakable sizes.

Zyban's manufacturer does mention that liver disease, heart failure, age, and some medications may prolong Zyban metabolism, which involves the activity of liver enzymes, primarily cytochrome P450 2B6 (CYP2B6). Variation in liver enzyme activity is very common, even in people without medical illnesses or taking other medication. This is why some people respond at low dosages. This is also why they encounter side effects at manufacturer-recommended dosages.

Zyban, like Wellbutrin, has a fairly long half-life, meaning that with each dose it builds up in the system. For this reason, increasing from 150 to 300 mg a day (a 100% jump!) after three days may be far too fast for many people. Wellbutrin is often increased more gradually and by much smaller amounts.

Although the manufacturer recommends seven to twelve weeks of treatment with Zyban, the long-term results with this approach appear to be very poor. However, one report suggests that continuing Zyban on an ongoing basis may be more effective in maintaining smoking cessation. The manufacturer is conducting a study using Zyban long-term, and the results should be available soon. In the meantime, if you are successful in stopping smoking with the help of Zyban or Wellbutrin, but relapse after discontinuing the medication, you might consider restarting the drug and staying on it. It may turn out that continuous treatment with Zyban/Wellbutrin is the most effective approach for smoking cessation.

One more word of caution. Other than psychiatrists, most doctors have had little experience in prescribing Wellbutrin and therefore may be completely unprepared for many of the problems that Zyban at the manufacturer-recommended dosages may present. If you decide to try Zyban, make sure that you are working with a physician who's had experience in dealing with the wide range of interindividual variation in dosage and side effects with Wellbutrin.

Finally, despite the disappointing results from the manufacturer's studies with Zyban, it's a fact that smoking and chewing tobacco are perhaps the most prominent and pernicious public health problems in America. They are habits directly associated with cancer, heart disease, ulcers, and other major disorders. Efforts to help people quit their nicotine addictions should be commended—that is, if the treatment does more good than harm.

The jury has only just convened regarding Zyban. So far the data is unimpressive, but it's early. Let's hope that the ultimate verdict on Zyban, perhaps after some experience with lower doses and longer treatment periods, is more positive.

PART 3

Medications for Digestive Disorders

TEN

Medications for Ulcers, Esophagitis, and Heartburn

In-Depth Analyses

H2 Blockers:
    Zantac (ranitidine)
    Axid (nizatidine)
    Pepcid (famotidine)
    Tagamet (cimetidine)

Proton-Pump Inhibitors

    Prilosec (omeprazole)

Brief Comments

    Prevacid (lansoprazole)

About Ulcers, Gastritis, and Esophagitis and the Medications That Treat Them

ULCERS

Stomach and intestinal symptoms account for a third of all visits to primary care physicians. Ulcers are one of the more common disorders that are diagnosed.

Ulcers are crater-like sores, or erosions, in the lining of the upper gastrointestinal tract. The most common site is the duodenum, the first section of the small intestine, and the information presented in this chapter will pertain specifically to duodenal ulcer disease. Ulcers also occur in the stomach and lower parts of the intestine, and the treatment of these is often but not always the same as for duodenal ulcers.

Ulcers hurt because the exposed, underlying tissue of the intestinal wall becomes irritated by and reacts to stomach acid and, in some cases, to acidic or spicy foods. Here again, considerable variation exists between individuals in the amount of pain and sensitivity caused by duodenal ulcers. In fact, some ulcers are silent, causing no pain, finally revealing themselves via signs of blood loss such as anemia, blackened stools, or outright hemorrhage. Although most duodenal ulcers are mild and quickly controlled with proper medical treatment, all ulcers are considered serious because of the possibility of bleeding and, in a small percentage, death.

The cause of most duodenal ulcers is unknown. Some, but not all, are related to excessive stomach acid. In recent years, increasing attention has been paid to a bacteria, *Helicobacter pylori*, as being a contributing factor, if not the primary cause, of many ulcers. Studies have shown that a high percentage of ulcer sufferers tend to get recurrences of their ulcers when treated only with the acid-blocking agents discussed in this chapter, whereas those who are also treated with antibiotics to eradicate Helicobacter have a much smaller incidence of recurrence. This discovery has led to a better outcome in permanently curing ulcers, and it has also allowed people previously dependent on acid blockers to discontinue these drugs.

GASTRITIS

Gastritis is the irritation of the stomach lining. It may be mild or severe, brief or chronic. Under normal conditions, the stomach lining has mechanisms for protection against irritants such as alcohol, smoking or chewing tobacco, or spicy or acidic foods, as well as the hydrochloric acid that the stomach itself secretes. However, the stomach's inherent barriers can be worn down by chronic abuse.

Medications can also provoke gastritis. Foremost among these are aspirin and other anti-inflammatory drugs, but Prozac and other antidepressants, cortisone and other oral steroids, some antibiotics, and many other drugs can cause stomach irritation.

As with ulcers, an increasing amount of evidence suggests that the bacterium *Helicobacter pylori* may be associated with chronic gastritis.

Severe or chronic gastritis is usually treated by a modified diet, avoidance of alcohol, nicotine, and other irritants, one of the medications reviewed in this chapter, and if Helicobacter is implicated, antibiotic therapy.

ESOPHAGITIS

Esophagitis is the result of irritation of the esophagus, the tube-like structure that carries food from the throat to the stomach. In esophagitis, a more serious form of heartburn, acid from the stomach rises into the esophagus, which unlike the lining of the stomach has no natural protective barrier.

Esophagitis can be a very painful condition, not only greatly limiting foods, but causing pain on swallowing. Normally, a valve protects the esophagus from acid encroachment, but sometimes the valve leaks (reflux esophagitis) or part of the stomach has risen above the diaphragm into the chest cavity (hiatal hernia), making the valve incompetent. Sometimes these problems can be corrected surgically, but if not, esophagitis can be nasty. "It's harder to cure than a duodenal ulcer," says one doctor, and he's right.

TREATING ULCERS, GASTRITIS, AND ESOPHAGITIS

From the mid-1970s until the early 1990s, the treatment of these conditions centered on a group of medications known as the H2 antagonists. These drugs include Axid (nizatidine), Pepcid (famotidine), Tagamet (cimetidine), and Zantac (ranitidine), all top-selling drugs.

H2 antagonists block histamine, a chemical produced in many tissues of the body. However, unlike the better known antihistamines used for allergies, H2 antagonists exert their most pronounced effects on the cells that stimulate the release of stomach acid. When the acidity within the stomach and duodenum is reduced, the ulcers become less irritated and heal.

Since 1990, a new family of stomach-acid-inhibiting drugs has come on the scene: the proton-pump inhibitors Prilosec and Prevacid. These medications are more specific in their effects on the acid-secreting cells and are able to reduce acid secretion more effectively than the H2 blockers. Testimonials abound from people who've had only mixed results with Zantac or Tagamet who have received quick and complete relief with Prilosec.

FINALLY, LOW-DOSE H2 BLOCKERS

When I first began writing this chapter, all H2 blockers were available only by prescription. Now all can be purchased in lower-dose, nonprescription forms.

Tagamet has been around for about twenty years, Zantac about fifteen. For all this time, the evidence has been considerable for the effectiveness of doses substantially lower than the manufacturer recommended and doctors prescribed. The approval of lower-dose, nonprescription H2 blockers means that the evidence was strong enough for FDA approval.

The mystery is that it's taken so long for lower-dose H2 blockers to be recognized. After all, Zantac's PDR write-up has long stated that a daily dose of 200 mg, a third less than the recommended 300 mg a day, had proven equally effective in healing duodenal ulcers in repeated studies. With Axid, the 1996 PDR states that a dose of 100 mg a day, 67% lower than the recommended 300 mg, is only slightly less effective.

The nonprescription doses of these drugs are lower—Zantac 75 and Axid AR each contain 75 mg of their respective drug. All of the nonprescription H2 blockers are approved for treating mild indigestion or heartburn, not ulcers, esophagitis, or severe gastritis. Whether these nonprescription drugs will prove useful for the latter conditions, at least in medication-sensitive individuals, remains to be seen. Whether many physicians will even consider them for medication-sensitive patients is also an issue. In the past, few physicians have noticed the low-dose data on H2 blockers contained in the PDR, and instead most have routinely prescribed the general one-size-fits-all doses recommended by the manufacturers.

At the very least, the nonprescription H2 blockers offer an increased degree of dose flexibility. Prescription Zantac, Axid, and Pepcid are offered only in once-a-day and twice-a-day dosages. Even when used twice a day, these drugs often don't last twelve hours. By using the nonprescription forms of these drugs, the same daily dosages can be obtained via a four times a day regimen, which may be superior in consistently suppressing stomach acid in some people. That's what some physicians already do with Tagamet, which comes in a wider range of prescription dose sizes, in prescribing it four times a day.

H2 BLOCKERS AND SIDE EFFECTS

H2 antagonists are usually well tolerated, but side effects and drug interactions do occur. The most common side effect is headaches; constipation, nausea, malaise, rashes, and others may also occur.

Tagamet, because of its effect on liver enzymes, is the most prone to drug interactions, with Zantac next, and Axid and Pepcid least. Tagamet also appears to cause more side effects, including impotence (reversible when the medication is stopped) in a small percentage of males. For these reasons, I was surprised when Tagamet HB was approved for nonprescription usage—certainly Pepcid AC, Axid AR, and Zantac 75 are better choices. Nevertheless, perhaps because it was the first drug in this class and is therefore most familiar to many physicians, Tagamet remains the second most prescribed H2 antagonist behind Zantac.

Most of the side effects caused by H2 blockers are dose related, so dose plays a key role in the occurrence and control of side effects.

H2 BLOCKERS AND THE ELDERLY

The elderly metabolize and eliminate these drugs more slowly than younger adults, yet the recommended initial doses are the same for older individuals as for younger persons. Several studies have commented on the failure of physicians to reduce doses of Zantac and Tagamet for elderly patients, especially those who are small, frail, or sickly or are on other medications, thereby exposing them to higher risks of side effects. For example, Tagamet may cause mental confusion that can be (and sometimes is) mistaken for Alzheimer's disease. This and most other H2 antagonist side effects that develop in elderly individuals are dose-related.

DOSING WITH H2 BLOCKERS

Because the greatest flow of stomach acid occurs during the night, the entire dose may be taken at bedtime. Some individuals, however, develop symptoms during the day, and regimens of twice to four times a day are sometimes used. Again, people vary, and the best regimen and optimum dose should be determined by working closely with your doctor.

During treatment, many people also use antacids such as Maalox or Riopan. Tagamet absorption is believed to be impaired when taken with antacids, Zantac less so, and Axid and Pepcid are purportedly not affected.

Because of their popularity, H2 antagonists are very familiar to most physicians, who routinely prescribe the often one-size-fits-all dosages recommended by the manufacturers. Many physicians are not aware of the substantial information on the effectiveness of lower doses of these drugs. Medication-sensitive individuals and others concerned about drug-related side effects may have to educate their physicians about the data and alternatives presented in this chapter in order to discuss the possibility and appropriateness of low-dose H2 antagonist drug therapy.

Nonsmokers, who respond to H2 antagonists better and at lower doses than smokers, may represent another group that can benefit from low-dose H2 antagonist treatment.

THE PROTON PUMP INHIBITORS: PRILOSEC AND PREVASID

A new era in the treatment of upper gastrointestinal diseases began in late 1990 when Prilosec (omeprazole) was released. Designed specifically to stop the mechanism for releasing acid into the stomach, Prilosec quickly demonstrated its prowess in treating duodenal ulcers. As one patient put it, ''I've been taking Tagamet or Zantac for ulcers for two decades, and I never got complete relief. With Prilosec, it was just a matter of days.''

Moreover, Prilosec showed remarkable effectiveness when prescribed for gastritis and, especially, esophagitis, conditions with which the H2 blockers are far less successful. Indeed, the main concern with Prilosec and with Prevacid, which was released a few years later, is that they inhibit stomach acid so strongly that prolonged usage may be dangerous. Stomach acid is, after all, an important component of the digestive process. Prolonged acid suppression by Prilosec resulted in stomach tumors in some animal studies. Fortunately, similar problems have not been reported in humans whose conditions have required long-term Prilosec therapy.

The reported incidence of side effects with proton-pump inhibitors have been low. Most side effects with these drugs are dose related.

THE ROLE OF BACTERIA IN
GASTRIC DISEASE

The recurrence of supposedly healed duodenal ulcers and the intransigence of chronic gastritis has long puzzled physicians. Whether H2 blockers or proton-pump inhibitors are used, recurrences are common after the medication is discontinued. This is why many people have remained on maintenance doses of these drugs for years.

Research over the last decade has drawn attention to an old adversary—bacterial infection. Slowly at first, the evidence has now become unequivocal that the bacterium *Helicobacter pylori* is associated with the development and recurrence of duodenal ulcers. The evidence connecting Helicobacter to chronic gastritis is also mounting.

Studies have shown that by eradicating Helicobacter with antibiotics, most long-term ulcer sufferers are apparently cured for good. Eradicating Helicobacter isn't easy, and it's taken several years to ascertain the best approach. Presently, it appears that the most effective regimen includes Prilosec in concert with Biaxin (clarithromycin), an antibiotic. Other combinations utilizing H2 blockers and/or different antibiotics, sometimes also with bismuth preparations such as Pepto-Bismol, have been used with lesser yet still substantial degrees of success.

Despite all of these efforts, Helicobacter reinfection occurs in a substantial percentage of patients. One reason may be that an important reservoir of Helicobacter persistence is often overlooked. Helicobacter can survive in dental plaque during antibiotic treatment; then it is swallowed in saliva and can reestablish itself in the stomach. Using a mouthwash that inhibits Helicobacter both during and after antibiotic therapy may increase your chances of avoiding a recurrence of an ulcer or gastritis.

COST FACTORS

Dosage decisions should never be based on cost factors. However, with the emergence of nonprescription forms of Zantac, Axid, Pepcid, and Tagamet, costs can be reduced without altering dosages. Despite the potential for substantial savings, most medical insurers do not cover nonprescription drugs; perhaps in time they will reconsider this position.

NONPRESCRIPTION H2 BLOCKERS OR ANTACIDS?

The release of the H2 blockers in nonprescription form has been accompanied by massive advertising campaigns extolling the virtues of these drugs and their superiority over antacids. We should question, however, this increased reliance on systemic drugs to handle symptoms of mild heartburn or indigestion, especially when nonsystemic, locally active antacids may be equally effective for many people. In other words, if Maalox or Tums or other antacids work well for you, switching to H2 blockers isn't warranted. Indeed, antacids work within seconds or minutes, while H2 blockers take much longer. I usually recommend calcium (Tums, Titralac) or magnesium (Riopan) antacids rather than those containing aluminum compounds. Liquid antacids work more quickly than tablets, although the difference may be small.

A few H2 blocker advertisements are particularly irksome because they seem to encourage dietary overindulgence, the effects of which will supposedly be neutralized by H2 blocker preparations. This message should be vigorously challenged. People have enough trouble maintaining good dietary habits; encouraging dietary indiscretion combined with drug usage isn't likely to improve things. Indeed, it has been suggested that some people have become dependent upon H2 blockers to control gastric symptoms that effective dietary methods might solve. Now that H2 blockers are even more available with fewer controls, people should be forewarned that even at nonprescription doses, these are not necessarily innocuous drugs, and they should be used with care and restraint.

In-Depth Analysis: Zantac (Ranitidine)

For many years Zantac has been America's favorite anti-ulcer remedy, ranking No. 5 in outpatient prescriptions in 1996. "Some days, it seems that every other prescription we fill is for Zantac," one pharmacist told me.

As mentioned above, Zantac is most effective in the treatment of duodenal ulcers. It's sometimes effective in treating gastritis, less so in esophagitis.

The PDR-recommended dosage for treating duodenal ulcers with prescription Zantac is 300 mg a day, administered via 150 mg twice a day or all 300 mg at night. The maintenance dose, once the ulcer is healed, is 150 mg at bedtime. There are no specific elderly doses, so they're apparently the same as for younger adults.

Prescription Zantac is produced as 150- and 300-mg caplets, and as 150-mg effervescent tablets and granules. Zantac has also been combined with bismuth citrate; the combination is called Tritec and is meant for usage with the antibiotic Biaxin in treating ulcers associated with *Helicobacter pylori*.

In 1996, Zantac 75 appeared as a nonprescription, lower-dose form of Zantac. Offered for the relief of mild heartburn and indigestion, each pill contains 75 mg of Zantac. The manufacturer-recommended dosage is one or two pills per day.

MOST FREQUENT SIDE EFFECTS

Zantac side effects include headaches, constipation, nausea, dyspepsia; rarely, malaise, dizziness, drowsiness, insomnia, mental confusion, hair loss, blurred vision, joint or muscle pain, rash, impotence (reversible), enlarged breasts in males (reversible), cardiac arrhythmias, altered blood cell levels, allergic reactions. It is not recommended for use in pregnancy or by nursing mothers.

LOW-DOSE PRESCRIPTION ZANTAC

For years, Zantac's package insert and PDR description contained this addendum to its dosing guidelines: "Smaller doses have been shown to be equally effective in inhibiting gastric acid secretion in US studies, and several foreign trials have shown that 100 b.i.d. [twice a day] is as effective as the 150-mg dose."

Indeed, Zantac's package insert and PDR description offer a chart that compares the effects of 100 and 150 mg of Zantac on suppressing stomach acid. The results with these two doses were virtually identical, with 100 mg edging out 150 mg on two of three measures.

Other references concur. *Drug Facts and Comparisons*, which many pharmacists consider their best medication resource, states: "100 mg twice daily is as effective as the 150 mg [twice daily] dose."

Unfortunately, no pharmacist I've spoken to has ever received a prescription for 100-mg Zantac. No physician I've asked has ever noticed the information in the PDR about this lower Zantac dose. Perhaps it's because no 100-mg pill was ever made available.

Will nonprescription Zantac 75 now fill this void? This preparation is approved for minor conditions, not the more serious ulcers, gastritis, and esophagitis for which prescription Zantac is used. Yet if 100 mg (twice a day) of Zantac is as effective as the currently recommended 150 mg dosage, would Zantac 75 mg be sufficient for some elderly or medication-sensitive individuals? For nonsmokers, who often require lower doses, or for mild conditions?

Ulcers, in particular, can be serious. The usage of lower doses should be discussed with your physician. However, if you are medication-sensitive, for gastritis and esophagitis, starting with Zantac 75 may be worth considering. You can start at the nonprescription dose of 75 mg twice a day, but if it isn't sufficient, under your physician's guidance you may be able to increase to three times a day and, if necessary, four times a day. Zantac 75 four times a day is 300 mg, the equivalent of the manufacturer-recommended prescription dosage.

Even with ulcers, nonprescription Zantac 75 can provide increased flexibility. Prescription Zantac can be used only twice daily, but one of the reasons that Tagamet remains a popular, although more side-effect-prone drug, is that it can be used four times a day, a regimen that seems to work better for some people. Zantac 150 mg, although prescribed twice a day, often doesn't last twelve hours; you may obtain a better, more consistent response with Zantac 75 three or four times a day. If Zantac 300 mg at bedtime or Zantac 150 mg twice a day isn't working, discuss this alternative with your physician.

ZANTAC AND THE ELDERLY

The manufacturer-recommended doses of Zantac are the same for older adults as for younger people. Research, however, demonstrates that the metabolism and elimination of Zantac is prolonged in older individuals, meaning that a given dose of Zantac may linger longer and/or reach higher blood levels in elderly than in younger persons. Studies also show that doctors don't adjust Zantac dosages according to elderly patients' age or body weight, despite the fact that both are risk factors for overmedication or drug interactions.

Thus, although Zantac has been on the market for over a decade, a recent study criticized the lack of information about optimal dosing with Zantac in relation to the physiological changes of aging. Others have called for the routine use of lower Zantac doses with the elderly: "If you are over 60, you should generally be taking less than the usual adult dose of ranitidine [Zantac]."

But previously, no lower-dose Zantac pill was available. Now Zantac 75 can be purchased without a prescription. It's usage and effectiveness for serious gastrointestinal illness has not been established, but it may earn a place in treating elderly individuals who cannot tolerate standard dosages.

RECOMMENDATIONS

Duodenal ulcer disease, as well as the other conditions for which prescription Zantac is used, can be serious. Using a dose of Zantac that is effective is the first priority; avoiding overmedication is the second.

Although multiple studies and the PDR provide ample evidence that low-dose, 100-mg Zantac twice a day is highly effective, physicians have heretofore relied upon the available although higher 150- and 300-mg doses. Now nonprescription Zantac 75 is available, but its role in serious conditions is not established.

In routine cases, the manufacturer's dosage recommendations should be applied because they have the benefit of being the most studied and the most likely to be effective for the largest number of people. For milder types of gastritis or esophagitis, or with elderly or medication-sensitive or other high-risk individuals, Zantac 75 may offer a reasonable alternative. Nonsmokers also usually require less medication and may benefit from a lower-dose approach.

Even when prescription dosages are required, nonprescription Zantac 75 can provide increased dose flexibility. Prescription Zantac is utilized either once or twice a day, but with some people the medication doesn't last twelve hours, and breakthrough discomfort occurs as the medication wears off. Using Zantac 75 four times a day may be more effective without any reduction in dosage. Zantac 75 three times a day may also be sufficient, while at the same time lowering the amount of medication by 33%. (Over the years, dosing three and four times a day with Tagamet, which has been available at lower prescription doses, has proven useful in some cases.)

Effervescent Zantac tablets and granules and Zantac syrup can be used similarly. By using half the standard amount, 75 mg instead of 150 mg, these products can be used three or four times a day. In addition, unlike nonprescription Zantac 75, their costs may be covered by your health insurance.

In-Depth Analysis: Axid (Nizatidine)

Axid is a top-selling ulcer remedy, ranking No. 67 in outpatient prescriptions in 1996. Like Zantac, Axid is prescribed for duodenal ulcers, gastritis, and esophagitis; it's most effective in ulcer treatment.

The manufacturer-recommended dosage of Axid for duodenal ulcers is 300 mg a day initially administered either as 150 mg twice a day or all 300 mg at bedtime. The maintenance dose, once the ulcer is healed, is 150 mg at bedtime. For esophagitis, it's 150 mg twice a day. Lower doses are recommended for people with impaired kidney functioning. The dosage for the elderly is the same as above unless kidney functioning is impaired. Prescription Axid is produced in 150- and 300-mg capsules.

In 1996, Axid AR appeared as a nonprescription, lower-dose form of Axid. Offered for the relief of mild heartburn and indigestion, each pill contains 75 mg. The manufacturer-recommended dosage is one or two pills per day.

MOST FREQUENT SIDE EFFECTS

Axid side effects include headaches, drowsiness, dizziness, fatigue, sweating, anemia, or diarrhea. Rare side effects are indigestion, constipation, weakness, fever, drowsiness, anxiety, nervousness, rash, liver irritation, mental confusion, enlarged breasts in males (gynecomastia; reversible with discontinuation of medication), or allergic reaction. Axid is not recommended for use in pregnancy or by nursing mothers. Drug interactions occur, but less frequently than with Tagamet or Zantac.

LOW-DOSE PRESCRIPTION AXID

The medical literature contains three studies demonstrating the effectiveness of low-dose Axid. A dose of 100 mg at bedtime provided very similar rates of ulcer healing as the recommended 300-mg dose. The 1996 PDR contains this acknowledgment: "Lower doses, such as 100 mg h.s. [at bedtime], had slightly lower effectiveness [than the recommended, 300% higher, 300-mg bedtime dose]." Indeed, studies have shown that doses of 25 mg twice a day are significantly more effective than a placebo. In one study, among nonsmokers this very low dose was nearly as effective as 150 mg twice a day.

Despite these findings, Axid has not been available in pills lower than 150 mg. With the arrival of 75 mg Axid AR, greater dose flexibility is now possible. Even at prescription doses, 75 mg Axid AR taken three or four times a day may be more effective for some people than twice-a-day Axid 150 mg, a dose that doesn't always last twelve hours.

AXID AND THE ELDERLY

The manufacturer recommends reduced doses for elderly individuals with impaired kidney functioning. But even with normal kidney blood tests, the kidney functioning of a 75-year-old may be reduced 50% or more compared to younger adults. This can lead to higher and more prolonged blood levels of Axid, placing elderly individuals at greater risk of side effects and drug interactions. Here, too, the arrival of 75-mg Axid AR may provide greater dose flexibility.

RECOMMENDATIONS

Duodenal ulcer disease, as well as the other conditions for which Axid is prescribed, can be serious. Using a dose of Axid that is effective is the first priority, but effective treatment also depends on avoiding overmedication and side effects. Because the manufacturer's recommended initial dose has the benefit of being the most studied and most likely to help the greatest number of people, this dose should be given primary consideration, especially with individuals with serious conditions and/or lacking a history of medication sensitivities.

On the other hand, Axid doses of 25 and 50 mg twice a day were shown to be effective in several studies. This suggests that nonprescription 75 mg Axid AR, although not approved for ulcers, gastritis, or esophagitis, may prove sufficient if you are medication-sensitive or a nonsmoker.

Prescription Axid is utilized either once or twice a day. However, for some people the medication doesn't last twelve hours, and breakthrough discomfort occurs as the medication wears off. Using 75 mg Axid AR four times a day may prove more effective without any reduction in dosage. Axid AR three times a day may also be sufficient, while at the same time reducing the amount of medication by 33%.

In-Depth Analysis: Pepcid (Famotidine)

Pepcid is a top-selling ulcer remedy, ranking No. 38 in outpatient prescriptions in 1996. Pepcid is prescribed for duodenal ulcers, gastritis, and esophagitis; it's most effective with duodenal ulcers.

For duodenal ulcers the PDR suggests an initial dose of 40 mg a day taken as 20 mg twice a day or 40 mg at bedtime; once the ulcer is healed, the maintenance dose is 20 mg at bedtime. For esophagitis, 20 mg twice a day; for severe cases, up to 40 mg twice a day. Elderly doses are the same as those for younger adults, except for those with severe kidney function impairment.

Prescription Pepcid is produced as 20- and 40-mg tablets.

In 1995, 10-mg Pepcid AC was introduced as a nonprescription treatment for mild heartburn and indigestion. The recommended dosage is one or two pills per day.

MOST FREQUENT SIDE EFFECTS

Pepcid side effects include headaches, dizziness, constipation, or diarrhea. Rare side effects are weakness, fatigue, numbness, drowsiness, insomnia, anxiety, nausea, dry mouth, indigestion, rash, liver irritation, joint or muscle pain, fever, hypertension, ringing in ears (tinnitus), cardiac arrhythmias, altered blood cell levels, or allergic reactions. Pepcid is not recommended in pregnancy or for nursing mothers. Drug interactions occur, but less frequently than with Zantac or Tagamet.

LOW-DOSE PEPCID

The medical literature contains several studies demonstrating the ability of 10 and 20 mg of Pepcid to suppress stomach acid. For example, a 1988 study in the *American Journal of Gastroenterology*, stated: "The results obtained in the present study provide evidence that low doses of famotidine [Pepcid 20 mg] markedly inhibited night gastric acidity and should, therefore, prove efficacious in the therapy and maintenance of duodenal ulcer patients." In these studies the degree and duration of acid suppression varied considerably between individuals, meaning that Pepcid-sensitive persons may do fine at lower doses, whereas others may require the standard recommended amount of Pepcid.

Nonprescription 10-mg Pepcid AC provides new flexibility with this drug. Even at prescription doses, Pepcid AC taken three or four times a day may work better for some people than prescription Pepcid 20 mg twice a day because the latter dose doesn't always last twelve hours.

PEPCID AND THE ELDERLY

The manufacturer-recommended dosages of Pepcid are the same for elderly individuals as for younger adults, unless kidney function is severely impaired. However, virtually all elderly persons exhibit some degree, usually 50% or more, of diminished kidney function. Depending on the illness and its severity, lower doses of Pepcid, 10-20-30 mg a day, may be useful. Ten-mg Pepcid AC may offer extra dose flexibility.

RECOMMENDATIONS

Duodenal ulcers, gastritis, and esophagitis can be serious. Using a dose of Pepcid that is effective is the first priority, but effective treatment also depends on avoiding overmedication and side effects. Because the manufacturer's recommended initial dose has been the most studied, and because it provides the most reliable degree of stomach acid suppression beyond eight to ten hours, this dose should be given primary consideration with individuals with serious conditions and/or lacking a history of medication sensitivities.

However, studies suggest that lower doses may be sufficient for the medication-sensitive or others at risk for side effects. Although it doesn't appear that Pepcid has as yet been specifically studied in nonsmokers, studies with similar drugs suggest that nonsmokers may respond at lower doses.

Prescription Pepcid is utilized either once or twice a day. However, for some people the medication doesn't last twelve hours, and breakthrough discomfort occurs as the medication wears off. Using 10-mg Pepcid AC four times a day may prove more effective without any reduction in the manufacturer-recommended daily dosage. Pepcid AC three times a day may also be sufficient, while at the same time reducing the amount of medication by 33%.

In-Depth Analysis: Tagamet (Cimetidine)

Tagamet, the first H2 blocker, was introduced for general usage in 1977; this marked the beginning of a new era of duodenal ulcer treatment. Since then, newer and, in the opinion of many physicians, better stomach acid suppressors have been developed (e.g., Axid, Pepcid, Prilosec, Zantac). Still, despite its higher rates of side effects and drug interactions, Tagamet and its generic, cimetidine, remain top-selling medications.

The manufacturer-recommended initial dosage for duodenal ulcers is 800 mg at bedtime (600 mg for those with impaired kidney functioning); once ulcers are healed, the maintenance dose is 400 mg. Other effective doses are 400 mg twice a day and 300 mg four times a day. For esophagitis, 800 mg twice a day or 400 mg four times a day. The elderly dose is the same as that of younger adults. Because antacids can interfere with the absorption of Tagamet, they should not be taken within one hour of a dose of Tagamet.

Prescription Tagamet is produced in 200- and 300-mg coated tablets, in 400- and 800-mg breakable tablets, and in a syrup.

In 1996, 100-mg Tagamet HB was released as a nonprescription remedy for mild heartburn and indigestion. The manufacturer-recommended dosage is one or two pills per day.

MOST FREQUENT SIDE EFFECTS

Tagamet is considered more prone to producing side effects and drug interactions than other H2 blockers. Side effects include headache, diarrhea, drowsiness, fatigue, dizziness, mental confusion, and enlarged breasts in males (gynecomastia/reversible with discontinuation of drug). Less frequent side effects are impotence (reversible), reduced sperm counts, liver irritation, drop in blood pressure (hypotension), anxiety, lethargy, increased or decreased heart rate, joint or muscle pain, rash, fever, altered blood cell levels, and allergic reactions. Tagamet is not recommended in pregnancy or for nursing mothers. Tagamet interacts with numerous drugs; it can enhance the effects of benzodiazepines such as Dalmane and Xanax, calcium channel blockers such as Calan and Cardizem, beta blockers such as Inderal, cardiac drugs such as quinidine, tricyclic antidepressants such as Elavil, and others including Novocain and Coumadin. Tagamet can diminish the effects of Digoxin, tetracycline, iron compounds, and others.

LOW-DOSE TAGAMET

Doses 50% lower than those currently recommended by the manufacturer have shown significant effectiveness in healing duodenal ulcers. Interestingly, when Tagamet was first released, the recommended dose was 300 mg four times a day (1200 mg/day). Years later, based on experience with the general population, the manufacturer lowered its suggested dose 33% to the currently recommended 800 mg at bedtime. Some physicians, however, continue to prefer the 300 mg four-times-a-day regimen, because it provides better round-the-clock acid control. The problem is that the latter regimen requires a 50% higher daily dosage. Similar four-times-a-day dosing can be achieved without increasing total daily dosage with 200-mg Tagamet tablets. If you are medication-sensitive, 100-mg Tagamet HB may be sufficient. Three-times-a-day dosing may also be enough for some people. The labeling for nonprescription Tagamet HB is for one or two pills per day; any usage above this amount should first be discussed with your physician.

LOW-DOSE TAGAMET AND THE ELDERLY

Elderly individuals tend to metabolize Tagamet more slowly than younger adults, producing higher and more prolonged Tagamet blood levels that increase the risks of side effects and drug interactions. For example, the dementia known as Tagamet-induced confusional state is not uncommon. "A 74-year-old man and his wife both feared that he was developing Alzheimer's disease," a psychiatrist told me. Still the head of a corporation, the man had been showing signs of progressive memory loss over three years. He finally sought help after an episode of confusion forced him to stop in the middle of a presentation to the board of directors. "The memory tests revealed definite cognitive and memory deficits. The diagnosis was looking like Alzheimer's. Then I asked about other medications. He'd been taking Tagamet. How long? About three years. When I told them that his condition might be due to the Tagamet rather than Alzheimer's, they hugged me and cried. The Tagamet was discontinued, and the memory deficits disappeared." The doctor added, "I've seen five of these cases; this one surprised me because it developed at standard Tagamet doses." I replied, " 'Standard doses' means the same dose for everyone. Maybe this man needed less." The doctor paused a moment, then said, "Obviously he did."

Tagamet-induced dementia, although devastating, can be overlooked. As Dr. Steffi Woolhandler said in 1994 (as quoted in *The New York Times*): "A lot of the problem is that doctors frequently ascribe the side effects of drugs to old age. . . . If a patient loses memory or balance, they say it's old age." The occurrence of Tagamet-induced confusional state is directly related to dosage. Yet excessive dosing isn't unusual. For this reason, some have called for lower Tagamet doses for elderly patients: "If you are over 60, you should generally be taking less than the usual adult dose of cimetidine.''

RECOMMENDATIONS

Duodenal ulcer disease, gastritis, and esophagitis can be serious. Using a dose of Tagamet that is effective is the first priority, but effective treatment also depends on avoiding overmedication and side effects. Because the manufacturer's recommended initial dose has been the most studied, this dose should be given primary consideration with individuals with serious conditions and/or lacking a history of medication sensitivities.

On the other hand, the low-dose data suggests that with medication-sensitive individuals and/or mild conditions, initiating treatment with the 50% lower, 400-mg bedtime dose of Tagamet may be reasonable. Small or elderly individuals may also represent populations with whom starting with a lower dose may be considered. Nonsmokers may also respond at lower Tagamet doses.

Not everyone responds to a single nighttime dose of Tagamet. Some people require one or more doses during the day to provide protection against stomach acid released in response to meals or stress. The availability of Tagamet in several sizes including 100-mg nonprescription Tagamet HB allows for very flexible dosing according to individual needs.

Tagamet is the oldest and most side-effect-prone medication of the H2 blockers. With the recent availability of other H2 blockers at lower, nonprescription doses, Tagamet no longer offers any advantage over Axid, Pepcid, or Zantac.

If you intend to use one of the nonprescription H2 blockers for mild heartburn or indigestion, Axid AR and Pepcid AC are less likely than Tagamet HB to cause side effects or undesirable drug interactions.

In-Depth Analysis: Prilosec (Omeprazole)

Introduced in 1990, Prilosec has quickly become recognized as perhaps the most effective drug available for treating duodenal ulcers. In addition, it has proven to be the first truly effective drug treatment for esophagitis. For treating *Helicobacter pylori*–related ulcers or gastritis, Prilosec is usually chosen to augment the effects of antibiotics. For these reasons, Prilosec has become increasingly favored for treating upper gastrointestinal disorders and in 1996 ranked No. 12 in U.S. outpatient prescriptions and exceeded $1 billion in sales.

Prilosec represents the first member of a new class of stomach acid suppressors, the proton-pump inhibitors. By preventing gastric cells from releasing hydrochloric acid, these drugs decrease stomach acid far more efficiently than Zantac and the other H2 blockers—hence Prilosec's superior effectiveness.

The PDR-recommended dosage of Prilosec for treating duodenal ulcers or esophagitis is 20 mg a day for four to eight weeks. Elderly dosage is the same. Prilosec is produced in only one size, a 20-mg sustained release capsule.

MOST COMMON SIDE EFFECTS

Prilosec is usually well tolerated. Side effects may include headaches, malaise, nausea, constipation or diarrhea, abdominal pain, or joint pains. Early studies with rats on high doses of Prilosec for prolonged periods resulted in the occurrence of abnormal stomach cell development; therefore, the PDR recommends Prilosec only for short-term (four to eight weeks) usage with most conditions. However, subsequent to its release Prilosec has been used long-term in severe cases; so far, no association with increased cancer has been reported.

LOW-DOSE PRILOSEC

Numerous studies before and after Prilosec's release have demonstrated its effectiveness at 10 mg, which is 50% lower than the recommended dosage. For example, in a 1989 study, 75% of duodenal ulcer patients healed with 10 mg a day of Prilosec. The 1996 PDR confirmed the acid-suppressing and ulcer-healing capabilities of this dose.

Clinical experience also supports the effectiveness of lower doses. "Prilosec is a good medication," a gastroenterologist told me, "but I think the dose sometimes is too strong. It works so fast in so many patients, I suspect a lower dose would work nearly as well with less risk. As soon as my patients show sufficient improvement, I have them switch to an every-other-day dose, which is essentially 10 mg a day. Prilosec has a very long duration of action, so just one capsule every other day is sufficient for some people."

PRILOSEC AND THE ELDERLY

The recommended initial dose is 20 mg a day, same as younger adults. Yet in a 1992 study, it was found that elderly patients metabolize Prilosec far more slowly that younger adults: "The average reduction in omeprazole [Prilosec] clearance with age was 58%." The result was "an approximately 2-fold increase" in the peak blood concentrations of the drug and a markedly prolonged duration of action. Moreover, this study was conducted with healthy seniors; less healthy individuals or those taking other medications would likely demonstrate even higher Prilosec blood concentrations and slower clearances. Another study examined several Prilosec dosages in elderly subjects. The briefness of the study, seven days, favored the higher doses, but the 5- and 10-mg dosages performed well: more than half of the subjects responded impressively to the lower doses. Moreover, the subjects were healthy males, while the typical elderly patient is female, has other medical problems, and takes several medications; all of these factors lend toward lower doses.

RECOMMENDATIONS

Prilosec is a very effective medication, so effective that it is gradually supplanting top-selling H2 blockers like Zantac and Tagamet. Yet Prilosec is, as one pharmacist put it, "a big gun." Prilosec works by interfering with the sodium/potassium balancing systems within cells. Although the acid-producing cells of the gastric lining are particularly sensitive to Prilosec's effect, the drug does penetrate other cells of the body. As a doctor told me, "Any drug that affects the sodium/potassium balance is bound to have effects throughout the system." Nonetheless, most physicians I've asked report relatively few problems with Prilosec.

Most of Prilosec's pre-release research studies were conducted over very short time frames that may not have revealed long-term side effects. As mentioned above, post-release long-term usage—six to seven years—has apparently not been associated with any untoward effects. However, it remains to be seen if further usage reveals problems. Prilosec greatly reduces the acid content of the stomach. It is not known whether prolonged acid suppression causes changes in digestion, the normal bacterial flora of the digestive system, or the cells lining the gut.

Short-term pre-release studies also tend to favor higher dosages. Nevertheless, low-dose, 10-mg Prilosec performed well, well enough to be suitable for many people. Indeed, 10-mg Prilosec performed so well, it's possible that even lower doses may be effective in a small percentage of people, especially elderly or other medication-sensitive individuals.

Because Prilosec is produced only as a 20-mg capsule, flexible dosaging is difficult. An every-other-day approach provides an average dosage of 10 mg a day. Every-other-day dosing works with Prilosec because of its very long duration of action.

Standard Prilosec dosaging is 20–40–60 mg a day, but by utilizing Prilosec's long duration of action, intermediary doses of 30 or 50 mg a day can be attained (e.g., an average dose of 30 mg = 2 Prilosec capsules one day, 1 Prilosec capsule the next).

If you've developed side effects with Prilosec, reducing your dosage as described above may remedy the problem without interfering with Prilosec's effectiveness.

Other Medications

PREVACID (LANSOPRAZOLE)

Closely related to Prilosec, Prevacid is a proton-pump inhibitor used for treating ulcers, gastritis, and esophagitis. Like Prilosec, its effectiveness for duodenal ulcers and, especially, esophagitis appears to be significantly superior to Zantac and other H2 blockers. In 1996, Prevacid ranked No. 155 among the top 200 prescribed medications in the United States.

The incidence of side effects with Prevacid is generally low. The most common are diarrhea, nausea, abdominal pain, joint pain, and rash. It is manufactured as 15- and 30-mg capsules. The Recommended dosage for duodenal ulcers is 15 mg a day; for esophagitis, 30 mg a day. Prevacid is recommended for short-term usage because, like Prilosec, high doses given to rats for long periods produced abnormal gastric cell development. Regarding lower doses: 15 mg a day for esophagitis, 50% lower than recommended, may be sufficient for many people. The 1996 PDR states that at 15 mg a day, 88% of subjects with esophagitis healed after four weeks, 91% after eight weeks. Long duration of action may allow every-other-day dosaging with some people.

PART 4

*Drugs for Lowering Cholesterol and
Controlling Hypertension*

ELEVEN

Cholesterol-Lowering Medications

In-Depth Analyses

Mevacor (lovastatin)
Pravachol (pravastatin)
Zocor (simvastatin)
Lescol (fluvastatin)

About High Cholesterol and Cholesterol-Lowering Drugs

Cholesterol and its relationship to heart disease have become important public health issues. An awareness of dietary cholesterol and saturated fats is now part of our cultural consciousness. On any given day, articles can be found in popular magazines about ways to lower dietary cholesterol and saturated fats. The supermarket shelves are loaded with fat-free and low-fat products. And pharmacies carry an array of cholesterol-lowering drugs.

By far the most prescribed, most effective, and best tolerated cholesterol-lowering medications are the statins: Mevacor (lovastatin), Pravachol (pravastatin), Zocor (simvastatin), and Lescol (fluvastatin). More important, this group of drugs now has been proven to prevent the formation, slow the progression, and sometimes cause actual regression of narrowing of arteries (atherosclerosis, formerly called arteriosclerosis). By doing so, these drugs significantly reduce the incidence of coronary artery disease, heart attacks, strokes, and cardiac death.

The first statin was Mevacor, released in 1987 and the top-selling statin through 1995, when it ranked No. 28 among America's top 200 drugs in outpatient prescriptions. In 1996, Zocor claimed the No. 21 position, while Mevacor retreated slightly to No. 32. Meanwhile, from 1995 to 1996, Pravachol climbed from No. 57 to No. 41, and Lescol from No. 110 to No. 63. Together, the statins are one of the most prescribed groups of drugs in America. And because they are available only as brand name, not generic, drugs with costs of about $1.50 to $3 per pill—which patients must take daily for the rest of their lives—these medications are tremendously profitable for their manufacturers. In 1996, Zocor alone exceeded over $1 billion in sales.

THE IMPORTANCE OF SAFE LEVELS OF TOTAL CHOLESTEROL AND LDL-C

Our growing awareness about the harmful effects of excessive cholesterol and saturated fats, and the development of low-fat and fat-free foods, is good because high cholesterol kills. Coronary heart disease affects about 12 million Americans and is the No. 1 cause of death for both men and women in the United States.

Treatment alone costs more than $100 billion each year, with $60 billion paying for hospital costs. According to one journal article, "Patients with documented coronary heart disease and elevated LDL-C cholesterol [the low density, or "bad cholesterol"] levels are 12 times more likely to die of coronary heart disease than are people with healthy levels of LDL-C cholesterol."

Over the last decade, attempts to educate the public about the need for healthier diets has produced results: total dietary fat intake has dropped from 36% to 33% and saturated fat from 13% to 11%. Average total blood cholesterol among U.S. adults has gone from 213 in 1978 to 205 in 1990, and the percentage of the population with dangerously high levels of total cholesterol (greater than 240) has fallen from 26% to 20%. Most of all, the mortality rates from coronary heart disease have declined steadily.

A lot has been accomplished in a relatively short time, but 52 million Americans still have cholesterol levels requiring at least dietary change, and millions also require medication therapy. In the group of 35- to 44-year-olds, about 50% have undesirable cholesterol levels of 200 or more, levels associated with increased risk of coronary and other atherosclerotic vascular diseases such as strokes. They're not alone; overall, 96 million Americans have cholesterol levels of 200 or above.

DO YOU NEED TREATMENT?

Whether you require treatment for high cholesterol depends on several factors, but the primary one is your blood level of LDL-C.

The total level of cholesterol in blood is comprised of several components. These include HDL-C (high density lipoprotein-cholesterol), LDL-C (low density lipoprotein-cholesterol), and VLDL-C (very low density lipoprotein-cholesterol)—the three types of lipoproteins that carry cholesterol through the bloodstream. HDL-C is the "good cholesterol" that can provide some protection from cardiovascular disease. LDL-C and VLDL-C are the harmful cholesterols that foster atherosclerosis. Another substance, triglycerides, can also foster the narrowing of arteries and heart disease. Statin medications lower LDL-C, VLDL-C, and triglycerides, and often increase HDL-C, producing the precisely desired effect.

More than any other factor, your LDL-C blood level is the most important indicator of risk and has become the main focus of treatment. Additional risk factors involved in deciding if you need to lower your total cholesterol or LDL-C levels are: male gender, obesity, diabetes, hypertension, smoking, family history of premature atherosclerosis-related heart disease, and if your HDL-C level is below 35 mg/dl. (Levels of total cholesterol, HDL-C, LDL-C, and VLDL-C are measured as milligrams per decaliter, mg/dl.) If your HDL-C is 60 or above, it is considered protective and offsets one risk factor.

Desirable and At-Risk Levels of LDL-C and Total Cholesterol. (Adapted from S. Grundy, et al., Circulation, 1997

PREFERRED LEVELS

With one or no risk factors*: LDL-C below 160.

Even with an LDL-C below 160, some physicians prefer that your total cholesterol also should be below 200.

With two or more risk factors: LDL-C below 130.

People with known coronary or other atherosclerosis-related disease (secondary prevention): LDL-C below 100.

MILD TO MODERATE RISK GROUP

With one or no risk factors: LDL-C of 160–190.

Even with a LDL-C below 160, some physicians believe a total cholesterol of 200–240 represents a mild to moderate risk.

With two or more risk factors: LDL-C 130–160.

HIGH RISK GROUP

With one or no risk factors: LDL-C above 190.

Even with a LDL-C below 190, some physicians believe a total cholesterol above 240 represents a high risk.

With two or more risk factors: LDL-C above 160.

People with known coronary or other atherosclerosis-related disease (secondary prevention): LDL-C above 100.

---

*Risk factors: Age (males 45 or older; females 55 or older, or menopausal without estrogen therapy), obesity, diabetes, hypertension, smoking, an HDL-C level below 35, or a family history of early coronary heart disease. An HDL-C level above 60 offsets one risk factor.

Target levels of LDL-C have been established for people who haven't had coronary heart disease or other atherosclerosis-related problems. Treating these people before such problems develop is called primary prevention, which is the goal of the prodigious efforts toward public education about cholesterol and heart disease.

If you are in the primary prevention group and have fewer than two additional risk factors, your target LDL-C is 160 or less (see box). If you have two or more additional risk factors, your target LDL-C is 130 or less.

In other words, if your LDL-C level is above 130 but below 160 with two or more risk factors, or above 160 but below 190 with no risk factors, or your total cholesterol level is above 200 but below 240, your risk is considered mild to moderate. Initial treatment is usually dietary. Regular exercise, stress reduction, and if necessary, weight loss are also recommended. If after six months of nondrug therapy you haven't achieved the desired total cholesterol/LDL-C levels, medication therapy is then considered.

If your LDL-C is above 160 with two or more risk factors, or above 190 with no risk factors, or your total cholesterol is above 240, your risk is high. Treatment is often initiated with both diet and medication.

If you have already developed coronary or other atherosclerosis-related disease, the need for total cholesterol and LDL-C control is even more compelling. Treatment of this group is called secondary prevention, and the allowable levels of LDL-C are more stringent. If you are in this group, your target LDL-C is 100 or less. If the LDL-C is 101–130, dietary measures may be tried, but for an LDL-C above 130, drug therapy is usually mandatory.

DIETARY TREATMENT—SOMETIMES SURPRISINGLY EFFECTIVE

Because medication therapy is expensive, lifelong, and not entirely risk-free, you should make every effort to reduce your LDL-C level by nondrug methods. Dietary treatment consists of maintaining an appropriate intake of calories each day, with particular emphasis on limiting your intake of cholesterol, total fat, and most of all, saturated fat. Also highly recommended are regular aerobic exercise, stress reduction and, if necessary, weight loss.

For some people these measures may require a shift in lifestyle, but many people have already switched to low-fat foods and exercise regularly. Taking these steps a little further may make a big difference.

For example, one 40-year-old had a total blood cholesterol of 250. Already exercising regularly, he substantially reduced his cholesterol and fat intake, cutting back on cheese, one of his favorite foods, and no longer eating eggs. His total cholesterol dropped to about 215, a significant reduction but still too high. He scaled back even further, adopting the austere Pritikin diet, but his total cholesterol refused to go below 200.

At this point he told me that his mother's cholesterol was 250 and his maternal aunt's was over 300, and their father (his grandfather) also ran a high cholesterol and had died of heart disease. He therefore assumed his high cholesterol was at least in part genetic and therefore wasn't likely to drop further, but he still refused to take medication.

The following year, for other reasons he adopted a vegetarian diet. He ate far more vegetables than ever, but also ate nut butters and sesame seed dressings containing high amounts of good fats. When he next checked his blood cholesterol, it was 150. He didn't believe it and checked it again. The result was the same and remained so until he became weary of the diet a few years later. At that time he started eating fish, turkey, and chicken, as well as eggs once or twice a week, but still avoided red meat and cheese. His cholesterol rose, but only to 180, where it has stayed for several years. His total cholesterol and LDL-C levels remain in the preferred range—without his ever taking cholesterol-lowering medication.

The lesson we both learned was that genetics may have indeed played a role in his elevated cholesterol while he was on some diets including several routinely recommended for lowering cholesterol, but that when he was on a vegetarian diet and subsequently added low-fat meats and eggs, but still severely restricting saturated fat, his genetic predisposition had little impact.

HOW STATIN MEDICATIONS LOWER CHOLESTEROL LEVELS

The statins are so effective in reducing high total cholesterol/LDL-C levels that a 1996 editorial in the *American Journal of Cardiology* is headed: "The underused miracle drugs: the statin drugs are to atherosclerosis what penicillin was to infectious disease." Perhaps not every physician is this sanguine, but in the decade since Mevacor's arrival the statins have proven to be very effective medications, far superior to other cholesterol-lowering agents.

Mevacor, Lescol, Pravachol, and Zocor work by inhibiting cholesterol synthesis. They accomplish this by interfering with an enzyme involved in the formation of the cholesterol molecule. However, this mechanism of action may interfere with coenzyme A, a substance essential to normal cellular activity. This interference makes some authorities uncomfortable.

"Coenzyme A is a potent antioxidant which neutralizes free radicals and other cancer-promoting factors," says researcher Stan Mills. "Will interfering with Coenzyme A affect the body's ability to prevent cancer? Over a few days or weeks, probably not. But over many months and years, who knows?"

The medical literature contains few voices echoing Dr. Mills's concern, but the respected *Medical Letter on Drugs and Therapeutics* notes: "Cholesterol is a component of all human cell membranes; the long-term consequences of interfering with its synthesis and the synthesis of related compounds are unknown." The letter further mentions that trials of up to six years have not detected an increase in the incidence of cancer. Nevertheless, the impact of ten, twenty, thirty years, or a lifetime of treatment remains unknown. Indeed, the people who have been taking statins the longest are serving as our experimental group for long-term side effects of these drugs.

SIDE EFFECTS WITH STATIN MEDICATIONS

Clearly, the statins are better tolerated than any other group of cholesterol-lowering drugs. Most physicians I've asked say that their patients encounter few problems with statin drugs. The PDR-listed side effects include muscle pain or headaches as occurring in 3% to 10%; nausea, indigestion, abdominal pain, heartburn, constipation, diarrhea, flatulence, skin rash, anxiety or insomnia in less than 5%.

Other physicians disagree. "Far more than half of those I see on these medications complain of side effects," states one doctor. Another states, "Many people—far more than 10%—get muscle aches from these drugs." A local pharmacist who closely monitors his clients concurs: "Most of them get side effects, usually muscle discomfort or gastrointestinal problems that don't seem to diminish with time. Eventually, many of them discontinue their medication." Indeed, in one study, about 50% of people taking cholesterol-lowering drugs quit therapy after one year and only 25% were still receiving therapy after two years.

There also is no debate that all statin medications have occasionally been associated with serious side effects. Serious, infrequent side effects include liver irritation or injury; thus, manufacturers recommend blood tests at regular intervals. Statins have also been associated with a severe type of acute muscle degeneration (rhabdomyolysis) that, in rare instances, has led to kidney failure and death. Although muscle degeneration of this severity is unusual, many people get muscle soreness or pain, and blood tests may show mild muscle breakdown. These symptoms are usually transient, but even mild muscle pain, especially when accompanied by fever or fatigue, should receive prompt medical evaluation. A lupus-like syndrome (reversible upon discontinuation) has also been related to statin drugs. This is one reason why virtually all authorities agree that up to six months of dietary therapy without medication should be tried first for all but the most severe types of cholesterol problems. Even when diet alone is insufficient in reducing an elevated total cholesterol or LDL-C, it should be remembered that drug therapy is meant to augment, not replace, continued dietary and other efforts.

Most statin side effects are directly related to dosage—the lower the dose you require, the less the likelihood or severity of side effects.

Statin medications are usually taken once daily with the evening meal or at bedtime. Statins are more effective when taken later in the day, possibly because the body produces cholesterol mainly at night. However, taking a high dose at one time produces higher peak blood levels of medication than half doses taken eight to twelve hours apart. Side effects often are a function of peak blood levels of a drug, so if you find that a single nighttime dose of statin medication causes unpleasant side effects, shifting to a twice-a-day regimen may eliminate the problem without lowering your total daily dosage.

THE IMPORTANCE OF USING THE VERY LOWEST EFFECTIVE STATIN DOSAGE

Medication therapy for elevated total cholesterol or LDL-C is a lifelong affair. If you stop your medication, your total cholesterol and LDL-C gradually return to their original levels.

The standard approach with statin drugs is to start patients at the manufacturer's recommended initial dose. For Mevacor, Pravachol, and Lescol, the usual starting dose is 20 mg a day; for Zocor, it's usually 10 mg a day. Your blood lipid levels (total cholesterol, HDL-C, LDL-C, and VLDL-C) are checked in four to six weeks. If your total cholesterol or LDL-C level is still too high, the dosage is increased in a stepwise manner. The steps are relatively large: for Mevacor, Lescol, and Pravachol, it's usually from 20 to 40, and if necessary, to 60 and then 80 mg a day; for Zocor, from 10 to 20, and if necessary, to 40 mg a day. In essence, jumps of 100%, 50%, and 33%, respectively. No medical reference I've seen has suggested, for example, increasing from 20 to 30 mg a day of Mevacor, Lescol, or Pravachol, or from 10 to 15 mg a day of Zocor.

Neither has any reference I've seen recommended the converse—lowering the dosage of patients who respond well at the initial manufacturer's dose. If your total cholesterol or LDL-C has fallen to within target levels, few physicians will actually try to gradually reduce your dosage. This is because the manufacturer-recommended starting doses are generally assumed by physicians to be the lowest effective doses. Few physicians are aware of the numerous studies showing that low doses are more than satisfactory for many people.

Using the very lowest effective dosage of any statin medication is important for several reasons:

1. Most side effects with statin drugs are dose-related. Studies vary, but in one study 21% to 33% of patients encountered at least one side effect with a statin medication at the manufacturer-recommended initial dosage.
2. Serious, occasionally fatal side effects have occurred with these medications. Again, dosage may play a key role.
3. If you are prescribed statin medication (or any other type of cholesterol/LDL-C-lowering drug), you will be taking it for many years, perhaps life. Yet the effect of ten, twenty, thirty, or more years of continuous usage of these drugs is unknown.
4. Common sense and medical science agree that with any medication, whether the treatment is short-term or long-term, the very lowest effective dosage should be used.

Another reason for starting with low doses of Mevacor, Pravachol, Zocor, or Lescol is that the majority of side effects seem to occur at the beginning of treatment. Starting with a lower dose may allow your body to gradually adjust to treatment with less initial impact, thereby lowering the tendency toward adverse reactions. It also gives you and your physician a chance to see what can be accomplished with low-dose therapy.

Some physicians may consider this a waste of time, but in one study of people with mild to moderately elevated levels of LDL-C, 37% were able to reduce their levels below 160 with just 10 mg a day of Lescol, half the initial recommended dosage. Similar results have been seen with low-dose Mevacor, Pravachol, and Zocor, as you will read in the specific analysis of each of these drugs.

LOW-DOSE THERAPY COMBINING TWO CHOLESTEROL-LOWERING DRUGS

If medication side effects prevent you from taking a statin medication at sufficient dosage to lower your total cholesterol or LDL-C to your target levels, there are other alternatives. One of the most interesting combines a very low dose of a statin drug with a low dose of another type of cholesterol-lowering agent.

Cholestyramine is a resin that binds cholesterol in the intestine and thereby prevents its absorption into the body. In one study cholestyramine was used at a dose of 8 mg a day—the standard dose of this drug is 12 to 24 mg a day. The cholestyramine was given in concert with 10 mg a day of Lescol, half the manufacturer-recommended initial dosage. This combination was very well tolerated and more effective than 20 mg of Lescol alone. The combination treatment reduced LDL-C levels an average of 25% to 30%. At the end of the study, 63% of those taking the drug combination achieved the desired LDL-C level, as compared with 43% of those taking 20 mg of Lescol. The authors commented: "We have shown that the addition of [cholestyramine] resin to low-dose (10 mg/day) statin therapy with fluvastatin [Lescol] was more effective in lowering cholesterol than doubling the statin dosage."

COST FACTORS

Although cost should never be the primary factor in determining medication selection and dosage, the reality is that statin medications are very expensive, and many people, including Medicare beneficiaries, are not covered for prescription costs. Thus, affordability is important, and lower doses can produce substantial savings. In some cases, these savings may mean the difference between continuing and discontinuing treatment.

Using lower doses reduces costs, especially if you use a pill cutter to split larger pills (such as splitting a 20-mg tablet of Mevacor to obtain two 10-mg doses). Mevacor, Pravachol, and Zocor are produced as tablets. Lescol is made in 20-mg and 40-mg capsules; your pharmacist may be willing to make 10-mg capsules for you.

Prices vary considerably between these drugs, with Lescol being about 30% to 40% less expensive than the others. The reason for this is that Lescol, the last statin to reach the market, is competing with already well-established competitors.

RECOMMENDATIONS

First, let's be clear: high levels of total cholesterol or LDL-C are dangerous. These factors are clearly associated with higher risks of coronary artery disease, cardiac death, and other types of arteriosclerotic disease such as strokes. If you have an elevated total cholesterol or LDL-C, you should immediately adopt the necessary dietary measures, exercise regularly, and maybe lose some weight, as outlined by your physician. If after six months your efforts don't lower your blood lipids to your target levels, don't hesitate to take medication. The quote comparing statin drugs to penicillin may be an exaggeration, but not by much. Yet only one in four people who require treatment for high cholesterol or LDL-C actually are receiving it.

As certain as it is that high cholesterol or LDL-C levels are dangerous, it's equally clear that lowering these factors saves lives. Since 1993, studies have repeatedly shown that reducing elevated total cholesterol or LDL-C levels reduces the incidence of coronary disease, heart attacks, and cardiac death. According to a 1995 study, ''For every 10 percentage points of cholesterol lowering, CHD [coronary heart disease] mortality was reduced by 13%.''

There's another reason not to hesitate to take statin medication if you need it. For example, the full effect of 10 mg a day of Mevacor on total cholesterol and LDL-C levels is apparent after four to six weeks, but the effect of the medication on blockages of the coronary or other arteries doesn't reach full effect for six to twenty-four months. That's why treating healthy people with elevated cholesterol or LDL-C levels is called primary prevention: the goal is to inhibit the atherosclerosis that precedes angina, heart attacks, and strokes. Between diet and, when necessary, medication, prevention of this type is possible for the first time in history.

When starting a statin medication, decisions about dosage should be made carefully. If you have a history of encountering medication side effects, or if you are small or elderly or just want to be sure to determine the very lowest effective dosage, discuss with your physician the possibility of starting with a dose that is below the manufacturer's recommendation. Although most patients may ultimately require standard doses, a surprising percentage do fine with lower doses.

Even if you eventually need a standard dosage, starting low may allow your system to accommodate to the drug without encountering the side effects that sometimes make these medications difficult to tolerate. And increasing gradually via intermediary doses may allow you to take, for example, 15 rather than 20 mg a day of Zocor—25% less of a medication whose long-term side effects remain unknown.

Some lower doses are easily obtained. Mevacor and Pravachol come in 10-mg tablets, and 5 mg of Zocor can be purchased. Other low doses require using a pill cutter: 5 mg of Mevacor and Pravachol, and 2.5 mg of Zocor. An intermediary dosage such as 15 mg a day of Zocor can be attained with either three 5-mg tablets, one 10-mg and one 5-mg tablet, or one and a half 10-mg tablets. The last method is the least costly. For some people, using a pill cutter to achieve some lower doses is worth the effort and cost savings. For others, it's more convenient to take standard amounts even if it means a higher dose.

Because reducing high total cholesterol/LDL-C with statins or other cholesterol-lowering drugs is lifelong, expensive process, little is lost by taking four to six weeks to determine the very lowest statin dosage that is effective for you. At the same time, if you ultimately require a higher dose of these drugs, don't hesitate to take it. The dose must fit the individual, and low, moderate, and high dosages all have their place according to individual tolerance and need.

Most physicians are unfamiliar with the data about the effectiveness of low-dose Mevacor, Lescol, Pravachol, and Zocor. Most drug references contain little or no information about the use of lower doses in healthy individuals. Hopefully, your physician will be open to trying an initial low-dose approach, but many will be skeptical. Don't hesitate to exercise the knowledge you have gained on this subject. If that's not enough, you can support your viewpoint by showing him the studies cited in this chapter and in the reference section at the end of the book. Quality studies in leading journals are usually quite persuasive for all but the most stubborn of doctors.

In-Depth Analysis: Mevacor (Lovastatin)

From 1987 through 1995, Mevacor was America's favorite medication for lowering total cholesterol and LDL-C (low density lipoprotein-cholesterol). In 1996 it ranked No. 32, behind its rival Zocor at No. 21, on the list of the top 200 prescribed outpatient medications.

Mevacor's continued popularity is attributable to three factors: (1) Mevacor was the first and for many years the only statin medication available; (2) Mevacor's development was a breakthrough in the treatment of elevated total cholesterol and LDL-C levels; (3) Mevacor, like other statin drugs, not only reduces blood levels of total cholesterol and LDL-C, but also has been shown to slow the development of atherosclerosis and to reduce the incidence of coronary artery disease and cardiac death. In some cases Mevacor has produced actual reduction in the degree of blockage of coronary arteries.

According to the manufacturer, the usual recommended initial dose of Mevacor is 20 mg a day with the evening meal. Up to 1995, this was the recommended starting dosage for *everyone* except people taking immunosuppressive drugs (such as transplant patients); for them, 10 mg was suggested.

In the 1996 and 1997 PDRs, Mevacor's dosage recommendations included a new statement about using a lower dose of 10 mg a day for people requiring reductions in LDL-C of less than 20%. For those needing LDL-C reductions of 20% or more, 20 mg a day remains the recommended initial dose. However, this recommendation appears to ignore Table 1 of Mevacor's PDR description, showing that the average LDL-C reduction among study patients taking 10 mg a day of Mevacor was 21%. Obviously, many subjects must have achieved LDL-C reductions substantially higher than 20% for the *average* reduction to have been 21%.

Mevacor's package insert and PDR write-up provide no specific dosage guidelines for elderly individuals. Seemingly, 20 mg a day is the recommended initial dosage, the same as for younger adults.

IMPRESSIVE FINDINGS WITH A LOWER DOSE OF MEVACOR

After Mevacor's release, several studies were published using 10 mg a day of Mevacor, half the manufacturer-recommended starting dose. In each study the 10-mg dosage performed impressively. A 1994 study published in the *Journal of the American Medical Association* (JAMA) demonstrated the effectiveness of 10 mg a day in postmenopausal women. A 1990 study showed its effectiveness in cardiac transplant patients.

The most impressive low-dose Mevacor study was published in 1991 by A. Rubenstein and others. A 10-mg dose of Mevacor was given to 28 subjects with moderately elevated cholesterol levels of 200 to 240. (Most people with elevated cholesterol are in the moderately elevated group.) In this study all 28 subjects had previously failed to reduce their cholesterol levels by dietary and other measures. After 20 weeks of Mevacor 10 mg a day, the average decrease in total cholesterol was 19% and in LDL-C 24%. In 24 of 28 subjects, cholesterol levels dropped below 200, the targeted response. Similar results were obtained in reducing LDL-C levels below the target level of 130.

These are not only excellent results in terms of achieving lower cholesterol and LDL-C levels, but, as the authors added: "Achievement of desirable values of cholesterol with 10 mg of lovastatin [Mevacor] was accompanied by less adverse effects and with significant financial saving. The calculated saving for lovastatin consumers in the USA could be an amount of $60,000,000."

These results suggest that 10 mg/day of Mevacor may be a preferable starting dose for many people with moderately elevated cholesterol or LDL-C levels uncontrolled by dietary means.

EVEN LOWER MEVACOR DOSES FOR HIGHLY MEDICATION-SENSITIVE INDIVIDUALS?

A publisher who reviewed this book takes Mevacor. Because he's had his share of medication-related adverse reactions, he's become extremely cautious about taking medications. Unfortunately, he also has an elevated cholesterol that dietary efforts failed to control.

His doctor prescribed Mevacor. The dose? The standard 20 mg a day, despite this man's impressive history of medication sensitivities. Accustomed to making his own decisions, the publisher broke the tablets into quarters. Taking only 5 mg a day, he lowered his cholesterol from 220 to 185 mg, a 16% reduction that satisfied both him and his physician. He accomplished this with 25% of the manufacturer-recommended initial dose and without encountering any side effects. Thus he has been able to stay on the medication and continue to obtain its benefits.

If average subjects achieved good results with 10 mg of Mevacor in the studies discussed above, it's not altogether surprising that a highly sensitive person might require even less. The subjects in the Rubenstein study were, other than having elevated cholesterol levels, healthy. If the study had included people with other illnesses or taking other medications, some of them may have proven responsive to an even lower dose of Mevacor. Indeed, the study subjects did so well with 10 mg a day of Mevacor that 5 mg a day, if it had been tried, might have been enough for some. Similarly, small people, those known to respond to lower than recommended doses of other medications, or those who like the publisher have a long history of adverse drug reactions may also demonstrate an increased sensitivity to low-dose Mevacor.

Neither the medical literature nor the manufacturer offer any studies involving Mevacor at 5 mg or other doses below 10 mg. This dosage certainly wouldn't be enough for the majority of patients, but if you are highly sensitive to medications or have developed side effects at higher Mevacor doses, a very low dose such as 5 mg might be enough for you.

MEVACOR AND THE ELDERLY

The manufacturer-recommended initial dose of 20 mg a day of Mevacor apparently applies to older adults. To date, little data exists on the effectiveness of low-dose Mevacor and elderly individuals. As mentioned above, a 1994 study with postmenopausal women showed 10 mg of Mevacor to be significantly effective. Not all of these women were elderly, but since dosage requirements often decrease with age, this finding suggests that if you are elderly, especially if you have only moderately elevated cholesterol or LDL-C, you may obtain a satisfactory response with fewer risks at 10 mg a day or less.

WHY LOW-DOSE MEVACOR IS UNDERUTILIZED

When Mevacor was first released, the smallest pill was 20 mg. In the Rubenstein study discussed above, one of the author's recommendations was that the manufacturer produce a 10-mg Mevacor pill. A year later, in 1992, a 10-mg Mevacor tablet was introduced. Unfortunately, according to several pharmacists I've contacted, only a small percentage of Mevacor prescriptions are written for this low dose.

"I ordered some bottles of 10-mg Mevacor once," one pharmacist told me, "but we had to return them because no one prescribed it. I get about thirty prescriptions a week for Mevacor. They're all 20 or 40 mg. I can't remember receiving one for 10 mg."

Some pharmacies I contacted did carry the 10-mg dose, but prescriptions for it were relatively few. One reason may be that it wasn't studied before Mevacor's release. In essence, prior to Mevacor's approval by the FDA and release for general usage, the lowest effective dose was never specifically defined. Twenty mg of Mevacor is the dosage with which most physicians started using Mevacor, so it remains their predominant choice.

APPLYING GRADUAL, LOW-DOSE METHODS FOR INDIVIDUALS NEEDING HIGHER MEVACOR DOSES

The highly respected *American Hospital Formulary Service* drug reference states: "The dosage of lovastatin [Mevacor] must be carefully adjusted according to individual requirements and response." However, because of their unfamiliarity with the 10-mg pill, physicians often miss the opportunity of using it in titrating Mevacor doses upward. For example, if you don't adequately respond to 20 mg of Mevacor, your physician will likely increase the dosage to 40 mg. That's a 100% jump. If that proves insufficient, the next dose is usually 60 mg—another 50% jump. It's done this way because almost all of the data doctors receive about Mevacor compares doses of 20, 40, 60, and 80 mg, without any mention of employing the 10-mg pill to adjust doses with intermediary steps such as 30, 50, and 70 mg. And Mevacor tablets are produced in 10-, 20-, and 40-mg sizes.

Dosage increases of smaller magnitude, from 20 to 30, or from 40 to 50 mg a day, etc., are less likely to provoke side effects. Also, they give you a chance to see if a relatively lower dose—30 mg instead of 40 mg, for example—is sufficient to meet your targeted total cholesterol or LDL-C levels. Because statin therapy is a lifelong process, using the very lowest effective dosage may be important in reducing the risks of as yet unknown long-term side effects, as well as in reducing costs.

RECOMMENDATIONS

There are many reasons to consider an initial trial of low-dose Mevacor for moderately elevated cholesterol or LDL-C. Studies using 10 mg a day of Mevacor have demonstrated significant effectiveness with this lower dose. This strongly suggests that for many people with moderately elevated lipids, 10 mg a day of Mevacor may be sufficient. Certainly if you have a history of drug reactions, or if you are small or elderly, are taking other medications, or simply want to be sure that you are taking only as much medication as your body needs, an initial trial with 10 mg should be considered. In selected cases, 5 mg a day may be tried. And if you try 10 mg a day of Mevacor and it isn't quite enough, there's no reason that you must jump 100% to 20 mg a day—15 mg a day may be just right.

Treatment with Mevacor is a long-term, usually lifelong process. Most of Mevacor's side effects are dose-related, and the long-term effects of decades of treatment remain unknown. It's worth taking an extra four to six weeks for you and your physician to ascertain the very lowest effective dose.

Of course, not everyone will respond adequately to Mevacor at lower doses. You may require 20 mg or more to reach the preferred levels of total cholesterol and LDL-C. If so, increasing by 10 mg at a time rather than the standard 20–40–60 mg approach may prove beneficial and cost-effective.

In-Depth Analysis: Pravachol (Pravastatin)

Pravchol is an effective cholesterol and LDL-C lowering drug, ranking No. 41 among the top-selling outpatient prescription drugs of 1996. Pravachol has been one of the most studied statins regarding its long-term effects on cardiovascular disease and cardiac mortality. The results have been impressive. Multiple studies involving thousands of patients for up to five years have demonstrated that Pravachol reduces the incidence of heart attacks, cardiovascular death, and strokes, as well as lessening the percentage of study subjects needing angioplasty and cardiac bypass surgery.

If you have moderately elevated cholesterol or LDL-C, dietary control and other nonmedicinal measures are the first steps of treatment. If after six months of these measures you have not been able to lower your total cholesterol/LDL-C to target levels, medication therapy should be considered. If you have highly elevated total cholesterol/LDL-C levels, initial treatment may include both dietary and drug therapies.

The manufacturer-recommended initial dose of Pravachol is 10 or 20 mg taken at bedtime. Maximum recommended dosage is 40 mg a day; 20 mg a day for the elderly. Ten mg a day is suggested for people with significant renal or liver dysfunction.

In actual practice, most patients are started at 20 mg a day of Pravachol.

LOW-DOSE PRAVACHOL

A 6-fold range of interindividual variation in the peak blood levels of Pravachol was detected among healthy individuals taking identical doses of Pravachol. That's a 600% variation in response from one person to the next. Among nonhealthy individuals, the range was up to 47-fold—that's 4,700%. In other words, the range of response to Pravachol may be highly variable from person to person. This suggests a wide range of effective doses—and that many people may respond to low doses of Pravachol. Several studies concur.

In a study published in *Cardiology* in 1994, 33% of subjects achieved LDL-C levels of 130 or less with 10 mg a day of Pravachol. In another 1994 study of over 1,000 patients with highly elevated cholesterol or LDL-C levels, 10 mg a day of Pravachol resulted in *average* reductions in total cholesterol and LDL-C of 24.5% and 33%, respectively. Statin medications generally have greater effects in people with higher levels of cholesterol or LDL-C; nonetheless, these findings were significant and impressive.

A 1991 study published in *Clinical Cardiology* compared doses of 5, 10, 20, and 40 mg a day of Pravachol. All doses significantly reduced total cholesterol and LDL-C levels. More surprising, "the 5 mg dose at bedtime produced an average reduction of 19.2% in LDL-C and 14.3% in total cholesterol." These numbers are impressive—and even more so when we remember that many study subjects attained reductions even larger than these averages. As expected, the higher doses of Pravachol produced greater reductions overall, but the results achieved with 5 and 10 mg a day may be all some people need to reach their target levels of total cholesterol and LDL-C.

APPLYING GRADUAL, LOW-DOSE METHODS FOR PEOPLE NEEDING STANDARD PRAVACHOL DOSAGES

The demonstrated effectiveness of 5 and 10 mg a day of Pravachol may also be useful if you require higher Pravachol doses for effective total cholesterol/LDL-C control. The usual approach is to start with 20 mg a day of Pravachol, and if that isn't adequate, to increase the dosage to 40 mg a day, a 100% increase. Even when patients are started at 10 mg, if this fails, dosages of 20 mg a day (a 100% increase), then 30 mg a day (50% increase) follow.

Biologically speaking, these are not small increases. Whether you start at 5 or 10 mg a day, if these aren't enough, why not try 15 mg before jumping to 20 mg a day? If you are prescribed 20 mg a day and that isn't enough, why not increase it gradually to 25 or 30 mg instead of leaping to 40 mg a day?

In the long run, if researchers discover that the use of Pravachol for ten or twenty or thirty years does have harmful side effects or drug interactions we haven't yet identified, using the very lowest effective dosage, even if it's 30 instead of 40 mg a day, may provide you with a better margin of safety.

PRAVACHOL AND THE ELDERLY

For elderly individuals, the Pravachol package insert and PDR description provide no specific dosage recommendations and very little information about the dynamics of this drug in older bodies. As mentioned above, however, the manufacturer does tell us that 6- to 47-fold ranges in variation of peak blood levels of Pravachol were detected in healthy and nonhealthy individuals, respectively. Because of declining kidney and liver function, the elderly generally metabolize medications more slowly than younger adults, and therefore are more likely to develop higher blood levels of Pravachol than younger individuals.

For these reasons, low-dose initial treatment with Pravachol should always be considered with elderly persons, especially those who are small or frail, have other medical illnesses, take other medications, or have histories of adverse reactions to other drugs. Treatment can be started with as little as 5 mg a day.

For the elderly who are healthy and robust, low-dose therapy may still be tried, especially if you have moderately elevated cholesterol or LDL-C. The initial dose can be 5 or 10 mg a day.

RECOMMENDATIONS

The *American Hospital Formulary Service* drug reference states: "The dosage of pravastatin [Pravachol] must be carefully adjusted according to individual requirements and response." Based on the results of studies and the very wide range of inter-individual variation in blood levels obtained with identical doses of Pravachol, 10 mg a day of Pravachol may be sufficient for many individuals. If you are small, frail, or elderly, have other illnesses, take other drugs, or are sometimes sensitive to medications, 5 mg a day may be enough. Ask your physician.

If you have moderately elevated total cholesterol/LDL-C and you want to be sure that you are taking the very lowest amount of Pravachol to reach your target total cholesterol/LDL-C, starting with 5 to 10 mg a day for six weeks makes sense. If these doses are insufficient, you can increase gradually by 5-mg gradations before going to the standard 20 mg a day dosage. For many people, 5–10–15 mg a day of Pravachol may be enough; for others, higher doses will be necessary. The only way to tell is to start low and increase gradually.

If you start at 20 mg a day and it isn't sufficient, you can increase by 5 or 10 mg at a time rather than jumping to 40 mg. On the other hand, if your physician started you with 20 mg of Pravachol and you responded extremely well, why not try reducing to 15 or even 10 mg a day?

If you are currently taking Pravachol and achieving target levels of total cholesterol and LDL-C, but are also experiencing side effects, reducing by as little as 5 mg a day may make a difference without raising your total cholesterol/LDL-C levels beyond the target range. Most Pravachol side effects are dose-related, so reducing your dosage by a small amount may make a difference. Also, the long-term effects of decades of treatment, which you are likely to require, are unknown. Using the very lowest effective dose exposes you to less risk.

Using lower doses of Pravachol may also substantially reduce costs. Using a pill cutter to split the 20-mg tablet for a dosage of 10 mg/day saves about $350 annually. Taking 30 instead of 40 mg a day provides similar savings. Pravachol is produced in 10-, 20-, and 40-mg unscored tablets.

In-Depth Analysis: Zocor
(Simvistatin)

In 1996, Zocor surpassed Mevacor as America's most prescribed total cholesterol and LDL-C-lowering medication, ranking No. 21 among the 200 top-selling outpatient prescription drugs. Along with Pravachol, Zocor has been one of the two most studied cholesterol-lowering drugs in regard to long-term impact on cardiovascular disease and cardiac death. Multiple studies have confirmed that Zocor reduces the incidence of heart attacks, cardiovascular death, and strokes, as well as lessening the likelihood of needing an angioplasty or cardiac bypass surgery.

If you have moderately elevated cholesterol or LDL-C, dietary control and other nondrug measures are the first steps of treatment. If after six months you have not been able to lower your total cholesterol/LDL-C to target levels, medication therapy should be considered. If you have highly elevated total cholesterol/LDL-C, initial treatment may include both dietary and drug therapies.

The manufacturer-recommended initial dose of Zocor is 5 to 10 mg in the evening. 10 mg a day of Zocor is recommended for people requiring reductions of 20% or more in their LDL-C levels. Five mg/day of Zocor is recommended for people needing smaller reductions (less than 20%) in total cholesterol/LDL-C and for the elderly. The recommended dosage range is 5 to 40 mg a day.

In actual practice, most patients are started at 10 mg a day of Zocor.

LOW-DOSE ZOCOR

Interestingly, although the 1997 PDR recommends Zocor 10 mg a day for those requiring LDL-C reductions of 20% or greater, just three pages before this recommendation is a table from a study comparing doses of 5, 10, 20, and 40 mg a day of Zocor. The subjects taking 5 mg a day *averaged* LDL-C reductions of 24%, so obviously many subjects achieved LDL-C reductions of 20% or greater with this low dosage. These same subjects reduced their total cholesterol by an average of 17% and raised their HDL-C by 7% with the 5-mg dose.

Supporting these findings are many other studies, including a 1989 study in *Clinical Therapeutics* in which subjects given 5 mg a day of Zocor attained average LDL-C reductions of 25%. Even more impressive, the medical literature offers several studies demonstrating the effectiveness of a mere 2.5 mg a day of Zocor, a fourth of the usual initial dose prescribed by physicians. In several studies, 2.5 mg a day of Zocor produced average reductions in LDL-C of 16.5% to 26.5%—individually, some subjects attained smaller and others achieved even greater reductions. In one study, 11% of subjects taking 2.5 mg a day of Zocor achieved LDL-C reductions of at least 40% and the overall mean reduction among these subjects was 19% to 23%. In the same study, 7% of subjects taking 5 mg a day of Zocor achieved LDL-C reductions of 40%, and the mean reduction with this dosage was 22% to 33%.

These data strongly suggest that many people will obtain satisfactory reductions in total cholesterol and LDL-C with Zocor doses as low as 5 and even 2.5 mg a day. For people for whom 5 mg isn't quite enough, 7.5 mg a day, a dosage that appears never to have been studied, may be sufficient.

APPLYING GRADUAL, LOW-DOSE METHODS FOR PEOPLE REQUIRING STANDARD ZOCOR DOSAGES

The proven effectiveness of 2.5 and 5 mg of Zocor may also be useful in adjusting doses if you require standard amounts, 10 to 40 mg a day, of Zocor. The typical method of initiating and increasing Zocor is 10–20–40 mg. Each increase represents a 100% rise in dosage—hardly gradual dosing. Zocor, like all statins, is a potent medication, and most side effects are dose-related.

If the usual starting dose of 10 mg a day doesn't lower your total cholesterol or LDL-C to target levels, ask your physician about increasing gradually by gradations of 2.5 or 5 mg, rather than jumping to 20 mg a day. Similarly, if you require more than 20 mg a day, doses of 25, 30, or 35 mg may work for you instead of immediately going to the maximum Zocor dosage of 40 mg.

In the long run, if it's found that using statin medications for ten or twenty or thirty years does cause harmful side effects or drug interactions we haven't yet identified, using the very lowest effective dose for you, even if it's 30 instead of 40 mg a day, may provide you with an extra margin of safety.

ZOCOR AND THE ELDERLY

In general, elderly individuals metabolize statin medications more slowly than younger adults, which may result in higher and more prolonged drug effects—and side effects. In general, therefore, lower doses of Zocor should be effective for many (but not necessarily all) elderly persons.

In a 1990 study, elderly subjects (average age 69) receiving 2.5 mg of Zocor demonstrated significant average reductions in total cholesterol of 16.7% and LDL-C of 22.5%, but in another study the results were less impressive.

Although the effectiveness of 2.5 mg of Zocor in the elderly population may not be unequivocally established, this low initial dose should be considered for elderly persons who are sensitive to medications, have other illnesses, are taking other medication, or have liver/kidney impairments. If this dose proves inadequate, increasing by as little as 2.5 mg at a time will ensure the use of the very lowest, safest effective dose.

If you are elderly and healthy and have little history of medication reactions, the starting dosage should be 2.5 mg a day or the manufacturer-recommended 5 mg a day.

RECOMMENDATIONS

The demonstrated effectiveness of 2.5 and 5 mg of Zocor suggests that these doses may be useful in selected individuals, especially in initiating treatment for moderately elevated cholesterol or LDL-C. Low-dose Zocor makes particular sense if you are small or elderly, have other medical problems, take other medications, or have had previous problems with side effects. Or if you just want to be sure that you are taking the very lowest dosage necessary.

Although the results with Zocor 2.5 mg are impressive, it should be noted that substantial variability was seen in individual responses. In a 1987 study 2.5 mg a day of Zocor lowered total cholesterol in different subjects by as little as 10% and as much as 23%, and reduced LDL-C by as little as 10% and as much as 26%. This means that some individuals may respond quite well with low-dose Zocor, while others will require higher doses. The key is that you are taking the very lowest effective Zocor dose that works for you, whether it's 2.5 or 10 or 15 or 40 mg a day.

Similarly, if you are already taking Zocor and experiencing side effects, you may find that by asking your physician to lower your dose by just 2.5 or 5 mg at a time, your side effects may diminish without decreasing the drug's effectiveness. Or if you have responded extremely well in lowering your total cholesterol or LDL-C with the standard 10- or 20-mg dosage of Zocor, you may want to try lowering your dose from 10 to 7.5 or 5 mg a day, or from 20 to 15 or 10 mg a day.

Because most of Zocor's side effects are dose-related and the long-term effects of decades of treatment remain unknown, using the very lowest effective dose exposes you to the least risk. A secondary benefit of using lower Zocor doses is that it reduces costs.

In-Depth Analysis: Lescol (Fluvastatin)

Lescol is the newest statin drug for lowering total cholesterol and LDL-C. Lescol is outsold by Zocor, Mevacor, and Pravachol, but because Lescol costs 30% to 40% less, it's closing on them. From 1995 to 1996, Lescol rose from No. 110 to No. 63 among the 200 top-selling outpatient prescription drugs in the United States.

Lescol is the first synthetically produced statin and is chemically distinct from the other three statins. For this reason, if you experience side effects with Mevacor, Pravachol, or Zocor, switching to Lescol may be a good choice. However, Lescol also can cause typical statin side effects such as gastrointestinal problems and muscle pain.

Because Lescol is the newest statin, studies clearly documenting its impact on the prevention of coronary disease and cardiac death have yet to be completed. However, two preliminary studies suggest that Lescol, like other statins, reduces the development of atherosclerosis and the incidence of coronary heart disease, heart attacks, cardiac death, and other vascular diseases such as strokes. Already established is Lescol's ability to lower total cholesterol, LDL-C, and triglyceride levels, and to increase HDL-C levels— the same effects achieved with Mevacor, Pravachol, and Zocor.

If you have moderately elevated cholesterol or LDL-C, dietary control and other nondrug measures are the first steps of treatment. If after six months you have not been able to lower your total cholesterol/LDL-C to your target levels, medication therapy should be considered. If you have highly elevated total cholesterol/LDL-C, initial treatment may include both dietary and drug therapies.

The manufacturer-recommended starting dose of Lescol is 20 or 40 mg with dinner or at bedtime. Dosage range is 20 to 80 mg a day; the 80-mg dosage is taken as 40 mg twice a day. The manufacturer provides no specific dosage guidelines for elderly individuals.

The usual starting dose of Lescol in actual practice is 20 mg a day. However, this dosage sometimes is less effective than comparative initial doses of Mevacor (20 mg), Pravachol (20 mg), and Zocor (10 mg) in reducing total cholesterol or LDL-C. For this reason, sometimes patients are started at 40 mg a day of Lescol.

LOW-DOSE LESCOL

The 1996 *American Hospital Formulary Service* drug reference states that "the dosage of fluvastatin [Lescol] . . . must be carefully adjusted according to individual requirements and response." Good advice—but not easily accomplished with Lescol, because it is made in only 20- and 40-mg capsules. To obtain a lower dose such as 10 mg, you will have to ask your pharmacist to make them for you. [Medical authorities discourage people from making their own, individualized doses of medications using empty gelatin capsules because of the possibility of dosing errors or of getting the powder in their eyes.]

A low dose such as 10 mg a day of Lescol may be useful if you are small, have other illnesses, are taking other medications, or simply want to be sure that you are taking the very lowest dose necessary to achieve your target cholesterol or LDL-C. For example, in one study 37% of subjects taking 10 mg a day of Lescol achieved their target LDL-C level of 160.

In another, 21% of subjects taking only *2.5 mg a day* of Lescol achieved LDL-C reductions of 15% or greater—a decrease that may be sufficient for some people. Thus, as with other statin drugs, the range of interindividual variation with Lescol can be broad. The only way to know what the very lowest effective dose of Lescol may be for you is to start low and see. If you have moderately elevated cholesterol or LDL-C, starting with 5 or 10 mg, then increasing gradually, if necessary, will allow you to find your specific dosage as well as to initiate treatment with a less side effect prone amount.

People with other illnesses and perhaps some who are taking other medications may also respond well and encounter fewer adverse effects with lower doses of Lescol. For example, people with reduced liver function showed a 2.5-fold (250%) increase in the bioavailability (active medication remaining in the system) of Lescol, meaning that they required much lower doses.

APPLYING GRADUAL, LOW-DOSE METHODS FOR PEOPLE NEEDING STANDARD LESCOL DOSAGES

Individual response to Lescol is highly variable. That's why some patients are rapidly increased from 20 to 40 mg, and if this isn't enough, to 60 and even 80 mg a day—increases of 100%, 50%, and 33%, respectively. Biologically speaking, these are not small increases.

Because Lescol is produced only in 20- and 40-mg capsules, it's hard to obtain smaller pills to provide more gradual increases.

To accomplish this, you can ask your pharmacist to fashion 10-mg capsules for you. This can be easily done. Some pharmacists charge for this service; others don't. With 10-mg pills, you can increase your Lescol dosage, if necessary, in more gradual steps including 30, 50, and 70 mg a day.

In the long run, if researchers discover that usage of statin medications for ten or twenty or thirty years does have harmful side effects, using the very lowest effective dosage, even if it's 30 instead of 40 mg or 50 instead of 60 mg, may provide you with a better margin of safety.

LESCOL AND THE ELDERLY

The Lescol package insert and PDR description provide no specific dosage recommendations for elderly individuals. We are left to assume that the starting dose is 20 mg a day, because that's the smallest pill available.

Elsewhere in the manufacturer's information on Lescol it states that blood levels of Lescol did not vary with age or gender. However, it also states: "Elderly patients (greater than 65 years of age) demonstrated a greater treatment response in respect to LDL-C, total cholesterol, and LDL/HDL ratio than patients less than 65 years of age." In other words, elderly patients respond more strongly to Lescol.

Why is this? Perhaps because liver function is usually diminished in the elderly, so a dosage of Lescol may last longer and work more effectively. Whatever the cause, the result is that the elderly may require less Lescol than younger adults. This may be especially true for elderly individuals who are small or frail, have other illnesses, take other medications, or tend to develop side effects to drugs.

RECOMMENDATIONS

Lescol is the newest statin medication. It is the first synthetic statin and is chemically distinct from Mevacor, Pravachol, and Zocor. Because of its newness, studies regarding the impact of Lescol on coronary artery disease, cardiac death, and strokes are not complete, but preliminary results suggest that Lescol will provide results similar to those of other statin medications.

The main reason that Lescol has rapidly challenged the other statins in sales is that it costs 30% to 40% less. On the other hand, Lescol is the only statin that is produced as capsules and in only two doses, 20 and 40 mg, greatly limiting dose flexibility.

Studies suggest that some people may obtain sufficient benefit from 10 mg a day of Lescol, and in one study 21% of subjects taking 2.5 mg of Lescol obtained reductions in LDL-C of 15% or more, a reduction that may be sufficient for some with mildly elevated cholesterol or LDL-C. Some elderly individuals may also respond to lower doses of Lescol. To use a low dose such as 10 mg a day of Lescol, ask your pharmacist about preparing 10-mg pills.

Certainly if you are small, frail, or elderly, have other illnesses, take other drugs, or are sometimes sensitive to medications, starting with a low dose of Lescol may be worth trying for six weeks. Not everyone will respond adequately, but the only way to know is to try it.

On the other hand, if you are started at the usual dosage of 20 mg a day and it isn't sufficient, you may want to increase more gradually than the standard approach of 40–60–80 mg a day, as needed. Again, if you can obtain 10-mg pills, you can increase in 10-mg increments, producing intermediary doses of 30, 50, and 70 mg a day, per your individual need.

Also, if your physician started you with 20 mg a day of Lescol and you respond extremely well, you may want to consider reducing to 15 or 10 mg. Again, such doses can be made from the standard 20-mg pill. Ask your physician.

Determining the lowest effective dose of Lescol for you is important because most Lescol side effects are dose-related. In addition, the long-term effects of decades of treatment of Lescol, more than any other statin, remain unknown. Using the lowest effective dose exposes you to less risk.

TWELVE

Antihypertensive Medications

Thiazide Diuretics

Hydrochlorothiazide (HCTZ): Esidrix,
HydroDIURIL, and Oretic
Hygroton (chlorthalidone)
Dyazide (triamterene-HCTZ) and Aldactazide
(spironolactone-HCTZ)

Beta Blockers

Inderal LA (propranolol)
Lopressor (metoprolol)
Tenormin (atenolol)
Zebeta and Ziac (bisoprolol)

Ace Inhibitors

Capoten (captopril)
Vasotec (enalapril)

Calcium Channel Blockers

Calan SR, Isoptin SR, Verelan (verapamil)
Cardizem (diltiazem)
Procardia (nifedipine)
Norvasc (amlodipine)

Alpha Receptor Blockers

Cardura (doxazosin)
Hytrin (terazosin)

Central Adrenergic Agonists

Catapres (clonidine)

About Hypertension
(High Blood Pressure)

*The selected [antihypertensive] agent should be prescribed
initially in less than full doses.*

—*Conn's Current Therapy 1993*

THE IMPORTANCE OF TREATING
HYPERTENSION

Most people are aware that hypertension (high blood pressure)
affects longevity, but they don't know the degree. Here's an example from *Conn's Current Therapy 1993*:

*A 35-year-old man with an arterial pressure of 130/90 will
die 4 years earlier than another 35-year-old man with the
same medical background but with normal pressure. If his
pressure is 140/90, he will die 9 years earlier, and if it's
150/100, he will die 17 years earlier.*

More than fifty million people have hypertension. "It is the most
common indication for visits to the physician in the United
States," according to a 1995 journal article.

This explains why the family of antihypertensive medications contains more top-sellers than any other drug group discussed in this book. In 1996, five of the top twenty U.S. outpatient prescriptions were antihypertensive drugs. If both brand-name and generic preparations are counted, twelve of the top hundred and twenty-three of the top two hundred were antihypertensive drugs.

Hypertension may be defined as an abnormally high pressure in the arteries. This high pressure causes increased wear and tear within the blood vessel walls, leading to the development of premature cardiac or kidney disease, strokes, or other circulatory problems. Lowering the pressure significantly reduces the risk of stroke and renal and cardiac disease.

Our national awareness of hypertension and its destructiveness is greater than ever. Yet recent data indicate that despite the brisk sale of antihypertensive drugs, less than one-quarter of people with hypertension in the United States are receiving adequate treatment. Among Mexican Americans, only 14% of those with hypertension are receiving adequate treatment; for Mexican American males, the proportion is a mere 8%.

One of the main reasons that so many people with hypertension go untreated is that except in extreme cases, hypertension is a silent condition until its later stages. Most people with hypertension feel fine. Without any symptoms, they are hardly motivated to change habits or take medication. If medication side effects develop, many drop out of treatment—about 50% according to statistics, because side effects from antihypertensive drugs often impair patients' quality of life. Other patients, fearing side effects, never even fill their prescriptions. Thus, medication side effects are one of the greatest barriers to effective treatment.

HYPERTENSION IN AFRICAN-AMERICANS

Hypertension is perhaps the single most serious medical problem of adult African-Americans. The frequency of hypertension in this group is among the highest in the world.

Hypertension is a common condition in all populations, but it occurs even more often in African-Americans—about 40% more often than other groups. According to one survey, among the black women who were studied, the prevalence of hypertension was 62.5%, whereas among Caucasians it was 20.6% and among Hispanics, 12.3%.

And according to a 1997 report: "Blacks have a higher prevalence, earlier onset, and greater severity of hypertension than do whites. They develop hypertension at a younger age and their hypertension is likely to be more severe." The result is that African-Americans are subject to a greater incidence of the diseases that hypertension produces: severe kidney disease, heart disease, and strokes.

One reason for the disproportionate occurrence of hypertension among African-Americans appears to be genetic. Recent research has suggested that a genetic abnormality on chromosome 10 may be involved.

Another factor may be severe socioeconomic stress, under which a greater segment of African-Americans live than whites. Lifestyle factors are also involved: African-Americans have a high incidence of smoking and obesity. However, Hispanic Americans share many of these factors, but their incidence of hypertension is similar to that of Caucasians. Therefore, genetic factors are considered primary in African-Americans. Still, lifestyle changes, particularly reducing the dietary intake of salt and other sodium-rich foods, can be very helpful in controlling hypertension in African-Americans.

African-Americans often respond to medication in a less predictable fashion than Caucasians. Many types of antihypertensive drugs are less reliably effective in African-American patients. However, the thiazides and other diuretics work particularly well with African-Americans and are usually the drugs of first choice in this population. Long-term follow-up studies have shown that diuretic-based therapies with African-Americans do reduce the incidence of hypertension-related morbidity and mortality.

DO YOU HAVE HYPERTENSION?

Hypertension is an excessive amount of pressure in the arteries, as determined by a blood pressure measuring device. Your blood pressure consists of two numbers—for example, 120/80. The first number is called the systolic pressure; the second number is the diastolic pressure.

The systolic pressure is the amount of pressure in the arterial system produced by a contraction of the heart. The diastolic pressure represents the amount of pressure between heartbeats, when the system is momentarily at rest.

The guidelines for the categorization of hypertension have been revised. Previously, the diastolic number was usually the most important in defining hypertension. The new model places equal emphasis on the systolic and diastolic measurements. A systolic pressure of 170 in a 70-year-old man was once considered normal. Today, it's considered high and treated.

In the new classification (see Table 12.1), a systolic pressure below 130 mm Hg (mm Hg = millimeters of mercury) is considered normal, 130–139 equals high normal, and above 140 equals hypertension. A diastolic pressure below 85 is normal, 85–89 is high normal, and 90 and above represents hypertension.

Table 12.1. Is Your Blood Pressure High?

In the new classification, both numbers (systolic and diastolic, respectively) of a blood pressure measurement are important. For example, if your blood pressure is 145/80, you have mild hypertension (Stage 1) because your systolic pressure is high. Or if your pressure is 128/96, you also have mild hypertension because your diastolic pressure is high.

(Adapted from ''The Fifth Report of the Joint National Committee on Detection, Evaluation, and Treatment of High Blood Pressure'' (JNC V), *Archives of Internal Medicine*, 1993, p 161)

CATEGORY	SYSTOLIC	DIASTOLIC
Normal Less than:	130	85
High normal	130–139	85–89
High blood pressure (hypertension)		
Mild (Stage 1)	140–159	90–99
Moderate (Stage 2)	160–179	100–109
Severe (Stage 3)	180–209	110–119
Very severe (Stage 4) Above:	210	120

A combined blood pressure of up to 130/85 is normal, 130–139/85–89 is borderline and warrants follow-up, and 140/90 or above is hypertensive and requires intervention. An optimal blood pressure is 120/80 or lower—as long as it isn't so low that it causes other problems.

Of those with hypertension, about 75% are classified as Stage I—mild hypertension, with an elevated systolic pressure of 140–160 or diastolic pressure of 90–100 mm Hg. The immediate risks in these cases are few, and medication treatment can be withheld for weeks or months while lifestyle alterations are implemented.

Interestingly, there is some debate among American and foreign specialists about whether all people with mild hypertension require treatment. The U.S. standards are the most rigorous in the world, requiring intervention that includes medication, if necessary, for pressures that aren't treated so aggressively elsewhere. For example, the threshold for treatment in Canada, Australia, and Britain is a diastolic pressure of 100. In Britain, treatment for elevated systolic pressure begins at 160.

Because so many people have pressures within the 140–160 systolic or 90–100 diastolic range, this means that many people with mild hypertension who receive treatment in the United States might not receive a similar recommendation elsewhere. The more aggressive approach adopted here is explained by the fact that increased risk of long-term damage from hypertension may begin with diastolic pressures as low as 80–89, and definite increased risk begins at 90–94.

Some authorities believe that rather than using a rigid standard, each person with mild hypertension should be evaluated individually. This includes considering your gender and age (males and the elderly are at greater risk), as well as health factors such as diabetes, or cardiac risk factors such as elevated cholesterol or family history of early cardiac disease.

Not debatable is the fact that as the blood pressure rises to higher levels, the risks increase exponentially. Blood pressures that are markedly elevated may initially require drug therapy as well as non-drug measures.

The usual goal in treating hypertension is to attain a pressure of 140/90 or lower. Some believe that a diastolic pressure of 85 should be achieved. For people with renal or cardiac disease, even lower pressures are suggested.

REDUCING HYPERTENSION WITHOUT MEDICATIONS

Underlying causes of hypertension must be considered first. Disorders such as hyperthyroidism or adrenal abnormalities, for example, may cause elevations in blood pressure. Medications such as oral contraceptives, high doses of steroids, and anti-inflammatory drugs, especially when used in the elderly, may sometimes produce hypertension.

If the elevation in blood pressure isn't caused by another disorder or external factors, then the condition is called primary or essential hypertension, which must be treated in its own right. Among the first steps of treatment are many nondrug approaches.

Lifestyle changes can sometimes do a lot to reduce blood pressure. Weight loss in overweight people is extremely important. The risk of developing hypertension is increased by 200% to 600% in people who are overweight, and weight loss is the single most effective activity they can do to reduce blood pressure. A modest loss of weight can sometimes make a significant difference.

Reducing sodium intake has long been a mainstay of antihypertensive treatment, although recently there has been renewed debate about the importance of salt (salt = sodium chloride) restriction. According to practicing physicians, reducing salt intake does appear to be helpful in some cases; up to 50% of hypertensives are salt sensitive. For such people, reducing sodium intake below 2 grams a day (= about 5 grams of sodium chloride, or salt) can have dramatic effects.

Of course, if 50% of people with hypertension are salt sensitive, then 50% aren't, so sodium control cannot be said to be an important factor in a unequivocal majority of hypertensives. Again, we encounter the issue of interindividual variation: for some, salt control may be essential; for others, of less value. The only way for you to know is to try it for a few months. If you are medication-sensitive or otherwise prefer to avoid taking medication, you will probably be glad to reduce the sodium in your diet if there's a 50% chance it allows you to avoid or minimize drug therapy. If you are African-American, sodium restriction is especially important because this group has demonstrated a high degree of salt sensitivity in hypertension.

A 1997 study has shown that increased potassium intake may also produce a mild reduction in both systolic and diastolic blood pressure. Physicians often prescribe potassium supplements such as potassium chloride, but these preparations can be irritating to the stomach and can cause nausea, gas, abdominal pain, or diarrhea. An alternative is to increase your dietary intake of vegetables and fruits. You may be aware that bananas are rich in potassium: 450 mg in a medium-size banana. Other fruits and vegetables also contain high quantities of potassium: 4 ounces of potato contain about 500 mg; ½ cup of beans, 330 mg; ½ cup of broccoli, 190 mg; one pear, 200 mg; 1 carrot, 155 mg.

Drinking more than three or four alcoholic beverages a day correlates with a higher likelihood of hypertension. Reducing daily alcohol intake to 24 ounces of beer, 8 ounces of wine, or 2 ounces of whiskey is recommended. Smoking is also a factor, so stop smoking if you are hypertensive.

Other important changes you can make in your life include stress reduction, regular aerobic exercise, and a healthy, low-fat diet.

Altogether, lifestyle changes are the only intervention necessary in 20% to 25% of people with hypertension. Yet, although all of these changes are beneficial and under the individual's control, not everyone is willing to make the effort. "The fact is that most of our patients would prefer a pill," a report concluded. "A pill is easier, and if it doesn't cause side effects and is affordable, it is certainly the way most people would choose to go."

This is unfortunate because even for those who in spite of lifestyle changes must still take medication, lifestyle changes can improve the chances of doing well on medication. As one specialist told me, "The easy part is prescribing the drug; the hard part is changing the behavioral aspects. But if you do a lot of things at the same time, you can use less medication."

Less medication means fewer side effects. Fewer side effects mean a better quality of life, an easier course of treatment, and fewer temptations to quit. Maintaining treatment means reducing the ravages of hypertension and living longer.

NEW APPROACHES IN
TREATING HYPERTENSION

A young man, age 30, was diagnosed with hypertension (140/100). His physician started him on Capoten (captopril) at 12.5 mg a day rather than the manufacturer-recommended initial dosage of 50 to 75 mg a day—i.e., a fourth to a sixth of the recommended starting dosage. Already exercising regularly, the man reduced his salt intake and tried coping better with his stress at work. When he went to the doctor again, his blood pressure was normal, and it stayed normal on subsequent visits. He remained on Capoten at the very low dose of 12.5 mg a day. He experienced no side effects.

Ultimately, most people with hypertension will require some drug therapy, but the ideal treatment approach for hypertension has still to be developed. More and more, low-dose medication approaches and the avoidance of side effects are becoming the cornerstones of hypertension management.

Many antihypertensive drugs can produce multiple effects within the human system. Side effects occur frequently and are a major reason why most people with hypertension aren't receiving treatment. A 1996 monograph from the Albert Einstein College of Medicine reported: ''The statistics do show that about half of treated hypertensive patients discontinue their therapy within a year.'' The main reason was side effects.

In addition, with antihypertensive drugs, silent side effects may occur such as alterations in blood levels of glucose, cholesterol, uric acid, and potassium caused by some diuretics. These dose-related changes, when not noticed and corrected, can become serious. Using the very lowest effective doses reduces the risks of most adverse effects.

''Overmedicating patients isn't good,'' a cardiologist told me. ''They come back tired, lethargic, light-headed, forgetful. Their heart rate's below 45, their blood pressure is too low. They really hate you. They think, 'He really doesn't treat me individually. He's too busy to be concerned.' That's why I always obtain a side effect profile, and I individualize the dosage, starting low.''

A start-low, go-slow strategy allows time to take corrective nonmedicinal measures such as reducing salt or losing weight before jumping to higher, perhaps unnecessary, drug doses. With this method, it may take several months to get hypertension under control, but because antihypertensive treatment is often lifelong, the time involved is worth the effort, especially if it results in using lower drug doses. Except in severe cases, the risks of going slow are few, the benefits many.

"My philosophy's real, real simple," a hypertension specialist told me. "I give just enough to make it work. I usually start by underdosing people. If their hypertension isn't horrible, and if you 'crawl up' with the dosage, you can avoid scaring people by over-medicating them and giving them side effects. Very often their blood vessels relax over a period of time and you wind up ultimately needing less medication."

"By going slowly," a local internist concurs, "I get better compliance, and I end up using less medication. I get the most control and the least side effects."

AN EMERGING METHOD: LOW-DOSE DUAL DRUG THERAPY

The traditional method of treating hypertension has been to increase the dose of one medication until the blood pressure is brought under control. This approach is now being challenged. A new method of using very low doses of two drugs is gaining ground.

The rationale for a dual-drug approach is compelling. Hypertension may be caused by a combination of physiological factors, and using multiple drug therapy may influence these factors more comprehensively. Moreover, using very low doses of two drugs appears to cause fewer side effects than higher doses of a single medication.

New studies support the dual-drug approach. In one large study, the dual-drug approach allowed the use of dosages only a fourth those of the same drugs when used alone. Side effects were fewer and quality-of-life measures were better with the combination low-dose method. Other studies have shown that whereas single drug treatment at moderate doses is successful in 30% to 40% of cases, when a low dose of the same drug is augmented by a low dosage of a second medication, the success rate rises to 75% to 80%.

THE STATE OF THE ART

Like many shifts in medical methodology, new approaches to medication filter down slowly. Most physicians practicing today were taught to use one antihypertensive drug, starting at the manufacturer-recommended initial dose and increasing it, if necessary, until the blood pressure is brought down to acceptable levels. The newer, low-dose approaches are gaining acceptance, but gradually. Yet, according to one specialist who uses a low-dose approach, most of his colleagues do not. The medical literature bears him out.

Perhaps the main impediment to physicians' changing their approach are the wide discrepancies in the recommended antihypertensive drug dosages between different drug references. For dosage guidelines, the great majority of physicians rely on the PDR, which contains the manufacturer-recommended dosages. Many nonprofessionals rely on bookstore references such as *The Pill Book*, although regular folks also buy the PDR—about half a million are sold through bookstores each year. But other, more highly respected drug references, as well as many practicing physicians, often suggest significantly lower initial doses than suggested in the PDR and *The Pill Book*.

For example, this is the case with hydrochlorothiazide (HCTZ), a diuretic frequently prescribed as the first medication in treating mild hypertension. The PDR suggests initial doses that are 100% to 800% higher than recommended by other drug references and many physicians (25 to 50 mg a day versus 6.25 to 12.5 mg a day). This inconsistency is so glaring that *The American Hospital Formulary Service, Drug Information 1996* makes a point of addressing it:

> *For the management of hypertension, the usual initial adult dosage of hydrochlorothiazide recommended by the manufacturers is 50–100 mg daily. . . . Alternately, when used as a step 1 or 2 [first or second choice] drug in the stepped-care [low-dose] approach to antihypertensive therapy, an initial adult HCTZ dosage of 12.5–25 mg daily has been suggested.*

These differences are not trivial. According to Dr. Michael Ziegler, professor of medicine at the University of California, San

Diego, "It has been obvious for many years that standard doses of hydrochlorothiazide for hypertension are much too large. . . . As I review many older studies it appears that very low-dose diuretic therapy decreased the incidence of heart attack and sudden cardiac death in hypertensives, while moderate-size doses provided no cardiac protection, and larger doses seemed to kill people."

Other barriers are time and economics. As one specialist explained: "The cases I see usually have failed elsewhere, especially with family medicine or other primary-care physicians. They're always pressured to see patients within ten minutes or so. There's little time to do a careful medication history, let alone explain how to adjust the dosage of the medications, so they often throw full dosages at patients. Compounding the problem is that there's often no opportunity for follow-up. Careful dosaging requires frequent follow-up. I have an advantage—specialists like me get more time. That's why I'm usually successful even with patients who've failed with two or three other doctors. Low-dose approaches almost always work—they just take time."

HYPERTENSION AND THE ELDERLY

Tenormin, a beta blocker, is frequently prescribed for hypertension. The usual recommended dose for elderly individuals is 25 mg, but that was too much for one 77-year-old man. Doing fine two years after open heart surgery, this man nearly fainted while dining out. He was rushed to the nearest emergency room and hospitalized for observation. Despite the fact that one of the side effects of excessive Tenormin is fainting, the medical staff gave him his usual 25 mg of Tenormin. They did this possibly because 25 mg of Tenormin is the so-called lowest dosage, and the hospital physician probably couldn't conceive that it could actually be the cause of the man's sudden drop in blood pressure. Fortunately, the patient spent the night lying down. The next morning the man's regular cardiologist saw the patient and immediately discontinued the drug. There have been no further fainting episodes.

Hypertension is common in the elderly population. Because of changes in the metabolism and elimination of medications, elderly individuals are often more sensitive than younger adults to the effects and side effects of antihypertensive drugs. The elderly are also more likely to be taking other medications, prescription and nonprescription, that may interact with drugs for hypertension. Furthermore, hypertensive medications by definition affect the cardiovascular system, and many drugs that the elderly use have direct effects on the heart.

For all of these reasons, initiating treatment with lower doses is important with all elderly persons, and except in severe cases, increases in dosage should be made very gradually. Again, when necessary, low-dose dual medication therapies may be safer than higher doses of single antihypertensive agents.

WHERE TO START

Physicians can choose from over six distinct groups of medications for treating hypertension, with over a dozen different drugs within some groups. This chapter discusses a selection of the most used drugs, but there are many more.

As with initial drug dosages and single versus dual therapy, the best approach to hypertension remains a work in progress. The 1995 Joint National Committee on Detection, Evaluation, and Treatment of High Blood Pressure (JNC V) recommended starting with a diuretic such as hydrochlorothiazide (HCTZ) or a beta blocker such as Tenormin (atenolol). However, ACE inhibitors such as Capoten (captopril) and Vasotec (enalapril), or calcium channel blockers such as Cardizem CD (extended-release diltiazem), Procardia XL (nifedipine), and Norvasc (amlodipine) are also frequently prescribed by physicians because of they are effective and generally well tolerated.

New evidence and recommendations emerge every year. A 1997 study found that thiazide diuretics, beta blockers, and ACE inhibitors may be better for initiating treatment than other groups. The International Society of Hypertension recommends that any of the five major drug classes—the four groups mentioned above plus the alpha receptor blockers—may be used initially.

A 1997 article in *The Practitioner* perhaps put it best: Tailored therapy is the preferred approach—"fitting the most appropriate drug to the individual patient. . . . The lowest possible doses of any drug should be employed.''

Whichever medication(s) is chosen, it should provide coverage twenty-four hours a day. This is why many physicians and patients prefer preparations taken just once daily. Usually they are taken with dinner or bedtime so that you will sleep through possible side effects, while the medication provides its peak response during the night and early the next morning, when cardiovascular problems most often occur.

The choice of the initial antihypertensive medication should also depend on the your individual characteristics: age, gender, race, size, other illnesses (e.g., diabetes, cardiac disease), medication sensitivity or history of side effects, willingness to make lifestyle changes or to take medication consistently. For example, some antihypertensive drugs are more preferable than others for women of child-bearing age. Beta blockers and thiazide diuretics may be problematic if you have elevated cholesterol or LDL levels (see Chapter 11). In diabetics, ACE inhibitors many be preferred, while beta blockers and thiazide diuretics may cause problems. Yet thiazide diuretics are the drugs of first choice for African-Americans.

Elderly patients often have other illnesses such as heart or kidney disease and are taking other medications that may conflict with some types of antihypertensive drugs. Antihypertensive drug therapy must be initiated even more carefully.

All of these factors must be considered in choosing the initial drug and dosage. No antihypertensive medication is likely to work if it is prescribed without considering individual factors or started at a dosage that causes side effects and patient discontent.

COST FACTORS

Low-dose antihypertensive therapy is cost-effective for two reasons. First and foremost, if it increases the number of people who start and maintain their antihypertensive treatment and thereby reduce the long-term ravages of hypertension such as heart disease, kidney failure, and strokes, the savings in the overall cost of medical care will be enormous.

Second, using less medicine is usually less expensive. For example, Capoten was the drug mentioned in a case described above. The PDR and *The Pill Book* list the initial dose as a 25-mg tablet two or three times a day. Some other drug references suggest starting treatment as low as 12.5 mg twice a day. A scored 25-mg Capoten tablet costs about $1.00. Using it according to the manufacturer's guidelines amounts to $2.00 to $3.00 a day; using half a tablet twice a day costs $1.00 a day. In the case of the young man who responded to just 12.5 mg a day of Capoten, the cost would be 50¢ a day.

If generic HCTZ is used at a dose of 12.5 mg/day, the cost is less than 15¢ a day using half a 25-mg tablet.

RECOMMENDATIONS

Treating hypertension is like running a marathon: it's a long haul, lifelong treatment for many. Even under ideal circumstances, if you have hypertension, you will likely go through periods of detesting your medication and yearning to discontinue it. Starting low and going slow allows you the time to accept the diagnosis, to adjust to taking medication on a daily basis (a difficult psychological adjustment for many), to make necessary lifestyle changes, and to establish a solid working relationship with your physician without the often disruptive obstacle of side effects.

Thus the initial goal of treatment isn't simply to control your hypertension. Equally important, it's to come to terms with your disorder and to embark upon treatment gently.

Your initial treatment should include the evaluation of such factors as obesity, stress, other illnesses and other medications, salt and potassium intake, as well as a thorough medication-sensitivity history. If you smoke or drink excessively, you and your physician should discuss their impact on your hypertension and consider ways of altering these behaviors. If you require medication, a start-low, go-slow approach provides time for lifestyle changes to add their effect. Over time, changes you make in your lifestyle may reduce the amount of medication you need, thus reducing side effects.

Most authorities recommend starting with a single medication at low dosage. There are many groups of antihypertensive drugs and many specific medications within each group. Most often, treatment is begun with a thiazide diuretic or beta blocker, although ACE inhibitors and long-acting calcium channel blockers are also frequently prescribed. This chapter describes the most prescribed drugs within the various groups. However, new approaches and new drugs for treating hypertension are continually emerging. If your specific medication is not described below, the general concept of initiating treatment with low doses still applies.

Every antihypertensive medication has the potential for side effects, most of which are dose-related. Choosing a specific drug should be a joint decision between you and your physician based not only on the drug's characteristics but also on your previous history with other medications and side effects. Whichever drug is selected, if you have mild hypertension, you may try low-dose therapy involving doses below those recommended by the manufacturer. Indeed, some authorities recommend starting with the very lowest dose with all medications in all cases.

As discussed above, dual-drug therapy involving very low doses of two antihypertensive drugs is gaining wider acceptance. Usually this approach is used if you don't respond to low-dose single-drug therapy. However, some physicians prefer to start with a combination pill containing very low doses of two drugs, believing that this approach ultimately allows the very lowest doses and fewest side effects, and it brings your blood pressure to desirable levels more quickly.

If you are hypertensive and medication-sensitive, you may have already run into problems with antihypertensive drugs. This may make you hesitant about any drug therapy. Your reluctance is understandable, but hypertension is too important to ignore.

The key for you is to start low enough, sometimes at dosages that some physicians would consider placebos. But as you have probably already learned from negative experience, doses that are too low for most people may be just right for you. Thus, your primary goal should be to find a physician who understands medication sensitivities, especially in regard to the reactivity that you and many others demonstrate with antihypertensive drugs.

As one physician explained, "After having side effects, people become sensitized. Some of them almost demand lower doses. I had two female patients lately, both very sensitive to drugs. They'd already run into problems elsewhere, and they insisted on starting at one-fourth dosages. If you want patients to be compliant, you've got to work with them. Besides, starting low gives their systems time to adjust. Ultimately both of these women required and were able to tolerate standard dosages, but it took trying several medications, adjusting when they hit side effects, and moving very slowly.''

The trend toward using lower, safer drug doses in treating hypertension offers you an opportunity to take an active part in your treatment. The first step is for you to impress upon your physician that you are medication-sensitive, or that you have had previous problems with drug-related side effects, or that you just want to start low enough to be sure to avoid problems with antihypertensive drugs and to allow lifestyle changes to work. This means that the physician you select must be open to using antihypertensive medications in lower, safer doses until your individual degree of sensitivity to the selected drug(s) is determined, and to make dose adjustments, if necessary, in a careful and gradual manner.

Or as a 1995 journal article put it:

> The message should come loud and clear that the most important concern is to detect and evaluate patients with hypertension, and then to institute a meaningful and mutually acceptable plan of treatment both for the patient and the physician. Flexibility is definitely encouraged.

Thiazide Diuretics

Diuretics reduce blood pressure by prodding the kidneys to excrete more fluid, thereby reducing the pressure within the arterial system. There are many types of diuretics, but the thiazides are the group most often prescribed for mild hypertension.

Esidrix, HydroDIURIL, Oretic—all are hydrochlorothiazide (HCTZ)—and Hygroton (chlorthalidone) are the best known and best-selling thiazide diuretics. In 1996, just one type of the many generic preparations of HCTZ ranked No. 91 among the top 200 drugs in U.S. outpatient prescriptions, and No. 7 among all generic drugs in 1995.

Thiazide diuretics are used alone or in combination with other antihypertensive drugs. Some drug references list thiazide diuretics as equal or more effective than any other group of antihypertensive drugs. For this reason, these authorities rank thiazide diuretics as the first choice in the drug treatment of hypertension.

Recent studies have shown thiazide diuretics to be particularly useful with African-American and elderly individuals, although somewhat less effective in young white males. Overall, thiazide diuretics are effective as single therapy in 50% to 60% of mild cases; when combined with another drug, 75% to 80% successful.

When antihypertensive therapy is begun with a drug from another group, and after a few months it becomes necessary to add a second medication, a very low dose of thiazide diuretic (e.g., 12.5 mg of HCTZ) is often chosen. Indeed, a 1996 newsletter reported a high rate of success in mild hypertension with a combination containing a very low dose of bisoprolol, a beta blocker, and just 6.25 mg of HCTZ.

Side effects with thiazide diuretics may include fatigue, frequent urination, a rash, and sexual dysfunction in a small percentage. Thiazide diuretics may increase blood levels of glucose and cholesterol, and therefore must be used carefully in diabetics and people with elevated cholesterol levels.

Thiazide diuretics, especially at higher dosages, can significantly reduce potassium in the blood. Potassium supplementation is usually recommended. To prevent potassium loss, thiazide diuretics are often combined with triamterene or spironolactone, drugs that cause the kidneys to retain potassium. Increased dietary potassium may in itself help reduce elevated blood pressure.

ESIDRIX, HYDRODIURIL, ORETIC (HYDROCHLOROTHIAZIDE)

The PDR descriptions for Esidrix, HydroDIURIL, and Oretic differ considerably in their dosage recommendations. The Esidrix and Oretic descriptions seem outdated, recommending initial doses of 50 to 100 mg a day. For HydroDIURIL, it's 25 to 50 mg a day.

Many authorities today cite initial doses as low as 12.5 mg a day, including the *AMA Drug Evaluations Annual 1995*,

Conn's Current Therapy 1995, and *The American Hospital Formulary Service, Drug Information 1996*, as well as the Joint National Committee on Detection, Evaluation, and Treatment of High Blood Pressure (JNC V). The differences in these recommended dosages aren't insignificant. The consequences of taking needless and excessive amounts of hydrochlorothiazide, as well as other antihypertensive drugs, may be profound.

Brand-name and generic HCTZ is manufactured in scored tablets beginning at 25 mg, so flexible dosaging is possible. By using half a 25-mg pill, doses of 12.5, 25, 37.5, and 50 mg can easily be fashioned for gradual dose increases, if needed. Generic HCTZ is inexpensive—a dosage of 12.5 mg a day costs less than 15¢.

HYGROTON (CHLORTHALIDONE)

Interestingly, the 1997 PDR contains little information and no dosage guidelines for this drug. Standard dosaging is 25 to 50 mg a day, but initial doses as low as 12.5 mg a day are recommended by some authorities.

DYAZIDE (TRIAMTERENE-HCTZ) and ALDACTAZIDE (SPIRONOLACTONE-HCTZ)

Dyazide contains 25 mg of hydrochlorothiazide (HCTZ) combined with 50 mg of triamterene. This combination provides the benefits of a thiazide diuretic (HCTZ) in controlling hypertension, while triamterene reduces potassium loss. Because of its effectiveness and convenience, as well as prolonged experience with this combination in patients, Dyazide and generic equivalents are very popular medications. In 1996, Dyazide ranked No. 111 in U.S. outpatient prescriptions; one type of generic HCTZ-triamterene (Geneva) ranked No. 18.

Another brand-name combination of triamterene-HCTZ is Maxzide; there are also many generic preparations. The amount of medication in these different products may vary, ranging from 25 to 50 mg of HCTZ and 37.5 to 75 mg of triamterene. Unfortunately, the amount of HCTZ in these combinations is high for the initial treatment of mild hypertension: many authorities recommend initial doses of 6.25 or 12.5 mg of HCTZ. Triamterene can be prescribed separately starting at 50 mg a day for its potassium-sparing effect.

Aldactazide is a brand-name spironolactone-HCTZ combination that is also frequently prescribed for treating hypertension. Spironolactone, like triamterene, reduces the amount of potassium loss caused by HCTZ. Aldactazide is produced in two sizes containing either 25 or 50 mg of both spironolactone and HCTZ. As with Dyazide, many generic preparations are also available. Again, the doses of HCTZ in these combinations are too high for the initial treatment of mild hypertension; doses of 6.25 or 12.5 mg of HCTZ are preferred. Spironolactone can be prescribed separately starting at 25 mg a day for its potassium-sparing effect.

Beta Blockers

Beta blockers are another group that medical authorities often recommended for first-step antihypertensive drug therapy. Some practitioners, however, prefer other types of antihypertensive drugs because of a high incidence of beta-blocker-induced fatigue, dullness, and depression in their patients.

Beta blockers effectively reduce blood pressure by blocking the effects of epinephrine (adrenaline) and norepinephrine (noradrenaline) on the arteries, as well as reducing the nerve stimulation on the heart. These effects cause a relaxation of the arteries and a reduction of pressure within the cardiovascular system.

There are many kinds of beta blockers; the drugs discussed in this chapter represent the most frequently prescribed. Beta blockers are also prescribed for myriad other uses, including some types of heart disease, migraine headaches, and mitral valve prolapse syndrome; the discussion here regards the use of beta blockers in hypertension.

Side effects with beta blockers include fatigue, light-headedness, dizziness, headache, a slowed heart rate, cold extremities, and mental depression; beta blockers must be used with caution in people with some types of pulmonary disease including asthma, cardiac disease, thyroid disorders, and diabetes.

When low-dose beta blocker treatment is insufficient for controlling hypertension, a low-dose thiazide diuretic, such as 6.25 or 12.5 mg of HCTZ, is frequently added.

INDERAL (PROPRANOLOL) AND INDERALLA (LONG-ACTING)

The granddaddy of the beta blockers, Inderal and generic propranolol continue to enjoy wide usage. Long-acting forms of this drug are often preferred because of the ease of dosage. With Inderal LA, the manufacturer-recommended initial dosage for hypertension is one 80-mg capsule daily. Other authorities suggest a starting dose of 60 mg a day.

Using regular Inderal, the manufacturer-recommended initial dosage is 40 mg twice a day (80 mg a day). Other authorities suggest 20 mg twice a day as an effective starting dosage.

The manufacturer offers no alternative dosage guidelines for elderly patients, but if 80 mg a day of regular or LA Inderal is the recommended dosage for younger adults, a lower dosage for the elderly is probably appropriate. Indeed, one internist told me, ''With older people, I sometimes use doses that appear homeopathic. With Inderal, I begin with 10 or 20 mg a day. That's all.''

LOPRESSOR (METOPROLOL)

The manufacturer-recommended initial dosage of Lopressor is 100 mg a day. Many authorities suggest an initial dose of 50 mg a day. Indeed, the *AMA Drug Evaluations Annual 1994* makes special note of Lopressor's wide variation in individual response: ''The effective dose varies widely and must be titrated on the basis of the therapeutic response.'' It also recommends starting treatment at 50 mg/day—50% less than the manufacturer-recommended initial dosage.

Lopressor is produced as 50 and 100 mg scored tablets.

TENORMIN (ATENOLOL)

Tenormin and atenolol are among the most prescribed medications in America. In 1996, Tenormin and three different types of generic atenolol ranked among the top 200 drugs in U.S. outpatient prescriptions. One of the reasons for Tenormin's popularity is that it was one of the first once-a-day beta blockers.

The PDR recommended initial dose of Tenormin is 50 mg a day; 25 mg a day for "some" elderly patients. Many authorities suggest starting at 25 mg a day with everyone. This dose may be too high for the elderly.

Tenormin is produced in 25-, 50-, and 100-mg tablets; these are not scored but can be cut in half; generic atenolol is made by many companies.

ZEBETA AND ZIAC (BISOPROLOL)

Zebeta is a beta blocker with effects similar to other members of this group. The manufacturer-recommended initial dose is 5 mg a day, but a lower dose of 2.5 mg a day is suggested for some patients. The 2.5-mg dose is less likely to provoke side effects when drug therapy is initiated.

Ziac is a top-selling, low-dose combination drug. In addition to Zebeta, it also contains the diuretic hydrochlorothiazide. Ziac is made in three sizes containing 2.5, 5, and 10 mg of Zebeta, respectively; all sizes are combined with a very low dose of HCTZ, 6.25 mg. If combination drug therapy is warranted, Ziac offers both a low-dose pill (2.5/6.25 mg) and considerable dose flexibility. Ziac tablets are not scored but can be split or cut with a pill cutter.

Ace Inhibitors

The ACE inhibitors are named for their ability to block an enzyme (the angiotensin-converting enzyme, or ACE) involved in blood pressure regulation. The ultimate result is a relaxing of the muscles within artery walls that control the diameter of the blood vessels and therefore the pressure within the system. Relaxing these tiny muscles reduces the pressure within the cardiovascular tree.

ACE inhibitors have proven to be effective and popular drugs because they are generally well tolerated. Although they have not been available as long as thiazide diuretics and beta blockers, which have been proven over time to reduce the risk of renal and cardiac disease and strokes in people with hypertension, evidence is mounting that ACE inhibitors do the same. They are certainly equally effective in reducing hypertension in many cases. Thus, many physicians prescribe ACE inhibitors as an initial medication in the single- or dual-drug therapy of hypertension.

Because they do not adversely affect blood levels of glucose or cholesterol, ACE inhibitors are often first-choice medications for people with diabetes or high cholesterol.

Most common side effects include persistent cough, diminished taste, dizziness, light-headedness, or a rash; ACE inhibitors are usually contraindicated in pregnant women.

CAPOTEN (CAPTOPRIL)

A frequently prescribed ACE inhibitor for hypertension, in 1995 Capoten ranked No. 31 among the most prescribed outpatient medications. After it became available as a generic in 1996, brand-name Capoten ranked No. 146 and one type of generic captopril ranked No. 168. The manufacturer-recommended initial dose is 25 mg either twice or three times a day—i.e., 50 to 75 mg/day. The elderly dosage is the same.

Earlier in this chapter I described the case of a young, fit, 180-pound man with a blood pressure of 140/100 given a very low initial dose of Capoten, 12.5 mg a day. Although only a fourth to a sixth of the manufacturer-recommended starting dose, this amount was sufficient, along with lifestyle changes such as reduced salt intake, to bring this man's hypertension under control. Several drug references support starting with low doses of Capoten—doses such as 12.5 mg once or twice daily. Capoten is produced in 12.5-, 25-, 50-, and 100-mg scored tablets, making flexible dosing easy.

VASOTEC (ENALAPRIL)

Vasotec is one of the most prescribed antihypertensive drugs in America, ranking No. 6 among all medications in outpatient prescriptions in 1996.

The manufacturer-recommended initial dose is 5 mg a day; the recommendation for the elderly is the same. Anecdotal reports, several drug references, and the Joint National Committee on Detection, Evaluation, and Treatment of High Blood Pressure (JNC V) suggest a starting dose of 2.5 mg. For people who are highly medication-sensitive or at risk for drug-related side effects, a dose of 1.25 mg can be made by splitting the 2.5-mg tablet.

When combined with another antihypertensive drug such as the diuretic HCTZ, a 2.5-mg dose of Vasotec is often employed.

Vasotec is manufactured in 2.5-, 5-, 10-, and 20-mg scored tablets.

Calcium Channel Blockers

The calcium channel blockers, or calcium antagonists, constitute another group of medications often used in treating hypertension. Generally, calcium channel blockers have been reserved for cases not controlled by single or combination therapy with thiazide diuretics, beta blockers, and ACE inhibitors. Or they are used if you have other illnesses or are taking other medication that contraindicate other types of antihypertensive medications.

Recently there has been some controversy over the significance of scattered reports of sudden death with these drugs, particularly

Cardizem (diltiazem). Controversy has also touched Procardia (nifedipine) because of reports that it may actually cause an increased incidence of cardiac problems in people with hypertension and coronary heart disease. Cardizem, Procardia, and Calan are produced in short-acting and long-acting preparations; a 1995 study found that people with hypertension taking *short-acting* calcium channel blockers had a 60% greater incidence of heart attacks than those taking other antihypertensive drugs. Studies published in 1990 and 1992 reported increased incidences of cancer and gastric hemorrhage with these drugs, although subsequent studies have not supported these findings.

For now, perhaps the best approach with calcium channel blockers in hypertension is that suggested by a 1997 report in *The Medical Letter on Drugs and Therapeutics*: ''Short-acting calcium-channel blockers, particularly nifedipine [Procardia], should not be used for treatment of hypertension. For previously untreated patients with hypertension, a diuretic, beta-blocker or ACE inhibitor is generally preferred over a calcium-channel blocker.'' The report also recommended that people taking short-acting calcium channel blockers should be switched to a long-acting form of the same drug; those already on long-acting calcium channel blockers could stay on them.

Calcium channel blockers work by inhibiting the movement of calcium ions in the muscle cells within the walls of arteries. The result is a relaxation of these muscles, a reduction in artery and capillary tension (resistance), and a decrease in blood pressure. Used alone, calcium channel blockers are effective in about 35% to 40% of cases; with the addition of a low-dose thiazide diuretic, approximately 75% to 80% respond.

Some calcium channel blockers such as Cardizem (diltiazem) and Calan (verapamil) have similar effects on the coronary arteries and the heart itself, so they are often employed in the treatment of angina and cardiac arrhythmias. Doses for treating angina and arrhythmias may differ from those for hypertension; the doses discussed here apply only to hypertension. Other calcium channel blockers such as Norvasc (amlodipine) and Procardia (nifedipine) XL have no effect on the coronary arteries or heart.

Side effects with calcium channel blockers include headache, light-headedness, constipation, dizziness, increased heart rate, palpitations, fatigue, gastrointestinal disturbances, constipation, and ankle swelling. The latter two problems may occur less often with Norvasc (amlodipine).

CALAN SR, ISOPTIN SR, VERELAN (VERAPAMIL)

Calan, Isoptin, and Verelan are different brands of the same medication, verapamil, which can also be purchased in generic form. Four of these preparations ranked among the top 200 outpatient drugs of 1996.

Calan SR, Isoptin SR, Verelan, and verapamil SR are all long-acting, extended-release drugs. Calan, Isoptin, and generic verapamil are also available in short-acting forms, but these should not be used for treating hypertension. Only the long-acting forms of these medications should be considered.

The usual doses recommended in the PDR are 180 to 240 mg a day initially; a dose of 120 mg a day is suggested for small or elderly or otherwise sensitive individuals. Many authorities suggest the latter dose for the initial treatment of all individuals.

Long-acting preparations of these drugs are produced in many pill types, but usually as 120-mg unscored tablets, and sometimes as 180- and 240-mg scored tablets. For individuals desiring to initiate treatment at a very low dosage, splitting a 180-mg long-acting tablet produces a 90-mg dose.

CARDIZEM CD AND CARDIZEM SR (LONG-ACTING DILTIAZEM)

In 1996, long-acting Cardizem CD ranked No. 14 among all medications in U.S. outpatient prescriptions. The manufacturer suggests a flexible range of initial dosages including 120, 180, and 240 mg a day utilizing twice-a-day Cardizem SR or once-a-day Cardizem CD. Cardizem CD is produced in capsules of 120, 180, 240, and 300 mg; Cardizem SR in capsules of 60, 90, and 120 mg.

In its recommendations for Cardizem CD, the PDR mentions that ''some patients may respond to lower doses.'' Some authorities recommend starting with a low dose of 120 mg a day of Cardizem CD in mild cases.

PROCARDIA XL (EXTENDED-RELEASE NIFEDIPINE)

In 1996 Procardia XL ranked as the No. 8 best-selling medication in U.S. outpatient prescriptions. Short-acting Procardia is not recommended for treating hypertension; only long-acting Procardia XL, which is specifically indicated for hypertension, should be used.

The manufacturer-recommended initial dose of Procardia XL is 30 or 60 mg once daily. The manufacturer emphasizes the need for careful dose titration in prescribing this drug. Procardia XL is produced in 30-, 60-, and 90-mg round, film-coated pills.

Several authorities recommend starting with the 30-mg dose. If you are medication-sensitive or otherwise at risk for drug-related side effects, start at the 30-mg dose.

NORVASC (AMLODIPINE)

Norvasc is a long-acting drug that is specifically recommended for treating hypertension. In 1996 it ranked No. 13 among the top 200 drugs in U.S. outpatient prescriptions.

The manufacturer-recommended initial dose is 5 mg once daily; maximum dose, 10 mg once daily. However, the manufacturer does note that some individuals respond to lower doses: "Small, fragile, or elderly individuals, or patients with hepatic insufficiency may be started on 2.5 mg once daily and this dose may be used when adding Norvasc to other antihypertensive therapy."

The Joint National Committee on Detection, Evaluation, and Treatment of High Blood Pressure (JNC V) and other authorities suggest 2.5 mg of Norvasc as the usual initial dose.

Norvasc is produced in 2.5-, 5-, and 10-mg tablets. The tablets are not scored but can be cut or split, so you can start with an even lower dose, such as 1.25 mg daily if you and your physician desire.

In mild hypertension, the initial dose of Norvasc should be

given at least seven to fourteen days to work before being increased to a higher amount. Increases in dosage, if necessary, can be made gradually rather than jumping 100% from 2.5 to 5 to 10 mg. By cutting the 2.5-mg tablet, you can fashion intermediate doses such as 3.75, 6.25, 7.5, and 8.75 mg.

Alpha Receptor Blockers

Alpha receptor blockers work by inhibiting nerve receptors on the small muscles in artery walls. This results in a diminished ability for the muscles to contract, thereby relaxing the arteries and lowering the pressure within the vascular system. Alpha receptor blockers may be more effective in lowering an elevated diastolic pressure (the second number of the blood pressure measurement) than an elevated systolic pressure (the first number).

Because of a high rate of side effects, alpha receptor blockers are usually reserved for cases that don't respond to diuretics, ACE inhibitors, or beta blockers. One drug reference cited a study in which 18 of 42 subjects taking alpha receptor blockers dropped out because of side effects. The most common side effects are dizziness, light-headedness upon sitting up or standing (postural hypotension), headache, lethargy, somnolence, increased heart rate (tachycardia), and stomach upset. Side effects may occur less often and be less severe with long-acting alpha receptor blockers such as Cardura and Hytrin, which can be taken before bedtime so that you sleep through the peak effect of the drugs.

Because of problems with side effects, this is one group of medications for which all drug references, including the PDR, seem to agree about using the very lowest initial dosage. Indeed, the manufacturer of Hytrin emphasizes the point: "This initial dosing regimen should be strictly observed to minimize the potential for severe hypotensive [low blood pressure] effects."

Alpha receptor blockers are often added as a second or third medications in a combination drug approach, thereby allowing for a very low dosage. They are often combined with diuretics or beta blockers, but they are not usually used with calcium channel blockers. Alpha blockers are also helpful for the benign prostate enlargement that occurs in many older men. For this reason, alpha blockers may be the first-choice drugs for men with both prostate enlargement and hypertension.

CARDURA (DOXAZOSIN)

Cardura was ranked No. 69 among the 200 most prescribed medications in the U.S. in 1996; the recommended starting dose is 1 mg at bedtime. The maximum dose is 16 mg. The dose for the elderly is the same as that for younger adults.

Cardura is produced in 1-, 2-, 4-, and 8-mg tablets. The tablets are scored, so if you are medication-sensitive or prone to medication side effects, you can start at an even lower dose such as 0.5 mg at bedtime.

Doses of Cardura should be increased very gradually and only after at least seven to fourteen days at the initial dose. If you require higher doses, you can use the scored 1-mg tablet to go from 0.5 to 1 to 1.5 before jumping to 2 mg a day. Similarly, rather than skipping from 2 to 4 mg a day, or 4 to 8 mg a day, you can use the 1- and 2-mg tablets to fashion intermediate doses such as 3, 5, 6, and 7 mg.

HYTRIN (TRAZOSIN)

In 1996 Hytrin ranked No. 31 among the top 200 prescribed medications in the U.S. The recommended starting dose is 1 mg at bedtime; the manufacturer emphasizes that higher initial doses should be avoided because of potential side effects. The usual necessary dosage is 1 to 5 mg at bedtime; the maximum dose is 20 mg a day. The dose for the elderly is the same as that for younger adults.

Hytrin is produced in 1-, 2-, 5-, and 10-mg capsules. Only after at least seven to fourteen days, if your hypertension is not improved, should the dose be very gradually increased. Rather than increasing from 2 to 5 mg a day, or from 5 to 10 mg a day, you can use the 1- and 2-mg capsules to fashion intermediate doses of 3, 4, 6, 7 mg, etc.

Central Adrenergic Agonists

This group of antihypertensive medications works in the brain to decrease sympathetic nervous system activity, thereby decreasing muscle tone within arteries and reducing blood pressure. Once extremely popular, the central adrenergic agonists have in recent years been displaced by newer drugs with fewer side effects. Today, central adrenergic agonists are usually employed when other medications aren't effective. They are often combined with other medications in order to keep the dosage low and side effects minimal.

Side effects are common with this group. As many as 20% to 30% of subjects dropped out in studies because of side effects, and in contrast to several other groups of antihypertensive drugs, the central adrenergic agonists caused a measurable decrease in the quality of life of a large percentage of subjects.

Side effects include dry mouth, drowsiness, dizziness, sedation, nausea, nervousness, light-headedness, weakness, fatigue, depression, subtle cognitive impairment, and rashes. Abrupt withdrawal of these drugs may lead to rebound hypertension, so they should be discontinued gradually under a physician's supervision.

CATAPRES (CLONIDINE)

The manufacturer-recommended initial dose of Catapres is 0.1 mg twice a day; an unspecified lower initial dose is recommended for the elderly. Since the smallest Catapres tablet is 0.1 mg and unscored, the lower dose likely means 0.1 mg once a day. Fortunately, generic clonidine is produced by many different companies in tablet form, which can be split.

Among other drug references, some agree with an 0.1-mg

twice-a-day initial dose, but others, including the Joint National Committee on Detection, Evaluation, and Treatment of High Blood Pressure (JNC V), suggest half that amount—0.05 mg twice a day.

Catapres is also produced as a patch that is affixed to the skin and supplies a continuous amount of medication through the skin. One patch supplies medication for a week. Three sizes of the Catapres patch are available, releasing 0.1, 0.2, and 0.3 mg a day, respectively. Conceivably, the patch should provide a more even, continuous level of medication to the body, and therefore perhaps a lower rate of side effects. The 0.1 mg/day patch does provide a low dose. Mild skin reactions to the patch occur in about 25% to 30%, but these are rarely troublesome enough to interfere with continued usage of the patch.

PART 5

Medications for Pain and Inflammation

THIRTEEN

Aspirin (Acetylsalicylic Acid) and Tylenol (Acetaminophen)

There are both theoretical and practical reasons to choose the lowest effective dose of aspirin. . . . The side effects of aspirin are mainly gastrointestinal, dose related, and reduced by using low doses.

—J. Hirsh et al., *Chest*, 1992

Many people who take aspirin do so to reduce their risk of having a heart attack. If you are one those who take an aspirin a day, you may be overmedicating yourself and unnecessarily increasing your risk of side effects.

Aspirin is a drug with many uses. Worldwide, over 50 billion doses of aspirin are taken each year. First introduced in 1899, aspirin reduces pain and fever and exhibits a powerful anti-inflammatory effect similar to medications such as Motrin, Naprosyn, and Relafen (all NSAIDs—see Chapter 14). Aspirin also inhibits the tendency of platelets to form blood clots. It is the latter effect that catapulted aspirin into the headlines in 1995–96 and accounts for much of aspirin's use today.

ASPIRIN AND REDUCED RISKS OF HEART ATTACKS

Beginning around 1991, attention became focused on studies reporting that aspirin usage was associated with marked reductions in the incidence of heart attacks. Most notable was the Physicians' Health Study, a carefully controlled, five-year study of over 22,000 healthy male physicians that showed a striking 44% reduction in the overall risk of having a heart attack with regular aspirin usage.

Another impressive aspect of this study was that the benefits were obtained with a very low dose of aspirin—325 mg (one regular-dose pill) every other day. This dosage was effective because, unlike the amounts required for pain relief or fever reduction, aspirin's antithrombotic (anti-clotting) effect can be accomplished with very low doses.

Aspirin inhibits platelets by blocking a key enzyme, cyclooxygenase, in the clot-forming mechanism. This effect is very rapid and persists with continued aspirin use. Recent studies have shown that even lower doses of aspirin may be equally effective as well as less prone to causing side effects.

WHO SHOULD TAKE ASPIRIN TO PREVENT CARDIOVASCULAR DISEASE?

Not everyone should take aspirin to prevent heart attacks, strokes, and other vascular disease. Studies have shown that aspirin's most significant preventive effects occur in males over age 50 and those with other risk factors such as smoking, high cholesterol/LDL blood levels, or a family history of early heart disease. Taking a low dose of aspirin also appears to be beneficial during a heart attack and in the months afterward.

The results are more equivocal with those with no risk factors. The results have also been less certain in women, although preventive aspirin usage is recommended in women over age 50 and those with significant cardiovascular risk factors.

Preventive aspirin usage doesn't appear to block the development of atherosclerosis (arteriosclerosis)—that is to say, the narrowing of arteries. Thus, the incidence of angina didn't drop in subjects in aspirin studies. Also, the incidence of cerebral hemorrhage, one type of stroke, increased slightly in some aspirin studies. Yet aspirin does reduce another, more common type of stroke, thromboembolism, and is now recommended for the immediate and ongoing treatment of this condition. And although aspirin has been shown to decrease the incidence of heart attacks, whether it reduces overall mortality is less clear.

Aspirin's antithrombotic effect is employed not only to prevent heart attacks in healthy individuals, but also for its proven beneficial effect in people who already have cardiovascular problems. Aspirin is often immediately administered to limit the damage of new heart attacks, and its usage is continued to prevent recurrences. It is also used in some types of angina, strokes, and other vascular disorders. In these instances, the recommended dosage of aspirin varies considerably with the disorder and should be determined by a medical expert.

ASPIRIN'S SIDE EFFECTS

No one disputes that aspirin frequently causes adverse effects, especially with frequent or high-dose usage. For example, those with rheumatoid arthritis taking high doses of aspirin often suffer from gastritis, gastric ulcers, and internal bleeding. One drug reference reported that gastrointestinal bleeding, often without symptoms, occurred in 70% of patients taking aspirin regularly. According to a physician quoted in a 1997 issue of *Newsweek*, "Last year [1996], 17,000 Americans died of gastric bleeding just from taking aspirin or other NSAIDs. . . . Most had no warning."

Most people do well with short-term aspirin, yet heartburn, nausea, and stomach pain do occur in about 20% of people regularly taking one aspirin daily or one every other day. Aspirin can also provoke unexpected (idiosyncratic) reactions in a small percentage of people: "One aspirin makes me throw up," one doctor told me. All of these side effects are dose-related.

Even if aspirin doesn't produce noticeable side effects for you, gastric injury may still occur. According to one journal article, "Gastric injury is evident within hours of ingestion of aspirin. . . . In other studies, administration of 650 mg [the regular strength dose] of aspirin produced endoscopically visible acute gastric mucosal injury in almost 100% of subjects." In other words, even if aspirin isn't causing overt symptoms, it may be causing changes internally.

Using lower doses helps, but studies have shown that even at very low doses taken on an ongoing basis, a significant increase in gastrointestinal bleeding occurs. Thus, the *AMA Drug Evaluations Annual 1995* warns: ''Overt bleeding from the upper gastrointestinal tract may occur when unbuffered aspirin is administered for long periods even at doses between 75 and 250 mg/day.''

Aspirin must also be used with caution in people with aspirin hypersensitivity, with a history of gastric problems, and with some types of hypertension and diabetes. Those taking anticoagulants such as Coumadin (warfarin) must be careful as well. Aspirin is generally avoided in pregnancy.

Aspirin is not advised in children and teenagers with the flu or chicken pox because of an increased association with a rare but serious condition known as Reye's syndrome, a severe, sometimes fatal, neurologic and systemic disorder. Aspirin-containing preparations should be avoided during flu season in youngsters because they already may be incubating the flu virus even though they as yet show no overt signs.

LOW-DOSE ASPIRIN

The discovery of aspirin's beneficial effect in preventing heart attacks means that millions of people will be taking aspirin regularly for a very long time. This in turn has raised concerns about aspirin's long-term side effects and has motivated a new round of dosage studies. As one leading drug reference put it: ''The toxic effects of aspirin appear to be dose-related; this is a major reason why clinical studies have attempted to find the lowest effective antithrombotic dose.''

People have told me that their physicians have recommended an aspirin a day; others, one every other day. These dosages work, but they may be unnecessarily high. Many studies have shown that lower doses are just as effective. Some reports have suggested that as little as 30 or 40 mg a day of aspirin is enough, with the full antithrombotic effect occurring within a week. Whether this tiny dosage is truly sufficient remains an issue of medical debate.

Not controversial is the effectiveness of aspirin doses such as 75 or 100 mg a day. In essence, one children's aspirin, which contains 75 to 81 mg, taken daily is sufficient to obtain aspirin's antithrombotic effect. Many physicians recommend this amount. Others recommend one children's aspirin just three or four days a week. It is important to know about the effectiveness and safety of these very low dosages because some packages of aspirin and some medical references don't mention it.

ASPIRIN FOR FEVER OR PAIN

For pain or fever, the usual aspirin dose most people know is 650 mg (two regular-strength, 325-mg pills) every four to six hours. However, there is considerable variation in individual response to the fever-reducing and pain-relieving effects of aspirin. Some people may require only one 325-mg pill; others may require the extra-strength dose of 975 to 1,000 mg. For some, the effect may last six or more hours; for others, four hours.

These same dosages are usually sufficient for minor inflammatory problems such as tendinitis, as well as sunburn and menstrual pain. For chronic or severe conditions such as arthritis, higher dosages may be necessary, but this should be decided with your physician.

THE IMPORTANCE OF USING THE LOWEST EFFECTIVE DOSES OF ASPIRIN

Is it important to use the very lowest effective dosages of aspirin? In addition to the side effects discussed above, aspirin usage raises other concerns. For example, a physician fell on his rump while skiing. When he returned to his room, he took aspirin for the pain. Aspirin's platelet-inhibiting action starts within an hour of ingestion. By evening, the bump on his rear had grown markedly; he'd bled into the wound. It took two months for the golf-ball-sized bruise to disappear, meanwhile causing constant discomfort, making jogging impossible, and nearly requiring surgery. He'd have been better off using an ice pack. If medication was required, acetaminophen (Tylenol) would have been a better choice because it doesn't affect platelet activity.

Even at low dosage, the ongoing usage of aspirin isn't without risks. A man taking one children's aspirin per day was in a car accident; he didn't experience any abdominal pain until he vomited two pints of blood. His hematocrit, a measure of blood cells, dropped to 16 (normal = around 42–50), and he required transfusions. Excessive bleeding is the reason that surgeons and dentists direct patients to discontinue aspirin seven to ten days before surgical procedures. The same is true for some other anti-inflammatory drugs.

The FDA has also raised concerns about the public's rush to take aspirin on an ongoing basis. According to the May 1994 *FDA Medical Bulletin*: ''The FDA is concerned that public awareness of new approved professional uses of aspirin—e.g., reducing the risk of myocardial infarction [heart attack] in patients with previous infarction or unstable angina pectoris—has grown without a commensurate awareness of the risk associated with such uses of aspirin.'' In other words, whatever the usage—pain, fever, inflammation, or the prevention of cardiovascular disease—use aspirin properly and in the very lowest effective dosage.

One way to reduce gastrointestinal injury with aspirin is to use safer preparations. Studies of buffered aspirin products generally have shown that these have few advantages over plain aspirin, but some people assert that they have done better with buffered products. You can try one of these or simply take aspirin with an antacid tablet or liquid. More impressive in studies has been enteric-coated forms of aspirin. Ecotrin is perhaps the best known product of this type. Enteric-coated aspirin doesn't dissolve in the stomach, thereby avoiding aspirin's acid-like effect on the stomach lining, but it still can cause some gastrointestinal problems through aspirin's systemic effects. Enteric-coated aspirin is available in regular (325 mg) and low-dose (81 mg) sizes; the latter is sufficient for aspirin's preventive effect.

ASPIRIN AND THE ELDERLY

Multiple studies have shown that elderly individuals taking aspirin are more prone to developing gastric symptoms and bleeding than younger adults. This occurs even at doses as low as 100 mg a day. Other adverse effects include easy bruising and nosebleeds. One article projected that if a thousand seniors without prior cardiovascular problems took low-dose aspirin, three cardiovascular deaths and six nonfatal cardiovascular problems (e.g., heart attack, stroke) would be prevented; yet thirty would develop clinically apparent gastrointestinal bleeding. For this reason, whether to use low-dose aspirin on a daily basis remains a delicate decision if you are elderly and have no history of cardiovascular problems. On the other hand, if you have had a previous heart attack or stroke, aspirin may help prevent or modify further episodes. This is a decision that you and your physician must make together. Aspirin is usually contraindicated in elderly people with gastritis, ulcers, or kidney failure.

FOR THOSE WHO CANNOT TOLERATE ASPIRIN

Aspirin isn't the only substance that inhibits platelet aggregation, the basis of aspirin's protective cardiovascular effects. If you develop gastric irritation, other side effects, or an allergy that make aspirin usage impossible, there may be other alternatives.

One man noticed that he was getting many more nicks while shaving. These nicks bled easily and were difficult to stop. Ordinarily, he rarely cut himself shaving. The only other time he'd experienced similar bleeding was when he was taking one aspirin daily, which he'd had to stop because of heartburn.

What was now causing the apparently similar clot-inhibiting response? This time he wasn't taking any medications, but was using a few nutritional supplements. Among them was an enzyme, bromelain, a natural component of pineapples and pineapple juice.

Bromelain is best known as a digestive enzyme, but several journal articles indicate that it has an inhibiting effect on platelet aggregation, thereby diminishing the clotting effect—the effect for which aspirin is taken to prevent cardiovascular problems. Although studies have confirmed bromelain's platelet-inhibiting effect, there are no studies proving that it provides the same cardiovascular protection of aspirin. Nevertheless, its effects on platelets appear similar, if not identical, to aspirin's, so for people who cannot take aspirin, bromelain may offer a suitable alternative. Bromelain doesn't appear to cause gastric irritation.

RECOMMENDATIONS

Aspirin is an unusually versatile medication, but it also can cause serious side effects. If you are sensitive to medications, one 325-mg aspirin every four to six hours may be sufficient for treating fever or mild pain. The standard dosage is 650 mg, and extra-strength aspirin is 975 to 1,000 mg. People with severe or chronic inflammatory disorders such as bursitis or rheumatoid arthritis may require a high dosage.

No matter the usage, always use the lowest effective dose of aspirin. Don't use aspirin at all if you don't really need it. For simple fever or pain, Tylenol (acetaminophen) is usually equally effective and less prone to causing gastric irritation. In children, particularly during flu season, aspirin should be avoided because of the possibility of Reye's syndrome.

For use in preventing heart attacks and some types of stroke, one children's aspirin (75–81 mg) has been shown to be sufficient in producing an antithrombotic effect. This lower dose is also less prone to producing side effects. This same dosage lately has been marketed in "adult low strength" preparations by several manufacturers. Check the label to be sure that you are getting the proper dose.

Take the very lowest effective aspirin dosage because even at as little as 100 mg a day, aspirin has been shown to cause a significant incidence of gastrointestinal bleeding. Enteric-coated formulations such as Ecotrin reduce the incidence of aspirin-related gastric irritation, although a small but significant risk still exists. Several enteric-coated aspirin preparations are available in the 81-mg dose.

Before starting preventive aspirin treatment, make sure that you truly require it. Such usage remains questionable for people under fifty and for those without any cardiovascular risk factors. Ask your physician.

For very rapid pain relief, buffered liquid forms of aspirin such as Alka-Seltzer Pain Reliever are quickly absorbed and therefore fast-acting. Aspirin is also available in suppository form for those wanting to reduce gastric irritation; some gastric irritation may still occur via aspirin's systemic effects.

If you take aspirin on a regular basis, be sure to report any persistent gastric irritation or pain to your physician. Any blackening of your bowel movements, which may indicate bleeding, should be reported.

Daily or every-other-day low-dose aspirin is usually well tolerated, but some people do develop problems. For simple pain or fever, Tylenol (acetaminophen) is usually equally effective and generally safer. If you have an inflammatory disorder such as arthritis, then you may require higher aspirin dosages; these dosages are usually associated with a high incidence of side effects, some serious and occasionally fatal. In this latter incidence, you may do better on other anti-inflammatory medications (see Chapter 14).

Tylenol (Acetaminophen)

Drugs such as aspirin, acetaminophen, . . . and ibuprofen have demonstrated a wide dose-effect range, extending approximately three to four times the minimally effective dose. . . . For example, acetaminophen has a dose-effect range from 300 to 2,000 mg.

—S. A. Cooper, *American Journal of Medicine*, 1984

Tylenol and its generic, acetaminophen, remain the first choice of the majority of physicians when mild pain relief or fever reduction is required. That's because acetaminophen is not only as effective as aspirin, ibuprofen, and other nonprescription anti-inflammatory drugs for these uses, but it works just as fast and causes fewer side effects, especially gastric problems. Unlike aspirin, acetaminophen doesn't affect platelet functioning or inhibit the ability of blood to clot, so it's safer to use with bruises and around surgery, but it doesn't provide any protective effect against heart attacks.

Taken regularly, acetaminophen is considered less likely to cause serious side effects than aspirin or other nonprescription anti-inflammatory drugs such as Motrin IB, Advil, Nuprin, and other ibuprofen preparations, and Aleve and Orudis KT. Nevertheless, there is some association of long-term acetaminophen usage with increased incidences of kidney damage. Similarly, some scattered reports link routine acetaminophen usage with serious, occasional fatal liver damage in people using moderate or heavy amounts of alcohol, or those fasting or dehydrated because of the flu or other illnesses.

Overall, acetaminophen is usually preferred over aspirin and other anti-inflammatory remedies for routine pain and fever. For conditions involving inflammation such as minor strains or tendinitis, anti-inflammatory drugs are generally more effective.

COMMON SIDE EFFECTS

Acetaminophen is generally well tolerated. Gastric irritation or nausea occur infrequently. Rashes or other allergic reactions are rare. As discussed above, frequent acetaminophen usage is associated with rare incidences of kidney failure and liver damage.

LOW-DOSE ACETAMINOPHEN

Studies have demonstrated that the pain-relieving amount of a single dose of acetaminophen ranges from 300 to 2,000 mg depending on the sensitivity of the individual. Surprisingly, many drug references include 325 mg as an effective dose of this drug. Unfortunately, most people overlook this alternative even when it's suggested.

For example, if you read the dosage guidelines on a box of regular Tylenol, it recommends *one or two* pills every four hours. Most people assume that two regular-strength Tylenol or acetaminophen (650 mg) is the standard dosage, but medication-sensitive individuals may respond to just one pill (325 mg). Another alternative is a single extra-strength pill, which is 500 mg. Again, people are accustomed to taking two extra-strength pills, but one may suffice for some individuals.

Using the very lowest effective amount of acetaminophen is important because of recent evidence about the association of a high utilization of acetaminophen and an increased incidence of kidney failure.

RECOMMENDATIONS

For general pain relief and fever reduction, Tylenol or generic acetaminophen are generally preferred over aspirin and other pain remedies. The effective range of acetaminophen is 325–500–650–1,000 mg, depending on your sensitivity.

Like all drugs, acetaminophen should be used only when necessary and in the lowest effective dosage. The use of one acetaminophen per day for over a year has been associated with an increased incidence of kidney failure, and modest amounts of acetaminophen in conjunction with moderate to heavy alcohol usage have been known to trigger liver failure. These reactions are believed to be rare, but the fact that they occur underscores the principle that any medication can have toxic effects in some individuals.

FOURTEEN

Anti-Inflammatory Drugs

In-Depth Analyses

Motrin (ibuprofen) and nonprescription Motrin IB, Advil,
  Nuprin, and other forms of ibuprofen
Voltaren and Voltaren-XR (diclofenac sodium)
Orudis, Oruvail, Orudis KT (ketoprofen)
Relafen (nabumetone)

Other Medications

Lodine, Lodine XL (etodolac)
Naprelan (naproxen)
Naprosyn, EC-Naprosyn, and Aleve (naproxen)
Cataflam (diclofenac potassium)

Brief Comments

Clinoril (sulindac)
Daypro (oxaprozin)
Disalcid (salsalate)
Dolobid (diflunisal)
Feldene (piroxicam)
Flurbiprofen (formally, Ansaid)
Indocin and Indocin SR (indomethacin)
Meclomen (meclofenamate)
Nalfon (fenoprofen)

Tolectin (tolmetin)
Toradol (ketorolac)
Trilisate (choline magnesium trisalicylate)

In-Depth Analyses

Cytotec (misoprostol): An Antidote for
NSAID Side Effects?
Colchicine: An Alternative Anti-
Inflammatory Drug

About Anti-Inflammatory Medications

*Dosage of [all anti-inflammatory drugs] must be carefully
adjusted according to individual requirements and response,
using the lowest possible effective dosages.*

—*The American Hospital Formulary Service
Drug Information 1994*

Anti-inflammatory medications are specifically useful for conditions such as arthritis, tendinitis, bursitis, and other ailments involving tissue inflammation. Their effectiveness has made them one of the most prescribed group of drugs in America and the world. Members include ibuprofen (generic Motrin), Relafen, Lodine, Daypro, Oruvail, naproxen (generic Naprosyn), and diclofenac (generic Voltaren), all of which ranked among the top 200 in U.S. outpatient prescriptions in 1996.

More than 100 million prescriptions for anti-inflammatory drugs were written in the United States in 1995. And this number doesn't include sales of nonprescription anti-inflammatory preparations such as Motrin IB, Advil, Nuprin, Aleve, Orudis KT, generic ibuprofen, and aspirin in its myriad forms.

Medically, anti-inflammatory medications are known as NSAIDs—*nonsteroidal anti-inflammatory drugs*, meaning they don't contain cortisone, which also reduces inflammation.

Inflammation can have both positive and negative ramifications. In healing an infection, the inflammatory response is the body's way of fighting off a foreign attack and healing the damaged tissue. After surgery, inflammation occurs as part of the process of healing, but it also can cause excessive scarring. In autoimmune disorders such as rheumatoid arthritis or lupus, inflammation can be terribly destructive to the body's own tissues.

Commonly Prescribed Anti-Inflammatory Medications (NSAIDs)

TYPE OF MEDICATION	PILL SIZES (MG)
Salycylic acids	
Aspirin (acetylsalicylic acid)	81, 325, 500
Disalcid (salsalate)	500 (scored), 750
*Ecotrin (acetylsalicylic acid)	81, 325, 500
Dolobid (diflunisal)	250, 500 (breakable)
Trilisate (choline magnesium trisalicylate)	500, 750, 1,000 (scored); liquid
Proprionic acids	
Ansaid (flurbiprofen)	50, 100
Daypro (oxaprozin)	600 (scored)
*EC-Naprosyn	375, 500
Motrin (ibuprofen)	300, 400 (unbreakable), 600, 800 (scored)
Naprelan (extended-release naproxen)	375, 500
Naprosyn (naproxen)	250, 375, 500, liquid
Nalfon (fenoprofen)	200, 300, 600 (scored)
Orudis (ketoprofen)	25, 50, 75
Oruvail (extended-release ketoprofen)	100, 150, 200
Acetic acids	
Cataflam (diclofenac potassium)	50

Clinoril (sulindac)	150, 200 (scored)
Indocin (indomethacin)	25, 50, liquid, suppository
Indocin-SR (extended-release indomethacin)	75
Lodine (etodolac)	200, 300, 400, 500
Lodine XL (extended-release etodolac)	400, 600
Tolectin (tolmetin)	200 (scored), 400, 600
*Voltaren (diclofenac sodium)	25, 50, 75
Voltaren-XR (extended release diclofenac)	100

Enolic acid

Feldene (piroxicam)	10, 20

Fenamic acid

Meclomen (meclofenamate)	50, 100

Nonacidic

Relafen (nabumetone)	500, 750 (breakable)

Nonprescription NSAIDs

Aleve (naproxen)	220
Ibuprofen: Advil, Motrin IB, Nuprin, generic ibuprofen, Medipren, Midol IB, and many other products	200
Orudis KT (ketoprofen)	12.5

*enteric-coated

Whether the inflammation is minor or severe, NSAIDs can be very helpful in reducing pain and swelling and sometimes promoting healing, which explains their wide popularity. Yet, like other medications, NSAID molecules go not only to the inflamed tissues, but also to other areas of the body, sometimes provoking unwanted effects. Many people take NSAIDs with no problem, but others develop side effects, some of which can be serious or lethal.

A SIDE-EFFECT-PRONE FAMILY OF DRUGS

Anti-inflammatory drugs account for the most frequently reported adverse drug reactions reported to medical authorities. The incidence of side effects with anti-inflammatory medications approaches 30% to 70% in frequent users. Most side effects are gastrointestinal problems which, quoting *Goodman and Gilman*, "may range from mild dyspepsia and heartburn to ulceration of the stomach or duodenum, sometimes with fatal results."

The medical establishment considers NSAID-related gastrointestinal injury a major medical problem in its own right. Gastrointestinal problems occur three times as often in regular NSAID users as in nonusers, and ulcer risk is increased up to five-fold. The risk of hospitalization for gastrointestinal problems is five times greater in NSAID users than in nonusers.

Moreover, the actual incidence of NSAID-induced side effects may be greater than reported, which is alarming enough. A 1992 study of arthritis patients revealed that gastric pathology was present in 70% of those studied, including people with no obvious symptoms. A 1994 study produced similar findings, yet only 45% of subjects with NSAID-related ulcers experienced any symptoms; 55% with ulcers didn't know they had them. A 1996 study agreed: "A large majority of patients with serious GI [gastrointestinal] complications do not have preceding mild side effects."

This is one of the big problems with NSAIDs—bleeding without pain. You may be taking an NSAID without any obvious problems, then hemorrhage without warning. People taking higher dosages or using NSAIDs for prolonged periods run the greatest risk, and the occasional or short-term use of NSAIDs is generally considered safe—but not absolutely so. As described by *Melmon and Morrelli*: "The onset of bleeding can occur as early as after very few doses." Indeed, the AMA warns that "a few life-threatening reactions have been reported after a single exposure to [NSAIDs]."

Avoiding needless NSAID usage is important for another compelling reason. Once you have developed an intolerance to NSAIDs, you may have difficulty with any future usage of these drugs. As a physical therapist told me, "People who developed stomach problems with NSAIDs ten or fifteen years earlier often have problems when we try to use them again." This doesn't happen in every case, but NSAIDs are important medications in many serious and painful medical conditions—tendinitis, bursitis, and arthritis, for example—and no other drugs serve nearly as well. NSAIDs are drugs you want to be able to use when you truly need them. The best way to ensure this is to use them only when really necessary—and in the very lowest effective dosage.

OTHER NSAID SIDE EFFECTS

Other common NSAID side effects include dizziness, nervousness, kidney damage, rashes, and ringing in the ears (see box on page 330). Numerous other side effects occur at lesser frequencies, but that doesn't make them any less serious. A 1996 journal article reported three cases of infertility associated with NSAID use. And bleeding from areas other than the stomach and intestine can occur from NSAID-related diminished platelet activity; this is especially true with aspirin products.

An example of a so-called mild side effect is mouth ulcers. Caroline, 45 and very healthy, pulled a rib muscle while doing her extensive exercise program. To minimize the pain and inflammation, she started Relafen 500 mg twice a day. Feeling little effect from this dosage and still hampered by her injury, on the third day she increased to 500 mg three times a day. On the next day, she developed a sore on the right side of her tongue that hurt her while she was eating and speaking. The following day, the sore was much worse despite antiseptic mouth rinses and a pain gel, and a new ulcer sprang up inside her lip. The sores were perplexing; she'd never had anything like this before. By the sixth day the sores were even worse and her speech was greatly impaired. This had a great impact on her life because she works with people doing health appraisals for a wellness program.

In the PDR, both glossitis (sore, inflamed tongue) and stomatitis (oral ulcers) are listed as infrequent side effects with Relafen and, indeed, with most NSAIDs. The cause is unknown. These side effects are usually considered mild, but they were anything but mild for Caroline. The sores hurt constantly, greatly impairing her work, and the pain necessitated sleep medication.

Finally it occurred to Caroline that the Relafen had been increased just when the eruptions began. She discontinued the Relafen and the sores disappeared within two days, never to appear again.

Common NSAID Side Effects

Gastrointestinal: Nausea, heartburn, stomach pain, indigestion, vomiting, gastric irritation, gastric or duodenal ulcer, bleeding, hemorrhage, abnormal liver tests. Gastrointestinal side effects are by far the most common NSAID side effects and can be mild or severe.

Cardiovascular: Edema (swelling of feet or other areas)

Skin and membranes: Rash, itching, dry mouth, mouth ulcers

Central nervous system: Headache, dizziness, nervousness, confusion, insomnia, depression, slurred speech, abnormal dreams, seizures

Special senses: Tinnitus (ringing in ears), hearing loss, visual changes

Blood: Increased bleeding tendency (aspirin-like effect inhibiting platelet function by some but not all NSAIDs)

Kidneys: Kidney damage, acute kidney failure

NONPRESCRIPTION NSAIDS— USE THEM JUDICIOUSLY

With the release of several new nonprescription NSAIDs such as Aleve and Orudis KT and their multi-million-dollar advertising campaigns, increased NSAID problems are inevitable. A former athlete I know, age 55, has hip problems that will eventually require hip replacement surgery. In the meantime, he takes Aleve twice a day every day. I asked him if he really needed the drug this often. "Probably not," he replied. "It's just easier to remember this way." And more likely to cause problems, too. In over 90% of studies examining the effects of regular *nonprescription* NSAID usage, gastrointestinal irritation or bleeding was significantly increased. This includes the people who take aspirin daily or every other day, even at tiny doses, for the cardiovascular benefits. In other words, NSAIDs, even in their nonprescription forms, shouldn't be taken lightly or without your being aware of their specific uses and dangers.

Presently, four types of NSAIDs are available on drugstore shelves: Aleve; Orudis KT; generic ibuprofen in Advil, Motrin IB, Nuprin, and many other preparations; and aspirin in its many forms.

Choosing among nonprescription NSAIDs can be confusing because manufacturers have poured hundreds of millions of dollars into advertising intended to sway you to buy their brand. How do you decide when you're told Aleve works longer, Orudis KT is stronger (requiring only 12.5 mg), and Motrin IB and Advil provide more medication (200 mg) per pill? In fact, little scientific data exist comparing nonprescription NSAIDs. Like prescription NSAIDs, the nonprescription products are generally equivalent in their effectiveness. However, whereas Orudis KT and the ibuprofen products are one-half the strength of standard doses of prescription Orudis and Motrin, respectively, Aleve is only slightly lower in dose than prescription Naprosyn (220 mg versus 250 mg). Aleve requires only twice-a-day dosing, which is easier to remember.

Most authorities consider aspirin the most gastric-irritating of all NSAIDs. If you prefer aspirin, it's probably best to use an enteric-coated preparation such as Ecotrin. Unfortunately, none of the other nonprescription NSAIDs are presently available in enteric-coated pills. Still, many people encounter fewer problems with, for example, plain ibuprofen than enteric-coated aspirin.

The important point about nonprescription NSAIDs is that they are quite effective for many people, even some with chronic or severe disorders such as rheumatoid arthritis or osteoarthritis. These drugs, therefore, offer a low-dose alternative to starting with prescription-strength medications. At the same time, you should remember that these drugs, even at nonprescription levels, can cause the same adverse effects as their prescription relatives. This is more likely if you take a nonprescription NSAID at the highest recommended dosage or for prolonged periods, but it can occasionally happen even at the lowest nonprescription doses.

Obviously, therefore, you shouldn't take nonprescription

NSAIDs needlessly. This is exactly what Michael, a repairman, did for months. Michael's pager beeps endlessly as he goes from job to job. Because he is self-employed, many of Michael's days don't end until after seven, and just as many end with headaches. What did Michael take for them? He told me, "I take Motrin all the time." But NSAIDs offer no advantages for noninflammatory pain such as headaches, aches from colds or the flu, muscle tension, or fever. Tylenol (acetaminophen) serves just as well and is generally considered safer. I told Michael to find a way to reduce his stress and in the meantime to try Tylenol, especially because he uses pain medication so often. Not that Tylenol is perfectly benign—it can cause kidney and liver problems—but overall it is considered potentially less harmful than NSAIDs.

At the same time, some people do obtain better pain relief with aspirin or ibuprofen than Tylenol, while others do better with Tylenol. There is a wide degree of interindividual variation. For most people, Tylenol is a better first choice. If you find that an NSAID truly works better, use it only when necessary and in the very lowest effective dosage.

OTHER NSAID USES

One of the acknowledged exceptions to using NSAIDs only for inflammatory conditions is in treating postoperative pain. Studies, most of them involving dental surgery, have shown that Motrin or Voltaren combined with codeine provides superior pain relief than either Tylenol, aspirin, or Motrin, or Tylenol plus codeine. The combined use of an NSAID with codeine appears to provide extra pain relief allowing for the use of lower, less side-effect-prone doses of each drug, particularly codeine.

Other exceptions are menstrual pain and migraine headaches. Studies show NSAIDs to be highly effective for menstrual discomfort. Both Tylenol and NSAIDs can be helpful with migraines; again, individual response varies greatly.

A more serious disorder that may be helped by NSAIDs is Alzheimer's disease. The evidence, although not conclusive, is beginning to mount that long-term NSAID usage (two years or longer) significantly reduces the incidence of Alzheimer's disease.

However, because long-term NSAID usage carries its own dangers and the effect of NSAIDs on Alzheimer's is neither proven nor understood, for now regularly using NSAIDs for this purpose would be premature and risky.

HOW NSAIDS WORK AND WHY THEY CAUSE GASTROINTESTINAL BLEEDING

NSAIDs cause gastrointestinal injury through the very same mechanism by which they reduce inflammation. NSAIDs block prostaglandins, a family of substances that mediate many processes in the human body. One of these processes is the inflammatory reaction. When prostaglandins are blocked, the inflammatory reaction is blunted.

But prostaglandins also play a role in maintaining the integrity of the stomach and duodenal. Prostaglandin 1 (PGE1) is required for the production of the buffers, mucus, and other mechanisms that protect the stomach lining from the hydrochloride acid it secretes in the process of digestion. When NSAIDs are used, PGE1 is reduced as much as 70%, thereby reducing the protective barriers of the stomach and duodenum. Stomach acid penetrates to the lining and causes injury.

PGE1 reduction is a systemic effect of NSAIDs; it occurs after the drug is absorbed into the body, no matter whether it is taken orally, intravenously, or by rectal suppository. That's why enteric-coated NSAIDs, which dissolve in the intestine instead of the stomach, still cause stomach injury. In addition, most NSAIDs are acidic, and unless they're enteric-coated, they directly irritate the gastric surface.

As research continues, new aspects of NSAID-related gastric injury are being uncovered. The process appears to be a complex one in which PGE1 plays a major but not solitary role.

WHICH IS THE BEST NSAID?

Numerous studies have been conducted to try to identify the safest NSAID among the currently available products. Because the various NSAIDs are generally equal in their ability to reduce inflammation, discovering the safest NSAID has long been a principal goal of the medical profession. Hundreds of studies have been conducted comparing an array of NSAIDs against each other in causing side effects, especially gastrointestinal problems, but these studies sometimes have produced differing, even contradictory, findings. A 1996 article in the *American Journal of Orthopedics* summarized it well: "There is a great deal of interpatient variability with respect to response to NSAIDs; it is currently difficult to predict which patient will respond best to which drug."

Overall, many authorities agree that aspirin and Feldene are the NSAIDs that cause the most gastric irritation. Indocin (indomethacin) and Clinoril (sulindac) are also believed to cause more gastric problems, and perhaps Orudis. Toradol is used only in select situations because of other side effects.

There is some evidence that Relafen (nabumetone) may be somewhat less gastric-toxic, but clinical reports have not always borne this out. Voltaren and Lodine also have performed better in some studies. In one analysis of twelve studies involving Motrin compared to other NSAIDs, Motrin caused fewer gastric problems, but this was because it was used at lower dosages. When compared at equivalent dosages, it caused as many problems as other NSAIDs.

When I talked to a number of orthopedists, rheumatologists, and internists, their preference leaned toward some of the newer NSAIDs, extended-release NSAIDs, and enteric-coated NSAIDs. Relafen, Voltaren and Voltaren XR, Oruvail, Naprelan, and EC-Naprosyn, and Daypro were the NSAIDs mentioned most. Recent studies have shown some superiority of some of these preparations, but individual tolerance and variability in response seems to play the largest role.

METHODS OF COUNTERING NSAID GASTROINTESTINAL INJURY

The buffering in some forms of aspirin is rarely sufficient to prevent gastric injury, but for brief therapy it's probably better to take buffered aspirin than plain. NSAIDs are sometimes prescribed with stomach acid-suppressing drugs such as the H2 blockers Zantac, Axid, and Pepcid. Sometimes these drugs are helpful in alleviating NSAID dyspepsia. However, a recent study found that sudden gastric bleeding without warning occurs more often in people using antacids or H2 blockers, so the wisdom of these approaches is now being reexamined. More effective and, so far, less questionable is the use of proton-pump inhibitors such as Prilosec for NSAID-related gastric pain, but even these don't always prevent gastrointestinal injury.

The reason acid-suppressing drugs don't necessarily prevent NSAID gastrointestinal injury is because NSAID-related PGE1 inhibition also reduces the blood flow to the stomach and the first segment of the small intestine, the duodenum. The reduced blood flow appears to be caused by the clumping of white blood cells (specifically, the neutrophils), which become stuck in the small vessels and capillaries. The diminished blood flow impairs the ability of the gastric and duodenal tissues to protect and repair themselves. (A similar mechanism is one of the causes of NSAID-related kidney damage.)

Interestingly, animal studies utilizing cardiac drugs similar to nitroglycerin that dilate the arteries, thereby reestablishing normal blood flow to the tissues, significantly reduced the occurrence of NSAID-caused ulcers. At this time, no studies utilizing this approach in humans have been published, perhaps because drugs that produce arterial dilation also often cause dizziness, lightheadedness, headaches, and other side effects. Research is under way to synthesize NSAIDs that don't diminish normal blood flow to the stomach. If this can be accomplished, it will serve as a breakthrough in solving perhaps the most frequent, pernicious drug side effect in medicine.

Another approach to reducing NSAID side effects has been the development of prostaglandin 1 enhancing drugs to counter NSAID effects on the gastrointestinal system. Currently, Cytotec (misoprostol) is the only PGE1 drug available in the U.S. Studies show that Cytotec does reduce and sometimes prevent the damaging effects of NSAIDs on the stomach and duodenum. However, Cytotec causes frequent side effects, and the manufacturer-recommended dosage is too high for a high percentage of patients. Many physicians find Cytotec more troublesome than helpful, but others claim better results. I know several arthritis sufferers who've found Cytotec extremely helpful, allowing them to stay on their anti-inflammatory medications.

Because NSAIDs are such crucial medications in chronic and often severe diseases such as rheumatoid arthritis, osteoarthritis, and ankylosing spondylitis, the search for a stomach-friendly NSAID has gone on for decades. Finally, several promising avenues are in the works. One area involves drugs known as COX-2 inhibitors. These NSAIDs will not block PGE1 and therefore will not cause gastrointestinal damage, but they will block PGE2, the slightly different prostaglandin that is involved in inhibiting inflammation (by blocking PGE2, NSAIDs block COX, or cyclooxygenase, a tissue-destructive enzyme). In late 1996, meloxicam, a reported PGE2 inhibitor, was released in Europe, but studies show that it does cause gastric injury and may not be significantly superior to current remedies. This may mean that meloxicam isn't a purer PGE2 inhibitor, or that the issue is more complex than we currently know. Other COX-2 inhibitors are under investigation.

Another approach is the development of nitric oxide–reducing NSAIDs, or NO-NSAIDs. In research studies in animals, these NSAIDs do not affect blood flow to the stomach and intestine. In fact, NO-NSAIDs appear to accelerate the healing of gastric damage caused by standard NSAIDs. In one study, healing occurred more quickly with the NO-NSAIDs than by simply stopping the standard NSAID and allowing the tissue to heal itself.

When a truly gastric-friendly NSAID is developed, it will hit the market with as much impact as the breakthrough antidepressant Prozac did in 1988–89. In fact it may have more impact, because many more people take NSAIDs than antidepressants, and NSAIDs cause far more damage. Indeed, as many as 10,000 deaths per year are reportedly caused by NSAIDs. Until a better NSAID is found, every method of reducing NSAID risk should be utilized, including identifying those who are at the greatest risk and using the very lowest effective NSAID dosages.

AVOIDING NSAID SIDE EFFECTS: WHO'S AT RISK?

The best way to deal with NSAID side effects is to avoid using them. First and foremost, don't use NSAIDs, including aspirin, unless they are specifically warranted. Don't use them for fever, the flu, or simple aches and pains unless Tylenol or generic acetaminophen doesn't work for you. The AMA agrees: "If no anti-inflammatory activity is required, acetaminophen is preferred."

Be sure to check every pain, headache, cold, flu, allergy, sleep, menstrual discomfort, or other nonprescription remedy you buy. Many of them contain aspirin or ibuprofen, often unnecessarily. Believe it or not, some forms of Alka-Seltzer contain aspirin.

If NSAIDs are required and you are over 60 years old, your risk of NSAID-related side effects is increased. One reason may be that elderly individuals produce less PGE1, the gastric protective prostaglandin. NSAIDs suppress PGE1, and if you have less to begin with, your gastric-protective mechanisms will be even further diminished. Also, older individuals metabolize medications more slowly than the young, resulting in higher and more prolonged blood concentrations of NSAIDs. That's why many authorities recommend starting with lower NSAID doses in the elderly. Starting with nonprescription NSAIDs may make sense in many cases.

If you are female, you may be more at risk with NSAIDs. The data isn't unequivocal, and if indeed a greater risk exists, it may be because women experience a higher rate of rheumatoid arthritis and other autoimmune diseases that often require prolonged NSAID therapy. Nevertheless, after accounting for these factors, women truly may be more vulnerable to NSAID side effects than men. If this is so, it may be because NSAIDs are usually prescribed at the same dosages for women as for men. Yet women are generally smaller than men, and therefore may be receiving relatively higher dosages, pound for pound. The incidence of most NSAID side effects is directly related to dosage. Again, depending on the nature and severity of your disorder, starting with dosages lower than recommended for prescription and nonprescription NSAIDs may be advisable if you are female, especially if you are medication-sensitive.

Frequent alcohol usage, which causes stomach irritation, can predispose to NSAID gastrointestinal injury. Smoking may also be a risk factor. Reducing alcohol consumption and stopping smoking will improve the health of the gastrointestinal system and help it to better resist NSAID injury.

If you have a chronic illness, especially one that causes substantial pain or disability and requires prolonged NSAID therapy, your risk of side effects is substantially increased. Although NSAID side effects can occur in anyone at any time, long-term usage decidedly increases the odds for gastric and other problems. Because of the greatly increased risk in this group, some authorities recommend using Cytotec from the outset with NSAIDs in cases that are likely to be long-term.

If you have liver or kidney disease, NSAIDs must be used cautiously and begun at lower doses. Many NSAIDs are metabolized by the liver, and NSAIDs have been shown to cause kidney injury and failure.

Mixing NSAIDs with other gastric-irritating drugs, such as cortisone or alcohol, substantially increases the risk of gastrointestinal problems. An increased risk of internal bleeding is also associated with the use of blood thinners (anticoagulants such as Coumadin) with NSAIDs. If possible, these medications should be discontinued or reduced when commencing NSAID therapy. Many people don't realize that aspirin is an NSAID, and mixing aspirin with Anacin or Excedrin or Motrin IB or Aleve or a prescription NSAID produces a combination that can readily cause gastric damage.

If you've had previous problems with NSAIDs, your risk is greater. You may do better by starting with a lower dose or trying a different NSAID.

If you have or have previously had gastric problems such as gastritis, esophagitis, or ulcers, you are a likely candidate for NSAID-produced gastrointestinal problems. If possible, the ulcer or gastritis should be treated before starting NSAIDs. You should also be checked for *Helicobacter pylori*, the bacteria now believed responsible for the majority of cases of ulcers and perhaps gastritis (see Chapter 10).

Helicobacter may increase the risk and/or the severity of NSAID-related gastrointestinal problems. Studies on this issue vary in their conclusions. However, although many people carry Helicobacter without any apparent problem, we know that Helicobacter does indeed cause severe gastrointestinal damage in others. We also know that NSAIDs reduce the natural protective barriers and normal blood flow of the stomach and duodenum, as well as alter white blood cell activity, thereby blunting the body's defense against infection. These NSAID effects certainly seem like an invitation for Helicobacter invasion in at least some people. As one journal article put it: "It is estimated that between 25% and 40% of all NSAID users and 30–50% of elderly patients taking NSAIDs could be infected with *H. pylori* and, as a result, are at special risk of developing peptic ulcers."

If you have stomach problems and Helicobacter is found, it may be wise to treat the Helicobacter before using NSAIDs. If you have stomach problems and Helicobacter isn't found, Cytotec or perhaps Prilosec should be considered when starting NSAID therapy.

In summary, factors that should be considered before starting NSAID therapy include size, age, gender, the nature and severity of your illness, preexisting liver or kidney disease, alcohol consumption and perhaps smoking, a history of abdominal problems such as gastritis or ulcers, previous problems with NSAIDs, other concurrent medications, and indications of the presence of *Helicobacter pylori*. Addressing these problems *before* NSAID problems begin is the ideal approach.

AVOIDING NSAID SIDE EFFECTS: THE IMPORTANCE OF LOWER DOSES

Perhaps the greatest risk factor in using NSAIDs is dosage. Nearly all NSAID side effects, including their sometimes severe and fatal effects on the gastrointestinal system, are dose related. This is why nearly every medical authority recommends using the very lowest dose of NSAIDs that is effective for each patient.

The problem is that most NSAID producers recommend only a narrow range of doses for a very diverse general population. A few NSAIDs are recommended at a one-size-fits-all dosage. A 250-pound football player and a 100-pound, 57-year-old woman may be started at the very same dosage of the same NSAID. This makes no sense. Neither does the fact that most NSAIDs come with no guidelines for specific lower dosages for the elderly.

The rationale for such limited dose recommendations, despite what we know about the wide range of interindividual variation, is articulated in the PDR guidelines for Voltaren: "the recommended strategy for initiating therapy is to use a starting dose likely to be effective for the majority of patients and to adjust dosage thereafter based on observation of diclofenac's beneficial and adverse effects.'' But if you're not in the majority, you're out of luck. The ''dose for the majority'' may well be overmedication for you. The way you find out is by getting side effects.

This was the case with Ella, who was 35 when she was diagnosed with rheumatoid arthritis in 1980. After she had experienced side effects with several anti-inflammatory drugs, her doctor prescribed Voltaren (diclofenac). The pills were 50 mg, and the instructions were to take one pill three times a day, the standard approach for her disease. For Ella, the first pill was too much.

''I felt wired,'' she recalled, the memory still vivid. ''It was as if all of my muscles were quivering, like bugs crawling around inside. It wasn't visible, my hands weren't shaking—it was just a terrible feeling, like I was going out of my skin.''

The reaction kept Ella awake all night. Unable to believe that one pill could affect her so, she tried the Voltaren again the next morning with the same result. Months later, after she had encountered difficulties with other NSAIDs, her doctor, doubting her first experience with Voltaren, encouraged her to try it again. Her reaction was a repeat of the first two times.

Her doctor's perplexity is understandable. The recommended dosage of Voltaren for treating rheumatoid arthritis is 150 to 200 mg a day—for everyone. He'd prescribed the medication correctly according to the information in the PDR—but not according to the individual nature of his patient.

As with all medications, interindividual variation can be considerable with NSAIDs. Most absurd about Ella's case is that Voltaren also comes in a 25-mg pill, but her doctor never considered trying this lower, less side-effect-prone dose despite Ella's repeated problems with the 50-mg pill. Why didn't he? Because many physicians tend to follow the standard guidelines without appreciating that lower doses can be very effective and much safer for many people—even when the situation makes it obvious. And Ella's doctor's job wasn't made any easier by the fact that the abundant data on the effectiveness of Voltaren at dosages of 50 and 75 mg a day, a third to half of the manufacturer recommended dosage, are not included in the PDR or other standard medical references.

If you are medication-sensitive, you should begin with an NSAID that you can start at lower doses and use flexibly. Some

NSAIDs are produced in only one size, but others come in a variety of pill sizes and/or breakable tablets.

The availability of a few nonprescription NSAIDs provides further opportunity for flexible, low-dose treatment. For example, the PDR recommends 400 mg as the standard initial dose of Motrin for most inflammatory conditions, and that's the dose that many physicians prescribe. But the 200-mg dose of ibuprofen was proven effective and used in Europe beginning in the 1960s, almost a decade before Motrin was introduced in the U.S. at higher prescription doses. A tablet of 200 mg is the nonprescription size of Motrin IB, Advil, Nuprin, and generic ibuprofen, and one tablet is quite enough for many people. "One Mutrin IB works fine for me," a woman told me. "If I take two [400mg], my stomach hurts and my ears ring." As one doctor told me, "I often tell my patients to start with a nonprescription NSAID. We can always raise the dose if needed."

Starting with a nonprescription-strength anti-inflammatory drug makes sense if you are medication-sensitive, elderly, or your inflammatory condition isn't severe. Some physicians are quite willing to suggest nonprescription NSAIDs in appropriate cases, but others may hesitate because patients sometimes get annoyed at the idea of paying for a doctor's visit only to be told to take a drug they could have bought at the drugstore. But if you raise the issue of starting at a nonprescription dose, you'll find that many doctors are open to discussing it.

If you start with a nonprescription NSAID or a lower than usual dosage of a prescription NSAID and you don't obtain a sufficient response, you can still use the lower dose pills to gradually increase your dosage rather than jumping 50% to 100% as often recommended in the PDR. Gradual upward titration of dosage allows you to arrive at the lowest effective dosage of medication necessary for your condition, a key to minimizing NSAID side effects.

DIFFERENT PEOPLE, DIFFERENT NSAIDS

Studies show that all NSAIDs are fairly similar in their ability to reduce inflammation. And all cause side effects. But when it comes to the individual, differences in response and adverse reactions are common.

A 65-year-old woman who developed a mild case of rheumatoid arthritis experienced severe stomach pain with Disalcid, a supposedly stomach-friendly aspirin derivative, but she has had no difficulty with Lodine.

A doctor I know developed tennis elbow. In the past he always used Motrin with good effect and no side effects. But a drug company sales representative had just given him some samples of a supposedly newer, better NSAID, Meclomen. He took one and became nauseated and vomited fifteen minutes later. He went back to Motrin and his tennis elbow improved without further problems.

Another doctor finds that Motrin makes him depressed, but he doesn't have that problem with other NSAIDs.

Interindividual variation is also reflected in the duration of effect of NSAIDs. For example, the pain-relieving effect of 200 to 400 mg of Lodine usually lasts four to six hours, but lasts eight to twelve hours in some people. Such variability is not uncommon and may allow for less frequent dosing, less overall medication, and therefore less risk of side effects.

In other words, different people can respond very differently to different NSAIDs. *Goodman and Gilman* note: "Large variations are possible in the response of individuals to different aspirin-like drugs [NSAIDs], even when they are closely allied members of the same chemical family. Thus, a patient may do well on one but not on another."

If you have side effects with a particular NSAID even at a low dosage, switch to another and try again. The advice of your physician may be very helpful. Most physicians have learned through trial and error which NSAIDs cause their patients the least difficulty.

NONACIDIC, ENTERIC-COATED, AND EXTENDED-RELEASE NSAIDS

Most NSAIDs cause direct irritation to the stomach, but there are a few exceptions. One of the newest NSAIDs, Relafen, reportedly causes little if any gastric irritation because unlike other NSAIDs, it isn't acidic and doesn't cause direct irritation to the stomach lining. For this reason, Relafen has been touted as safer than other NSAIDs. But Relafen ultimately exerts the same systemic NSAID effects, including PGE1 suppression and gastrointestinal injury. Clinically, some physicians feel they've had fewer problems with Relafen, but others are less convinced of Relafen's superiority over other NSAIDs.

Voltaren was one of the first NSAIDs to be manufactured as an enteric-coated pill. Several people have told me that after getting heartburn or stomach pain with other NSAIDs, they had no such problems with Voltaren. That's because Voltaren's enteric coating prevents it from dissolving in the acidic environment of the stomach, thereby avoiding direct gastric injury. Ecotrin, an enteric-coated aspirin, and EC-Naprosyn work similarly.

Several recent additions to the NSAID group include extended-release Lodine XL, Naprelan, Oruvail, and Voltaren XR. These preparations dissolve slowly and usually last twenty-four hours, allowing for a once-daily dosage, which is easy to remember. In addition to convenience, little or none of these drugs is released in the stomach; instead they dissolve mostly in the intestine. Much of the gastrointestinal injury caused by NSAIDs is due to direct irritation of the lining of the stomach and duodenum, but all NSAIDs also can cause gastric damage via their systemic effects, especially when used frequently or for prolonged periods.

Interestingly, if you are taking stomach-acid-suppressing drugs such as Zantac, Axid, Pepcid, Tagamet, Prilosec, or Prevacid, your stomach will be less acidic. Because enteric-coated and extended-release NSAIDs are designed to dissolve in the less acidic environment of the intestine, when combined with these acid-suppressing drugs, these NSAIDs may dissolve in the stomach, thus negating their purpose. Taking antacids at the same time as enteric-coated or extended-release NSAIDs may have the same undesirable effect.

The results of studies vary, but some indicate that enteric-coated or extended-release preparations may offer some advantage over standard NSAIDs, and the many favorable reports from patients are difficult to dismiss. Many of the physicians I asked were convinced that their patients experience less gastric irritation with these drugs. If you are medication-sensitive, have a sensitive stomach or have encountered NSAID gastric irritation previously, or you have a condition that will require the long-term use of NSAIDs, you may fare better with Relafen, an enteric-coated, or an extended-release NSAID.

SHORT-ACTING OR LONG-ACTING NSAIDS?

NSAIDs may be short-acting, such as four-times-a-day Motrin, or long-acting, such as once-a-day Relafen and Oruvail, or somewhere in between, such as twice-a-day Naprosyn or three-times-a-day Voltaren.

Once-a-day drugs are easier to remember. Once-a-day drugs may produce a more consistent, continuous medication effect than the peaks and valleys in blood levels seen with three- or four-times-a-day remedies. Once-a-day NSAIDs also may expose the stomach to direct NSAID irritation only once daily rather than repeatedly. Once-daily enteric-coated or extended-release drugs cause little direct gastric irritation. Yet all once-daily NSAIDs still can cause gastrointestinal damage through their systemic effects.

A disadvantage of once-a-day NSAIDs is that if a side effect develops, it will continue longer than with a short-acting NSAIDs. Once-a-day NSAIDs have long half-lives, meaning that they may build up in the systems of slow metabolizers or elderly individuals. Nevertheless, once-a-day NSAIDs are quite popular, and the success of Relafen, Daypro, and Oruvail has led other manufacturers to repackage older, shorter-acting NSAIDs into new, once-a-day, extended-release drugs such as Naprelan (Naprosyn) and Voltaren-XR.

The advantage of multiple dose drugs is that you can manage and adjust them more readily. If side effects occur, they will wear off more quickly and you can reduce the dose or discontinue the drug sooner. Their disadvantages are having to remember to take them repeatedly and subjecting the stomach to their irritating effects more often. Also, the blood level of these drugs is subject to more frequent peaks and valleys that may influence the medication effect. Studies show that people taking multidose drugs forget their medications more often than those on once-a-day remedies.

Generally, all NSAIDs are equally effective in reducing inflammation, so whether you choose a long-acting or short-acting drug isn't critical as long as you receive an adequate but not excessive amount of medication. The most important issue is finding an NSAID that works for you without provoking side effects.

NSAIDS AND THE ELDERLY

Because arthritis and other inflammatory conditions are the most frequent cause of physical limitation and disability in the elderly, NSAIDs are frequently prescribed to older individuals. A 1991 study found: "Patients over the age of 65 comprise about 12% of the U.S. population but consume 25% of all prescription medications and 40% of NSAIDs."

Unfortunately, the elderly are particularly vulnerable to NSAID side effects. They are more susceptible to NSAID-related ulcers and at greater risk for painless sudden bleeding. By one account, NSAIDs cause over 40,000 hospitalizations and 3,300 deaths annually due to ulcers in the elderly. As explained above, this is due to reduced levels of gastric PGE1, the protective prostaglandin, and a reduced ability to metabolize drugs that may lead to higher NSAID blood concentrations and increased side effects. This is why some authorities recommend short-acting NSAIDs which aren't as likely to build up and cause problems.

Lower doses work well for many elderly individuals. As a physician specializing in women's medicine told me: "I've got a lot of elderly patients who insist that nonprescription Motrin helps their arthritis. I believe them."

RECOMMENDATIONS

NSAIDs are extremely useful medications for the treatment of inflammatory conditions such as tendinitis, bursitis, and many types of arthritis. For these types of diseases, NSAIDs are unrivaled by any other group of drugs.

Despite massive advertising to the contrary, NSAIDs are not the first choice for noninflammatory problems such as simple pain, headaches, muscle aches, sinus pain, the discomfort of a cold or the flu, or fever. Tylenol (acetaminophen) is generally considered an equally effective and much safer choice.

NSAIDs provide benefit to tens of millions of Americans each year, but side effects, especially with high dosages or prolonged usage, can be severe and sometimes fatal. Gastric irritation, ulcers, gastrointestinal hemorrhage, and kidney failure occur with sufficient frequency to make NSAID side effects a recognized medical condition in their own right. These and most other NSAID side effects are directly related to dosage and duration of NSAID usage.

Therefore, for all but the most acute conditions, you should start NSAID therapy at a low dosage and adjust the dose gradually, if necessary, according to your response. Fortunately, many prescription NSAIDs are produced in breakable or smaller dose pills. Nonprescription NSAIDs offer additional low-dose alternatives.

Virtually every medical reference stresses the need to individualize NSAID treatment and to use the lowest effective NSAID dosage, yet most then simply offer the same narrow initial dosages suggested by drug manufacturers. Although many NSAIDs have been shown to be effective at lower dosages, most medical references contain little or none of this information. Consequently, some physicians simply follow the manufacturers' recommendations, prescribing similar dosages to all patients regardless of size, age, or medication sensitivity. Other physicians are more flexible and willing to begin with lower than recommended prescription doses or even nonprescription strengths, especially if you indicate a preference for low-dose therapy.

In addition to the variations in NSAID dosages required by different individuals, if you are medication-sensitive, you may find that a specific medication may last longer than the norm. The pain-relieving effect of aspirin lasts four hours in some people, six or more in others. Pain relief with Lodine usually lasts four to six hours, but up to ten to twelve hours in some.

If you are elderly, you may be especially sensitive to NSAID effects and side effects. Few manufacturers offer specific low-dose regimens for older individuals, but many medical authorities recommend starting with substantially lower doses.

Selecting an NSAID can be confusing because of the many choices: NSAIDs that are taken once, twice, three, or four times a day; enteric-coated NSAIDs; extended-release NSAIDs; nonprescription NSAIDs. Handling NSAID gastrointestinal irritation can also be complicated. Because NSAIDs are prescribed frequently, many physicians are well informed about the different types of NSAIDs and dealing with NSAID problems. Yet differences in opinion and approach exist, and only some physicians are aware of the effectiveness of lower NSAID dosages in medication-sensitive individuals.

If you require NSAID therapy, especially if you may need long-term treatment because of a chronic condition such as arthritis, you should be sure to work with a physician who will take the time to discuss the various choices, dosages, and dangers with NSAIDs. Preventing NSAID problems, especially gastrointestinal injury, is key, because once these problems begin, they can be difficult to control and sometimes dangerous, even fatal. Working to find the NSAID that works best for you at the lowest dosage, and therefore with the lowest risk of side effects, is worth the effort.

In-Depth Analysis: Motrin (Ibuprofen) Including Nonprescription Forms of Ibuprofen

Judy has had back problems for thirty years, since she was injured in a car accident in her teens. Over the years, she's seen a horde of specialists, tried all kinds of treatments, exercises, heat, ice, and about a dozen mattresses, yet her back still tightens and goes into spasms during the night, often awakening her with pain. What has helped her the most is one 200-mg Motrin IB, a non-prescription NSAID, just before bedtime.

Motrin (ibuprofen) was the first NSAID released in the United States. In its first years on the market, the PDR-recommended initial dose was 300 to 400 mg, three or four times a day as needed. Today, the recommended initial dose for pain is 400 mg every four to six hours; for arthritis, a total daily dosage of 1,200 to 3,200 mg a day using 300-, 400-, 600-, or 800-mg pills up to four times a day. Possible side effects of Motrin are listed on page 330.

Judy was wise to first try an anti-inflammatory drug at a low, nonprescription dose, because even this mild dose causes her some nausea. If she had gone to her physician and received a prescription dose, most likely 400 mg, her nausea would have been worse, and she may have had stomach pain or vomited. The reaction might have made her give up on the medication and continue to awaken with back spasms.

Instead, with low-dose Motrin IB Judy has had good results despite the mild nausea. But Judy was lucky; her timing was right. During its first decade on the American market, Motrin was available by prescription only, and there was no 200-mg Motrin IB. Why? That's a good question, especially since 200-mg Motrin had been established as an effective dose long before Motrin was approved by the FDA at higher doses.

IMPRESSIVE RESULTS FROM A LOWER DOSE OF MOTRIN

When Motrin was released in the United States in 1974 at higher prescription doses, numerous studies in Europe had already appeared in the medical literature establishing the effectiveness of low-dose Motrin. Yet when Motrin was approved here, a 200-mg pill wasn't offered and none of the data on its effectiveness was included in the PDR.

Even today, Motrin's PDR dosage guidelines still direct doctors to initiate treatment at the 100%-higher 400-mg dose, every four to six hours—that is 1600 to 2400 mg a day. There's not a word about the effectiveness of as little as 200 mg three times a day—only 600 mg a day.

Research also demonstrated the effectiveness of 300 mg of Motrin. Although this dose was initially recommended by the manufacturer, it's rarely prescribed. An industry insider told me, "Hardly anyone ever orders Motrin 300-mg tablets. Instead most doctors just prescribe 400 mg, 600 mg, or 800 mg." Indeed, a local pharmacist wasn't even aware that a 300-mg dose existed, explaining, "Since we never get any prescriptions for it, I assumed it didn't exist."

200-mg Motrin IB, Advil, Nuprin, Midol IB, and generic ibuprofen can be bought off the shelf. 300-mg Motrin requires a prescription, but it's still 33% lower than the standard 400-mg initial dose.

MOTRIN AND THE ELDERLY

If you are over 60, you metabolize Motrin (and other drugs) more slowly than younger adults. This leads to higher and more prolonged blood levels of Motrin. In addition, you may be more sensitive to the effects of Motrin and other NSAIDS, as well as more susceptible to their side effects. This is particularly true of gastrointestinal problems such as heartburn, gastritis, ulcers, hemorrhage, and kidney problems such as renal failure. For the elderly, many authorities recommend starting Motrin and other NSAIDs at dosages lower than those recommended in the PDR, which offers no specific geriatric dosages. Many older individuals obtain a sufficient response with the nonprescription dose of Motrin.

APPLYING GRADUAL, LOW-DOSE METHODS FOR ALL DOSAGE REQUIREMENTS

Prescription Motrin is no longer available as an adult-size brand-name product. However, generic ibuprofen continues to be produced by several manufacturers in 300-, 400-, 600-, and 800-mg sizes. Some are scored or breakable, others aren't. Brand-name Motrin is available in nonprescription children's size tablets of 50 and 100 mg, and a liquid containing 100 mg per teaspoon; these are generally available generically as well. And of course, Motrin IB, Advil, Nuprin, and many other forms of ibuprofen are available in the popular 200-mg nonprescription adult dose.

If you use various combinations of 100, 200, 300, 400, 500, 600, 700, and 800 mg, as well as in-between doses utilizing the 50 mg children's tablet, doses can be fashioned to fit your individual requirement without taking more medication than you need. Most Motrin side effects, including irritation or ulceration of the gastrointestinal tract, are usually related to dosage, so you should take the minimum dose necessary to treat your disorder.

RECOMMENDATIONS

Brand-name Motrin is no longer a top-selling prescription drug because it is readily available and much cheaper as generic ibuprofen, which itself ranks among the most prescribed drugs in America. In addition, the nonprescription forms of ibuprofen, which include generic ibuprofen, Motrin IB, Advil, Nuprin, and others, are taken by millions. Overall, Motrin/ibuprofen is probably still the most used NSAID in the U.S.

If you are medication-sensitive, elderly, small, taking other medications, or otherwise at risk for NSAID side effects, you should be aware that most Motrin side effects, including gastrointestinal problems such as stomach pain, ulcers, and internal bleeding, are often directly related to the dosage and duration of medication treatment. Depending on your disease, you should start with a low Motrin dosage. A nonprescription dose of 200 mg is available as Motrin IB, Advil, Nuprin, generic ibuprofen, and other products. Even lower doses are available in children's size preparations.

Even if you're not medication-sensitive or otherwise at risk for Motrin's side effects, you may find that nonprescription Motrin is sufficient for your needs. If not, you can gradually increase to an effective dosage instead of jumping to 400, 600, and 800 mg as many physicians prescribe. Ask your physician. Because of the frequency of NSAID side effects, use the very lowest dosage necessary to treat your disease.

This is especially true if you will be taking Motrin for more than a week or two. NSAID side effects are extremely common in people with conditions such as arthritis that require long-term NSAID therapy. Indeed, some physicians start such patients on Cytotec at the same time they prescribe Motrin or other NSAIDs. If you have a higher risk of developing NSAID side effects, you may want to consider Cytotec or the other protective measures discussed earlier.

In-Depth Analysis: Voltaren and Voltaren-XR (Diclofenac)

Unlike Motrin, you need a doctor's prescription to get any dose of Voltaren. This means that although the manufacturer-recommended dosages of Voltaren may be unnecessarily high for medication-sensitive individuals, you won't be able to get around this problem by buying Voltaren in a lower, safer, nonprescription dosage, because it doesn't exist.

Perhaps a nonprescription form of Voltaren will appear on drugstore shelves in the near future. This would be good because some people who've had gastric irritation with other NSAIDs have told me they've done well with Voltaren. That's because Voltaren is enteric-coated, so it dissolves in the intestine instead of the stomach, where many NSAIDs cause direct gastric irritation. Voltaren still has the same systemic tendency as other NSAIDs to cause gastrointestinal problems, but the enteric coating does seem to help some individuals.

Voltaren is a popular drug. According to the manufacturer, Voltaren was the No. 1 selling NSAID worldwide from 1982 to 1993. Six million prescriptions were written for Voltaren in the United States in 1992. In 1995 Voltaren ranked No. 84 on the 1995 list of top-selling drugs based on U.S. In 1996, when it became available as generic diclofenac, Voltaren dropped from the top 200 prescribed drugs, but diclofenac remained on the list. Voltaren is produced in 25-, 50-, and 75-mg enteric-coated tablets.

Voltaren is officially approved for treating osteoarthritis rheumatoid arthritis, and ankylosing spondylitis, but it is also frequently prescribed for tendinitis, bursitis, and other inflammatory conditions and pain syndromes. Possible side effects of Voltaren are listed on page 330.

IMPRESSIVE FINDINGS WITH A LOWER DOSE OF VOLTAREN

The manufacturer-recommended dosages of Voltaren range from 100 to 150 mg a day for osteoarthritis (the degenerative arthritis of injury or aging) to 150 to 200 mg a day for rheumatoid arthritis (an autoimmune disorder). Yet back in the 1970s and early 1980s, when the pre-release clinical trials of Voltaren were performed, 75 mg a day was the dosage tested in many studies, some extending over several years. The 75 mg a day Voltaren dosage was highly and significantly effective in these studies, and in one study 50 mg a day was effective.

Despite these findings, Voltaren is recommended at dosages of 100 to 200 mg a day for everyone. In the introduction to this chapter, I related the experience of Ella, a 35-year-old woman with rheumatoid arthritis. After she had experienced problems with other NSAIDs (a tip-off that she was sensitive to this group of drugs), her physician prescribed Voltaren at the standard initial dosage for rheumatoid arthritis of 150 mg a day. The first 50-mg pill she took caused profound side effects. Both Ella and her physician found her reaction hard to believe, but when she was given this dose another two times, her body again reacted.

Unfortunately, no one thought about simply trying a lower dose; Voltaren is produced in 25-mg pills. Why didn't Ella's physician consider this? Because there's no information in the PDR or in any other drug reference I've seen that mentions the effectiveness of low-dose Voltaren. Thus, few if any physicians are aware that Voltaren can be very effective at 50 to 75 mg a day.

As this case demonstrates, the range of interindividual variation with NSAIDs is wide. In fact, Voltaren's manufacturer agrees: "Diclofenac [Voltaren], like other NSAIDs, shows interindividual differences in both pharmacokinetics [actions within the body] and clinical response." A narrow range of dosages such as Voltaren's recommended 150 to 200 mg a day for all rheumatoid arthritis sufferers must be questioned, especially in light of the many studies demonstrating up to 80% of subjects deriving benefit for arthritis, tendinitis, and bursitis at doses of 75 mg a day.

A LOW-DOSE METHOD IGNORED

From 1987 through 1990, five papers were published addressing the heightened effectiveness of Voltaren when combined with B-vitamins in treating various types of pain. In a 1990 article, the authors note that although NSAIDs are effective in treating spinal pain, side effects are frequent and "a reduction of dosage would be to the patient's benefit." Citing studies demonstrating the enhanced effect of Voltaren when combined with vitamins B_1, B_6, and B_{12}, the authors tested the effectiveness of using lower doses of Voltaren with these vitamins. Their conclusions: "The results document the positive influence that B-vitamins contribute by . . . shortening the treatment time and reducing daily NSAID-dosage."

An elegant, simple, and cheap approach. Most of all, it allowed a reduction in dosage of NSAIDs, thus reducing the risk of side effects. Yet nowhere in my readings of medical references have I seen these studies mentioned.

VOLTAREN AND THE ELDERLY

If you are elderly, you metabolize drugs more slowly than younger adults. This means blood levels of the drug will be higher and more prolonged than usual—and for you there will be an increased risk of side effects.

In addition, elderly individuals are sometimes more sensitive to the effects of NSAIDs, so they don't require as large a dosage as younger people do. Nevertheless, the manufacturer's dosage guidelines for Voltaren in its package insert and PDR description contain no specific lower dosages for the elderly.

To reduce the risk of side effects with Voltaren, ask your physician to start with the 25-mg tablet, using it twice or three times a day, depending on your response. If this dose is insufficient, it can gradually be raised to a dosage that works. Because elderly individuals are at the greatest risk of NSAID-caused ulcers and bleeding, as well as fatalities, using the very lowest effective dosage of Voltaren and other NSAIDs is mandatory.

VOLTAREN-XR

Voltaren-XR is an extended-release preparation containing 100 mg of Voltaren. Over the last decade, once-a-day drugs have gained popularity with physicians and some patients because of the ease of usage. Because most of the medication dissolves in the intestine instead of the stomach, extended-release NSAIDs may cause somewhat less gastric irritation than standard NSAIDs. This is another reason that some physicians favor extended-release NSAIDs, enteric-coated NSAIDs, and Relafen. However, due to their systemic effects, gastric irritation and other typical NSAID side effects can still occur with Voltaren XR and similar preparations.

The difference between Voltaren and Voltaren-XR is simply ease of usage. Voltaren-XR is usually required just once daily, although in severe cases it may be used twice a day. Regular Voltaren is typically a three-times-a-day medication, and because it's manufactured in several sizes, it can be used more flexibly than Voltaren XR.

Nevertheless, Voltaren-XR, because of its prolonged effect and ease of usage, has become a favorite of some physicians. It is particularly useful for people with chronic arthritis or other painful conditions that require ongoing NSAID therapy. As one rheumatology nurse told me, ''Voltaren-XR is probably our most used drug.''

RECOMMENDATIONS

Multiple studies have demonstrated the effectiveness of Voltaren in dosages far lower than those recommended by the manufacturer and prescribed by doctors. Whereas patients are usually started on Voltaren at 50 mg twice or three times a day, doses of 25 mg twice or three times a day were effective in many pre-release studies.

If you are medication-sensitive, elderly, small, taking other medications, or otherwise at risk for NSAID side effects, you should be aware that most Voltaren side effects, including gastrointestinal problems such as stomach pain, ulcers, and internal bleeding, are directly related to the dosage and duration of Voltaren therapy. Depending on your disease, you should start with the very lowest effective Voltaren dosage. Discuss this with your physician.

Even if you're not medication-sensitive, but you want to use the lowest, safest dose of Voltaren, ask your physician to prescribe the 25-mg tablets. These will provide the flexibility you require to establish the dosage that's best for you. If you ultimately require doses of 100 mg a day or more, Voltaren-XR may be a convenient alternative.

If you may require Voltaren on a long-term basis, such as for arthritis, especially if you have had previous problems with NSAIDs or otherwise are at greater risk for NSAID side effects, you may want to discuss using protective medications such as Cytotec or Prilosec with Voltaren.

In-Depth Analysis: Orudis, Oruvail, and Orudis KT (Ketoprofen)

Orudis is generally considered equivalent to other NSAIDs in terms of efficacy and side effects, although in some studies ketoprofen actually caused more gastrointestinal problems than some other NSAIDs. "Many of my patients have had difficulty with Orudis," a rheumatologist told me.

"But," she added, "Oruvail is another story. So far, not a single patient I've prescribed it to has developed any gastrointestinal problems." Oruvail is an extended-release form of Orudis that dissolves in the intestine rather than in the acidic environment of the stomach. Oruvail causes less direct gastric irritation, although it may still produce gastrointestinal injury through its systemic effects. Still, Oruvail, like many of the newer enteric-coated and extended-release NSAIDs, appears to cause substantially fewer gastrointestinal side effects for many people.

Because of Oruvail's extended-release mechanism, it may also provide a more steady level of action. This explains why Oruvail has become one of the preferred NSAIDs among the physicians I surveyed. They aren't alone: in 1996 Oruvail ranked among the 200 most prescribed outpatient drugs.

MANUFACTURER-RECOMMENDED DOSAGES

The manufacturer-recommended initial dosage of Orudis for arthritis is 200 to 225 mg a day—50 mg four times a day or 75 mg three times a day. For Oruvail, 200 mg once daily. For menstrual pain, 25 to 50 mg of Orudis every six to eight hours. Maximum daily dosage: Orudis, 300 mg a day; Oruvail, 200 mg a day. Lower doses are suggested for small, elderly, or debilitated people. Orudis and Oruvail are offered in multiple pill sizes: 25-, 50-, and 75-mg Orudis capsules; 100-, 150-, and 200-mg Oruvail capsules. Possible side effects of this drug are listed on page 330.

LOW-DOSE ORUDIS AND ORUVAIL

Orudis' package insert and PDR description note that for pain relief, "Doses of 25 mg were superior to placebo. Doses larger than 25 mg generally could not be shown to the significantly more effective." Larger doses sometimes worked faster or lasted longer, but if you take 25 mg four times a day or even up to six times daily (every four hours), you will still be using only 100 to 150 mg a day.

With Oruvail, the manufacturer-recommended initial dose is 200 mg a day for arthritis. However, if you are small, elderly, medication-sensitive, or have had previous problems with NSAIDs, you may want to start with the smallest Oruvail pill, 100 mg. Oruvail 100 mg is the equivalent of 25 mg of Orudis four times a day. Although Oruvail may take a little longer to reach its peak effect, it will maintain its effect far longer. For some, 100 mg of Oruvail may last twenty-four hours, but others may need higher doses. Oruvail also comes in 150- and 200-mg sizes, so you can gradually increase your dosage according to your response.

Timing of the dosage is important if your pain is greater at a particular time of day. For example, if you have rheumatoid arthritis, your pain and stiffness may be greatest upon awakening. To obtain the maximum effect of Oruvail in the morning, you should take Oruvail with dinner or before bedtime with a snack.

If your pain is fairly constant and Oruvail 100 or 150 once

daily doesn't furnish adequate relief, Oruvail 100 mg twice a day may provide a more constant level of action than a single dose of 200 mg.

NONPRESCRIPTION ORUDIS KT

Another low-dose alternative is to use nonprescription Orudis KT, which contains 12.5 mg of ketoprofen. However, in comparison with other nonprescription NSAIDs such as Motrin IB and Aleve, Orudis KT offers no particular advantages, and some authorities believe that Orudis is more prone to causing gastric irritation than its competitors.

ORUDIS AND ORUVAIL AND THE ELDERLY

The Orudis package insert also mentions that blood levels of the drug are higher and remain longer in elderly individuals. The increases are even greater in women than men. Although the manufacturer does not recommend specific lower initial doses for elderly persons, its suggestion to start with lower doses makes sense. A dosage of 25 mg of Orudis two or three times a day, or 100 mg of Oruvail, may be adequate for many elderly people.

Again, as a group the elderly appear to be more prone to NSAID-related side effects, including silent gastric ulcers and spontaneous hemorrhaging, than younger adults. Therefore, using the very lowest effective NSAID dosage is essential. Because Orudis is considered more prone to causing gastrointestinal problems, other short-acting NSAIDs should be tried first. For long-acting effect, Oruvail seems to be well tolerated.

RECOMMENDATIONS

In summary, Orudis and nonprescription Orudis KT provide similar anti-inflammatory and pain-relieving activity as other NSAIDs. However, some authorities believe that Orudis may cause a higher incidence of gastric irritation than other NSAIDs.

There are many other short-acting prescription and nonprescription NSAIDs that may be used instead of Orudis and Orudis KT. However, because there is a great deal of variability between people in their response and tolerance to different NSAIDs, if you are already taking Orudis or Orudis KT and having good results with no side effects, switching to a different NSAID may not be necessary. Ask your physician.

For reasons that are unclear, long-acting Oruvail does not appear to share Orudis' gastric irritation tendency. Perhaps it is because very little Oruvail dissolves in the stomach, thereby minimizing its direct irritation on the gastric surface. In any event, anecdotal reports from both patients and physicians seem to indicate that extended-release Oruvail is highly effective and very well tolerated, even in people who've encountered gastric irritation with other NSAIDs. Oruvail comes in three dose sizes—100, 150, and 200 mg—for dose flexibility.

In-Depth Analysis: Relafen (Nabumetone)

One of the newer NSAIDs, Relafen was developed to provide effective anti-inflammatory effect with a reduced incidence of gastrointestinal side effects. Unlike other NSAIDs, Relafen is not acidic and doesn't cause direct irritation to the stomach lining. But Relafen does cause the same systemic gastrointestinal and other side effects seen with all current NSAIDs.

Some studies with Relafen showed a decreased incidence of major and minor side effects, but other studies reveal little difference between this drug and other NSAIDs. Some physicians feel that Relafen does cause fewer problems in their patients, but others aren't convinced. All of the physicians I asked listed Relafen among the NSAIDs they preferred. (Others they preferred included Voltaren and Voltaren-XR, Oruvail, and Naprelan.)

Whether due to a superior safety profile or to effective advertising, Relafen has quickly climbed in sales to a ranking of No.

42 in U.S. outpatient prescriptions in 1996. It's the top-selling brand name NSAID.

. Another reason for its popularity is that Relafen can be taken just once a day, making it easier to remember than multi-dose NSAIDs. And unlike some NSAIDs, Relafen doesn't decrease the clotting capability of platelets, so it can be used before and after surgery, whereas people taking aspirin or another platelet-inhibiting NSAIDs must stop their medication at least a week before surgery.

If there's a knock against Relafen, it's that some physicians believe Relafen's effect is weaker than that of other NSAIDs. For mild or moderate conditions, Relafen is sufficient, they say. But for severe pain or arthritis, several voiced a preference for Motrin in high doses, Voltaren, or extended-release types such as Oruvail, Naprelan, Lodine XL, or Voltaren-XR.

MANUFACTURER-RECOMMENDED DOSAGE

The manufacturer-recommended initial dose is 1,000 mg once daily *for everyone*. Dosages can be increased to 1,500 or 2,000 mg a day. The recommended dosage for elderly individuals is the same. Relafen is produced in 500- and 750-mg tablets that can easily be broken or cut. Possible side effects of Relafen are listed on page 330.

LOW-DOSE RELAFEN

Although the manufacturer-recommended initial dosage of Relafen is an one-size-fits-all 1,000 mg a day, in the PDR the manufacturer acknowledges that "there is considerable interpatient variation in response to Relafen." Pre-release studies focused on dosages of 1,000 and 1,500 mg a day. Hundreds and thousands were studied at these dosages, but only a handful at 500 mg and none at 750 mg.

If you are medication-sensitive or your condition is not severe or acute, you may want to try 500 or 750 mg a day of Relafen initially. Several physicians I know use these lower initial doses in smaller, older, and other medication-sensitive or high-risk patients. Be aware that it takes a few days for Relafen to reach its maximum effect; this is also true at higher dosages.

Although Relafen may be less irritating than other NSAIDs to the gastrointestinal tract, Relafen can cause gastric irritation and ulceration. It also causes other side effects, nearly all of which are directly related to dosage. If you take Relafen at a higher dosage or for a prolonged period, your risks of gastric and other side effects increase.

But side effects with Relafen, as with all NSAIDs, can also occur quickly. Leslie, a 32-year-old woman, was prescribed Relafen by her physician. Within a few days she began to feel increasingly anxious and agitated. Soon she began experiencing full-blown panic episodes that sent her to the emergency room. There she was examined, told there was nothing physically wrong (the implication being that her anxiety was psychological), and sent home with a prescription for Xanax, an anti-anxiety drug.

Leslie didn't believe her sudden, acute anxiety was emotional; nothing had changed or was particularly stressful in her life. She also didn't like taking a tranquilizer, which didn't help much anyway. But neither did Leslie like how she was feeling by now—"climbing the walls," as she put it.

Frustrated by her situation and unsatisfied with the medical input she'd received, Leslie stopped all of her medications—that is, the Xanax and the Relafen. Within two days, her anxiety had melted away.

In the PDR, nervousness and insomnia are listed as a side effect that occurs in about 1% of Relafen users. I suspect the incidence is higher. Anxiety and panic episodes are commonly overlooked side effects of NSAIDs.

Leslie's adverse reaction to Relafen is a classic example of overmedication. The standard, one-size-fits-all 1,000 mg a day dose was simply too much for her system. Within days, as her blood level of Relafen rose, her agitation emerged. With continued usage, panic attacks developed. These are not mild side effects, and they are directly related to dosage.

If Leslie had begun Relafen at a lower dose, she would probably have had a much better response. Unfortunately, only a small amount of information exists about the efficacy of 500 mg of Relafen, but it seems to indicate that this dose does have anti-inflammatory effects. No work seems to have been done at other low doses such as 600, 750, or 800 mg a day.

If you start at 500 mg a day but it isn't sufficient, you can increase to 750, 1,000, 1,250 mg, etc., by mixing the 500- and 750-mg Relafen tablets. You can increase even more gradually by splitting the pills. By using this method, you can arrive at a Relafen dosage that is no higher than absolutely necessary—the key to minimizing the risk of NSAID side effects.

RELAFEN AND THE ELDERLY

Relafen is prescribed at the same doses for older individuals as for younger ones. But studies show that the elderly metabolize Relafen more slowly and develop higher blood levels at equivalent dosages. It is well established that older individuals are often more sensitive to the effects and side effects of NSAIDs.

For all of these reasons, if you are over 60 you should consider starting with a lower dose of Relafen. As mentioned in the introduction to this chapter, several authorities recommend using lower doses of all NSAIDs in the elderly. Relafen is no exception.

NSAIDs can be dangerous in the elderly, who experience the highest rates of NSAID side effects, gastrointestinal reactions, hemorrhage, and death with these drugs. Starting with a lower, safer dose of Relafen, as with all NSAIDs, makes sense. If this dosage isn't sufficient, it can be gradually increased until an effective dosage is found. For example, you can start with 500 mg a day and, if necessary, increase to 750 and then 1,000 mg a day.

RECOMMENDATIONS

Although little study has been directed at lower doses of Relafen, it is clear that considerable variation exists in individual response to this drug. Relafen may possibly be a bit safer than some other NSAIDs in regard to gastrointestinal side effects, but it still causes problems in perhaps 20% of users. Severe side effects are most often associated with high dosage or prolonged usage, but sometimes side effects can emerge quickly, particularly if you are taking a dose that's too high for you.

If you are medication-sensitive, consider starting with 500 or 750 mg of Relafen rather than the recommended, one-size-fits-all 1,000 mg a day. It takes a few days for Relafen to reach its maximum effect; this is true with any dosage. Before making any changes in your Relafen dosage, discuss if with your physician.

Fortunately, Relafen is made in 500- and 750-mg tablets, so it's easy to use a lower dose. The pills are breakable, allowing even lower doses for those who are medication-sensitive or want to increase their doses by very small amounts.

Other Anti-Inflammatory Medications

LODINE AND LODINE XL (ETODOLAC)

Lodine's PDR write-up is in many ways exemplary. It makes repeated reference to the need to individualize dosage. It also informs us that the low 200-mg dose, which lasts four to five hours for most patients, may provide pain relief for eight hours in some patients. In another section, it states that doses of 200 to 400 mg, which usually last four to six hours, may provide pain relief in some people up to eight to twelve hours.

Unlike most PDR descriptions, this one provides you with specific, clear information about interindividual variation with this drug. My only criticism is that this data should be located at the beginning of the dosage guidelines where physicians and other readers would readily see it rather than lost amid the lengthy text. However, Lodine's description does offer this advice at the beginning of the dosage section: "As with other NSAIDs, the lowest dose and longest dosing interval should be sought for each patient." All PDR descriptions should be required to furnish this type of information on individual variability.

Several studies have shown Lodine to cause fewer gastrointestinal side effects than many other NSAIDs. Physicians seen to agree—Lodine was the third most prescribed NSAID and No. 68 among all drugs in terms of 1996 U.S. outpatient prescriptions.

Released in 1997, Lodine XL is an extended-release form of Lodine. Like other extended-release NSAIDs, it is designed to slowly dissolve in the intestine rather than the stomach. The result is a longer-acting drug that is even less likely to cause direct gastric irritation. Because regular Lodine seems to cause fewer gastric problems than other NSAIDs, Lodine XL may prove to be one of the least gastric irritating NSAIDs currently available.

The manufacturer-recommended dosage range for Lodine is 600 to 1,200 mg a day; for Lodine XL, 400 to 1,000 mg a day. Lodine is produced in 200- and 300-mg capsules, and 400-mg and 500-mg tablets that are unscored but can be split with a pill cutter. Lodine XL is made in 400- and 600-mg film-coated tablets that should not be cut or split.

The manufacturer provides no specific elderly dosages, but in the text about Lodine there are several references about the increased susceptibility of the elderly to NSAID side effects. If you are elderly, it may be presumed that the lower dosage range, such as 200 mg of Lodine three times a day or Lodine XL 400 mg once daily, is the best place to start.

For younger adults, these same initial dosages may be sufficient if you are small or medication-sensitive, have encountered NSAID side effects previously, or just want to start with the lowest possible effective amount. As mentioned above, in some people low doses of Lodine last longer or produce higher blood levels than average. Thus, lower doses may be sufficient in some cases. Lodine comes in multiple drug sizes for extra dose flexibility, allowing you to start with a low dose and, if necessary, increase gradually to determine your specific dosage need.

NAPRELAN (EXTENDED-RELEASE NAPROXEN)

A newer, longer-acting form of naproxen, Naprelan offers a once-a-day dosage. Designed to gradually dissolve throughout the gastrointestinal tract, the drug is designed to have an effect that lasts twenty-four hours. Because of the drug's convenient dosage and the familiarity of physicians with the basic compound, naproxen, the ingredient for the previous top-seller Naprosyn, Naprelan has quickly become a popular drug.

Naprelan is produced in 375- and 500-mg unbreakable tablets (splitting the tablet would ruin the sustained-release effect). The manufacturer-recommended dosage is two 375-mg tablets (750 mg) or two 500-mg tablets (1,000 mg) once daily.

Because of its gradual release effect, Naprelan may cause less direct gastric irritation than regular NSAIDs that aren't enteric-coated or extended release in form. Nonetheless, Naprelan, like all NSAIDs, still can cause significant gastric damage by its systemic effect. This and most of Naprelan's other side effects are dose related.

Naprelan's manufacturer acknowledges that ''Naprelan, like other NSAIDs, shows considerable variation in response. . . . The lowest effective dose should be sought and used in every patient.'' If you are medication-sensitive, you and your physician should consider initiating Naprelan at lower doses—375 or 500 mg a day. For those in whom 750 mg a day isn't quite enough, you can increase to 875 mg by combining a 375-mg and 500-mg pill.

NAPROSYN, EC-NAPROSYN, AND ALEVE (NAPROXEN)

One of the most popular NSAIDs in the U.S. in the 1980s and early 1990s, in 1993 Naprosyn led all NSAIDs in the U.S. in outpatient prescriptions and ranked No. 15 among all medications. In 1996, Naprosyn no longer ranked on the top 200 list, partly because Naprosyn's patent expired and generic naproxen (ranked No. 27 among all generic drugs) is being substituted. Another reason is competition from newer NSAIDs such as Relafen, Naprelan, Oruvail, and Daypro.

Naprosyn is produced in 250-, 375-, and 500-mg coated tablets, and as a liquid. Naprosyn recently has been released in an enteric-coated form as EC-Naprosyn, but only in 375- and 500-mg doses. Naprosyn also is available as nonprescription Aleve, which contains 220 mg of naproxen. Prescription Naprosyn is also marketed under the name Anaprox.

Naprosyn and EC-Naprosyn are taken twice a day and the recommended dosage ranges from 500 to 1,250 mg a day depending on the disease and its severity. Manufacturer-recommended dosages for the elderly are the same as for younger adults. Aleve is also a twice-a-day medication.

As with all NSAIDs, most side effects with Naprosyn, EC-Naprosyn, and Aleve are directly related to dosage. Lower doses cause fewer side effects. If you are medication-sensitive and your disorder isn't acute or severe, you and your physician should consider starting with nonprescription Aleve, which is 12% lower in dosage than the smallest Naprosyn pill. An alternative method of taking Naprosyn flexibly is to use Naprosyn liquid, but it is more expensive per dose than the tablets. If you find you require 375 or 500 mg twice a day of Naprosyn, you may want to switch to EC-Naprosyn.

Although the results of studies are equivocal, many physicians and patients feel that enteric-coated NSAIDs cause less gastric irritation. EC-Naprosyn may therefore be a better choice than regular Naprosyn, but only if you need the higher dose pills. Even enteric-coated NSAIDs cause side effects through their systemic effects. The key to reducing NSAID risks is to use the very lowest, effective dosage.

If you are over 60, many authorities suggest starting with dosages lower than recommended by NSAID manufacturers. Again, nonprescription Aleve may be a better initial choice because of its lower dose.

CATAFLAM (DICLOFENAC)

Cataflam (diclofenac potassium) is similar to Voltaren (diclofenac sodium). Their properties are identical, except that Cataflam is not enteric-coated like Voltaren, so Cataflam is more quickly absorbed after oral intake and therefore faster-acting. Made by the same manufacturer, Cataflam appears to have been developed to be marketed for pain relief, for which it is FDA approved. Cataflam is also approved for treating osteoarthritis and rheumatoid arthritis, like Voltaren. Cataflam is also prescribed for bursitis, tendinitis, and other disorders involving inflammation.

Cataflam trades one attribute for another with Voltaren. Cataflam works faster, but it doesn't possess the stomach-sparing advantage of being enteric-coated. If you have done well on

Voltaren, you cannot assume you'll have the same experience with Cataflam.

For treating arthritis, the manufacturer-recommended dosage of Cataflam is the same as for Voltaren: 100 to 150 mg a day for osteoarthritis; 150 to 200 mg a day for rheumatoid arthritis. For pain and menstrual discomfort, the recommended dose is 50 mg three times a day, or 100 mg initially followed by another 50 mg; maximum dosage, 200 mg a day.

If you are medication-sensitive, you may respond to a lower dosage of Cataflam. Lower doses were found effective in pre-release studies of this drug. Here's what one study found: "The investigators concluded that diclofenac [Cataflam], in low doses of approximately 75 mg daily, effectively reduces both menstrual pain and bleeding."

Unfortunately, Cataflam is made in only one size, a coated 50-mg pill that is difficult to break. Unless your pain is acute, Voltaren may be a better choice because it's available in a 25-mg pill and it's enteric-coated, thereby lessening some (but not all) of the stomach-irritating effects of these drugs.

Brief Comments

ASPIRIN (ACETYLSALICYLIC ACID)

(See Chapter 13)

CLINORIL (SULINDAC)

Clinoril is an older NSAID with a manufacturer-recommended dosage range of 300 to 400 mg a day depending on the disease. Clinoril is manufactured in 150- and 200-mg tablets that are taken twice daily. The tablets are scored, allowing flexible dosaging.

Most studies show Clinoril to have a similar side effect profile as other older NSAIDs, but some studies reveal a higher rate of gastrointestinal side effects. Clinoril has been associated with rare incidents of liver and pancreas damage. One patient of mine developed episodes of severe anxiety and a few panic attacks on standard doses of Clinoril. If you are medication-sensitive, you and your physician should consider starting Clinoril as low as 75 mg (half a 150-mg tablet) twice a day, increasing to 100 mg (half a 200-mg tablet) twice a day. Continued gradual increases can be made if necessary.

DAYPRO (OXAPROZIN)

A newer NSAID, Daypro offers the convenience of once-daily dosaging. Some physicians feel that Daypro causes fewer gastro-intestinal problems than older NSAIDs such as Motrin or Naprosyn. Daypro's popularity is reflected in its No. 74 ranking in U.S. outpatient prescriptions in 1996.

The manufacturer recommended dosage of Daypro is 1200 mg a day. A lower dose of 600 mg a day is recommended for smaller individuals and mild conditions. Maximum dosage is 1,800 mg a day. No specific dosages for the elderly are provided, but it is assumed that the 600 mg a day dosage is meant for this group. Daypro is produced in one size, a 600-mg scored tablet.

If you are medication-sensitive, you and your physician should consider initiating Daypro at 600 mg a day. Because the tablet is scored, you can begin as low as 300 mg to test your sensitivity and response. Although Daypro is usually taken once daily, the total dosage can be split into two doses, such as 300 mg with breakfast and dinner. By splitting the 600-mg pill, you can increase by 300-mg increments such as to 900 mg a day, thereby creating the lowest effective dosage for your disorder.

DISALCID (SALSALATE)

An aspirin derivative, Disalcid was designed to produce less gastric irritation than aspirin. Its side effect profile is generally similar to other older NSAIDs. The manufacturer-recommended dosage is 3,000 mg a day utilizing the 500- or 750-mg tablets in two or three doses. Lower doses are recommended for the elderly but are not specifically defined. Disalcid is produced in 500-mg capsules and scored tablets, and 750-mg scored tablets. It is also available as generic salsalate. Ask for the scored tablets, which allow flexible dosing. Disalcid and other aspirin products are not recommended for use in children and adolescents with viral syndromes such as chicken pox or the flu because of a possible association with the development of Reye's syndrome.

DOLOBID (DIFLUNISAL)

A derivative of aspirin, Dolobid is usually better tolerated than aspirin and perhaps equivalent to other older NSAIDs in terms of gastrointestinal and other side effects. The manufacturer-recommended dosage is 250 or 500 mg twice a day. The maximum dosage is 2,500 mg a day for acute treatment and 1,500 mg a day for ongoing therapy. Lower doses are recommended for the elderly: 500 mg initially, then 250 mg every eight to twelve hours. Dolobid is produced in 250- and 500-mg unscored tablets, but they are breakable for lower and more flexible dosaging. Also available as generic diflunisal. Dolobid and other aspirin products are not recommended for use in children and adolescents with viral syndromes such as chicken pox or the flu because of a possible association with the development of Reye's syndrome.

ECOTRIN (ENTERIC-COATED ASPIRIN)

See Chapter 13.

FELDENE (PIROXICAM)

Feldene has been the subject of controversy for several years. The Public Citizen Health Research Group has called for the FDA to ban Feldene because of its purported high incidence of severe and fatal gastrointestinal hemorrhage. While banning Feldene has been hotly debated, studies have shown it to be one of the more gastric-toxic anti-inflammatory drugs. Yet individual response can vary greatly; I've spoken to several people who've said that Feldene worked extremely well for them.

Feldene is a very long-acting medication that builds up in the system with continued usage. The manufacturer recommended dosage is 20 mg a day *for everyone*. The manufacturer notes that because Feldene accumulates in the body, its full effect may require a week or more of usage. Feldene is produced in 10- and 20-mg capsules.

If you are medication-sensitive, you and your physician should consider starting Feldene at the lower, 10-mg dose. However, because Feldene is such a long-acting medication and its full effects may not be seen for several days, this may be a drug that is difficult to evaluate and adjust according to individual sensitivity. Newer NSAIDs that are less likely to cause gastrointestinal irritation and are easier to adjust are better choices.

FLURBIPROFEN (ANSAID)

Previously marketed as Ansaid, flurbiprofen is only available in generic form at this time. An older NSAID, the usual dosage is 200 to 300 mg a day, taken in two or three 100-mg doses. However, dosages as low as 50 mg twice a day have been shown to be effective. Flurbiprofen is produced in 50- and 100-mg pills. Ask your physician to prescribe the 50-mg pills in order to begin at a lower dosage and to afford flexibility if an increase in dosage is necessary.

INDOCIN AND INDOCIN SR (INDOMETHACIN)

An older NSAID that can cause more side effects than many competitors, Indocin is usually reserved for situations in which it is specifically required. In addition to gastrointestinal side effects, Indocin also causes a high incidence of central nervous system reactions including headaches, dizziness, fatigue, and depression. In some rheumatologic disorders such as Reiter's syndrome, Indocin sometimes provides a better response than other NSAIDs. The manufacturer-recommended dosage is 25 or 50 mg twice or three times a day. The manufacturer notes the variability in individual response by defining the effective dosage range of 50 to 150 mg a day. The maximum recommended dosage is 200 mg a day. No specific dosages are listed for elderly persons, but if you are over 60, you should consider starting at 25 mg twice a day. If you are medication-sensitive, you and your physician should consider doing the same, starting at 25 mg twice or three times a day, depending on your response. Indocin is produced in 25- and 50-mg capsules. Indocin SR is a longer-acting 75-mg preparation that can be taken once or twice a day. Indocin is also produced in suppository and liquid form.

MECLOMEN (MECLOFENAMATE)

A newer NSAID, Meclomen appears to be similar to Motrin and other NSAIDs in its tendency toward gastrointestinal and other side effects. Diarrhea seems to be a problem for some taking Meclomen, occurring in 10% to 33% and severe enough to require discontinuation of the drug in about 4%. The manufacturer-recommended dosage is 200 to 400 mg a day taken in three or four divided doses of 50 to 100 mg. Meclomen is produced in 50- and 100-mg capsules. If you are medication-sensitive, starting at a lower dose such as 50 mg three times a day may be wise.

NALFON (FENOPROFEN)

An older NSAID, Nalfon is considered equivalent in its effectiveness and side effect profile to Motrin, Naprosyn, and other early drugs of this group. The manufacturer-recommended daily dosage range is 800 to 2,400 mg a day divided into three or four doses. Nalfon is available in 200- and 300-mg capsules, and 600-mg scored caplets. No specific elderly dosages are suggested. If you are medication-sensitive or elderly or otherwise at risk for NSAID side effects, treatment should be initiated at 200 mg or 300 mg three or four times a day.

TOLECTIN (TOLMETIN)

Tolectin is an older NSAID which is a generally similar in effectiveness and side effects to other early NSAIDs. However, *Worst Pills, Best Pills II* discourages the use of Tolectin because the drug has been associated with severe allergic reactions. The AMA does not recommend it for patients with known bleeding disorders.

The manufacturer recommended initial dosage of Tolectin is 400 mg three times a day. The dosage range is 600 to 1,800 mg a day. Dosages range from 200 to 600 mg three times a day. Tolectin is available in 200-mg scored tablets, 400-mg capsules, and 600-mg film-coated oval tablets. No specific elderly dosages are provided.

If you are medication-sensitive, elderly, small, or otherwise at risk of NSAID side effects, you and your physician should consider starting with the 200-mg tablet, using it twice or three times a day depending on how long its effect lasts. You may even split the 200-mg pill to start at an even lower 100-mg dose in order to test your response. If you require higher doses, increasing by 100 mg at a time can be accomplished by splitting the 200-mg tablet.

TORADOL (KETOROLAC)

A top-selling drug in 1993 (ranked No. 53 in outpatient U.S. prescriptions), Toradol was suspended from usage in several European countries after reports of severe, sometimes fatal bleeding from the gastrointestinal track or from wounds following surgery or severe injury. Today, Toradol is reserved for very short-term usage in severe pain, usually following surgery. Unlike other NSAIDs, Toradol can be administered intravenously or by muscle injection. Its pain-reducing effect can be dramatic. It is sometimes used before surgery to reduce inflammation and scarring postoperatively.

Toradol is produced in a 10-mg tablet, but its use is limited to people already given intravenous or intramuscular Toradol, and the total duration of Toradol treatment should not exceed five days.

TRILISATE (CHOLINE MAGNESIUM TRISALICYLATE)

Trilisate is an aspirin derivative designed to cause less gastric irritation than aspirin. Trilisate is generally similar to other older NSAIDs in terms of gastrointestinal and other side effects. The recommended dosage is 1,500 mg twice a day, although some people take all 3,000 mg once daily. Lower doses are recommended for the elderly: 750 mg three times a day. Trilisate is produced in 500-, 750-, and 1,000-mg scored tablets, and as a liquid. Also available in generic form. Trilisate and other aspirin products are not recommended for use in children and adolescents with viral syndromes such as chicken pox or the flu because of a possible association with the development of Reye's syndrome.

In-Depth Analysis: Cytotec (Misoprostol) An Antidote for Anti-Inflammatory Drug Side Effects?

Cytotec is a synthetic variant of prostaglandin, a naturally occurring compound in the human system. One of the functions of prostaglandin is to maintain the integrity of the stomach lining despite the erosive effects of food and stomach acid. Natural prostaglandin taken orally doesn't survive the digestive process, and taken intravenously produces many side effects. The development of synthetic Cytotec has overcome these difficulties.

Cytotec's greatest usefulness is in the prevention of the gastrointestinal problems incurred with the use of aspirin and other NSAIDs. With repeated or chronic use, side effects with NSAIDs are frequent and often serious, yet many arthritis sufferers require these medications in high doses for prolonged periods. The concomitant use of Cytotec with NSAIDs has been shown to markedly reduce the occurrence of gastrointestinal problems and to prevent recurrence of gastric or duodenal ulcers in NSAID-dependent patients.

Although Cytotec is specifically approved for usage with NSAIDs, it is also effective in the treatment of gastric and duodenal ulcers due to other causes. But it isn't as effective as the H2 inhibitors (Zantac, Axid, Pepcid, Tagamet) and, especially, the proton-pump inhibitors (Prilosec, Prevacid), which are more effective with fewer side effects. Cytotec is usually reserved for cases resistant to other approaches or may be combined with Zantac or other similar drugs to achieve an additive effect.

Because Cytotec itself can cause abdominal pain, it should be taken with meals. Cytotec taken on an empty stomach also may produce higher blood levels of the drug that may provoke increased side effects.

The biggest problem with Cytotec is diarrhea, which occurs frequently at standard recommended dosages. Because of this, abdominal cramps, and other side effects, some physicians have soured on Cytotec's usefulness. However, others continue to find it quite useful, and several people who developed NSAID-related gastritis have told me of obtaining excellent results with Cytotec, which allowed then to continue taking their NSAIDs.

MANUFACTURER-RECOMMENDED DOSES

The manufacturer recommended dosage is 200 mcg four times a day with meals. If this dose isn't tolerated due to side effects, 100 mcg four times a day. Elderly doses: same. Cytotec is produced in a 100-mcg tablet that can easily be split and a 200-mcg scored tablet. Not available as a generic drug.

MOST FREQUENT SIDE EFFECTS

Misoprostol side effects include abdominal discomfort, cramps, nausea, dizziness, and headaches. The greatest problem with Cytotec is its tendency to provoke persistent diarrhea. According to the PDR, this occurs in 14% to 40% of patients. Many physicians tell me that the rate is far higher; diarrhea is ''ubiquitous'' at recommended dosages according to *Conn's Current Therapy 1994*, and many people cannot tolerate Cytotec at any of the recommended dosages. Cytotec is absolutely contraindicated in pregnancy and nursing mothers.

LOW-DOSE CYTOTEC

The manufacturer-recommended starting dose of Cytotec is too high for a large proportion of patients, as demonstrated by the very high incidence of diarrhea and other troublesome side effects—which are directly related to dosage. That's why many authorities recommend starting at 100 mcg four times a day. If this dosage is insufficient to counter NSAID gastric irritation, it can be gradually increased by 25 to 50 mcg increments (125 mcg four times a day; 150 mcg four times a day) rather than immediately doubling to 200 mcg four times a day.

Studies of Cytotec at 100 mcg four times a day have repeatedly demonstrated its effectiveness in reducing NSAID-related gastric irritation and ulceration. In some, but not all, studies the 100-mcg dose was as effective as 200 mcg. Intermediate doses such as 200 mcg two or three times a day (50% and 25% less than the manufacturer-recommended dose, respectively) were also effective and may be of particular use with anti-inflammatory drugs taken once, twice, or three time daily.

In fact, a wide range of Cytotec doses have been proven effective in preventing NSAID-induced gastrointestinal pathology. This isn't surprising because subjects given repeated doses of Cytotec revealed a high degree of variability in blood levels of misoprostol acid, Cytotec's most active metabolite.

Indeed, in clinical studies, doses as low as 25 mcg of Cytotec taken with 650 mg of aspirin four times a day diminished aspirin-induced gastric irritation in some subjects. Similar protection was afforded by 50 mcg of Cytotec taken with high NSAID doses such as 800 mg of Motrin or 975 mg of aspirin four times a day. Although 25 or 50 mcg of Cytotec may not be enough for many people, for others it may be sufficient. Certainly if you develop intolerable side effects with 100 mcg of Cytotec, dropping to a lower dose makes sense.

RECOMMENDATIONS

If you are small, elderly, sensitive to medications, prone to side effects, or simply want to take the very lowest amount of Cytotec your body needs, you and your physician should consider starting Cytotec at a lower dose, choosing between 25, 50, 75, and 100 mcg three or four times a day depending on your medication history and your reason for using Cytotec. If, for example, you've already developed gastric irritation from NSAIDs, you may want to try higher Cytotec doses first, reducing only if necessary.

If side effects develop, stop the medication and restart at 25, 50, or 75 mcg. I've known people who have experienced abdominal cramps with 50 mcg of Cytotec, so obviously this dose was highly stimulatory to their gastrointestinal systems. The key with Cytotec is to find a dose that is sufficiently stimulatory to produce gastric protection without being so stimulatory to produce cramps or diarrhea.

If you smoke, you may require higher doses of Cytotec. Smokers also have a higher incidence of gastrointestinal problems with NSAIDs, so if you smoke and need frequent or regular NSAID therapy, it may be a good idea to start Cytotec at the first sign of any gastric problems or to use Cytotec preventively before gastric problems occur.

Colchicine: An Alternative Anti-Inflammatory Drug

Colchicine is an old medication that most doctors associate with the treatment of gout and don't consider for other inflammatory or pain problems. However, colchicine possesses potent anti-inflammatory properties that have been proven effective for a variety of disorders such as arthritis and disk disease.

Just like any other drug, colchicine may cause side effects, some of which can be serious. Its most common side effects are abdominal pain, cramps, and diarrhea, but not the gastric irritation, ulceration, and bleeding seen with other NSAIDs. For this reason, colchicine offers an alternative for people who encounter repeated or serious upper gastrointestinal problems such as gastritis, ulcers, or bleeding with better-known NSAIDs.

USUAL DOSAGE AND SIDE EFFECTS

Colchicine is available in 0.5-mg and 0.6-mg tablets. The dosage range is one to three tablets a day. Colchicine can be administered intravenously for acute, severe problems, such as herniated disks. Side effects include diarrhea, abdominal cramps, nausea; less common include muscle weakness, kidney damage, nerve injury, and bone marrow suppression.

LOW-DOSE COLCHICINE

Colchicine is frequently overlooked as an NSAID alternative for several reasons, one being that it is a generic drug and cannot be advertised and marketed very profitably. Another reason is side effects, most of which are dose-related. It is estimated that as many as 80% of patients encounter abdominal pain or diarrhea with colchicine at standard doses. Lower doses are an entirely different story, but the use of these doses has been limited by the availability of colchicine in only two, nearly identical sizes.

For low-dose colchicine, some physicians have turned to compounding pharmacies, pharmacies that operate like apothecary shops of old, producing custom-designed medications that are overlooked by or unprofitable for major pharmaceutical companies to manufacture. These pharmacies also prepare standard medications in dose sizes that are otherwise unavailable. With colchicine, doses such as 0.2 mg or 0.3 mg can be obtained. Some compounding pharmacies also mix the colchicine with an extended-release base, which slows down its absorption so that your body is not subjected to a sudden high impact from the medication. Instead the absorption and effect are more gradual and less prone to provoking side effects. For a compounding pharmacy near you, contact the Professional Compounding Centers of America, at 800-331-2498.

Depending on the situation and your sensitivity, virtually any dose of colchicine can be used at first. One patient started at 0.1 mg a day, increasing every few days until he obtained the desired anti-inflammatory effect at 0.3 mg twice a day. He encountered no side effects.

Like all medications, colchicine can cause long-term side effects when taken for prolonged periods. Yet some people who are prone to gout take colchicine, usually in combination with another medication, for years or decades with few problems.

RECOMMENDATIONS

If you derive benefit from standard NSAIDs such as Motrin, Relafen, Oruvail, Lodine, or from nonprescription ibuprofen, Aleve, aspirin, or others without repeated or serious gastric irritation, then continue using them. However, if you are one of the tens of thousands of people who have developed NSAID gastric problems and can no longer handle these drugs, colchicine may serve as a valuable alternative if you develop arthritis, bursitis, tendinitis, or disk problems.

Although colchicine does not cause the typical NSAID-related gastric irritation or bleeding, it can cause side effects. In fact it does so with great frequency at standard doses. At low doses, colchicine is much better tolerated. By starting low and, if necessary, gradually increasing the dose, an effective, well-tolerated colchicine dosage can usually be attained.

FIFTEEN

~

Notes on Narcotic
Pain Medications

When my son, Rory, was five, he jumped off of one of those children's climbing mazes, landed on the side of his foot, and broke his leg. The fracture was simple and clean, and the leg was placed in a cast. Nevertheless, Rory's pain was severe.

The orthopedist prescribed a codeine-containing remedy that could be repeated every four hours. Rory needed it. After about three hours, however, the effect of the pain medication began to wane, and Rory experienced considerable pain. We did everything possible to make him comfortable, but a newly fractured bone hurts. Yet I hesitated to give Rory the pain medication sooner for fear it would become addicting.

Fortunately, a emergency room physician lived up the street. He told me, "Don't hesitate to give Rory the medication every three hours if he needs it. His pain will subside with the swelling over the next three days, and his need for the medication will subside with it. Giving him a few extra pills isn't going to cause dependency that quickly. Besides, codeine and similar medications often don't last four hours—I don't know why orthopedists prescribe it that way. Probably because that's what it says in the PDR. Most of the time, using it every four hours for acute pain isn't frequent enough."

Rory did fine with the medication every three hours. We were greatly relieved. Over the next days, his pain diminished; the medication lasted longer and longer and soon wasn't required at all.

Here's another dosage story. Following an injury, a 40-year-old named Bill received a prescription for Vicodin from his physician. Vicodin, a top-selling codeine derivative, is usually a well-tolerated, effective narcotic pain medication.

Bill isn't medication-sensitive, but the dosage of Vicodin he received was too strong. He felt "spaced out, drugged," as he described it. With the next dose, he split the pill in half. This provided adequate pain relief without any side effects.

As these examples illustrate, interindividual variation is common with narcotic pain relievers. That's why many of these medications are produced in several sizes and, usually, as scored tablets in order to maximize dose flexibility. If you are medication-sensitive or are sensitive to alcohol or sedating drugs, be sure to tell your physician when considering a narcotic pain reliever.

Narcotic pain relievers are frequently prescribed drugs. Four different types ranked among the top 200 prescribed outpatient medications in 1996, with just one of the many forms of generic hydrocodone ranking No. 9, ahead of Prilosec, Mevacor, Claritin, Zoloft, Norvasc, Cardizem CD, Dilantin, and many other well-known medications.

There are considerable differences between different narcotic pain-relieving remedies. Some codeine and codeine-derivative preparations are combined with aspirin to enhance their pain-relieving effect. Others are combined with acetaminophen (better known as Tylenol). Codeine-and-aspirin-containing products may be prone to causing gastric irritation in some people. Codeine is more likely to cause nausea or vomiting than hydrocodone (Vicodin and others), and both seem to cause more of these side effects than oxycodone (Percodan, Percocet, and others). On the other hand, oxycodone is more prone to produce a dissociated, spaced-out reaction. Most of these medications are produced in a range of sizes. If you are medication-sensitive and require a narcotic pain reliever, ask about starting with the lowest dose and adjusting the dose depending on your response.

Another way to use the lowest amount of narcotic pain relievers is to combine them, when the situation warrants, with anti-inflammatory medications. Many of the studies utilizing a combination of these two types of drugs have been done with people undergoing dental surgery, and the results have been very impressive. Narcotic pain relievers and anti-inflammatory drugs seem to amplify each other, thereby allowing the use of low doses of each and reducing the risks of narcotic side effects. A commonly used combination is Motrin taken with codeine or Vicodin.

The opposite side of the coin in using narcotic pain relievers also involves interindividual variation. Hospice physicians often need to prescribe very high doses of these drugs to people with intractable pain, such as those with terminal cancer. As the pain increases, so does the amount of medication needed to blunt it. Tolerance and dependency often develop, which isn't unexpected, and in these cases the dosage of narcotic may reach extremely high levels. This isn't a problem if the reason for narcotic drug treatment is understood and a physician is providing close supervision.

However, as one hospice physician told me, many of her patients encounter great difficulty obtaining the amount of narcotic medication they need from their regular physicians, who are unaccustomed and uncomfortable with prescribing high and prolonged doses of these drugs. The result is that the hospice physician is swamped with having to monitor and prescribe for a large number of people who display a wide range of differing and often changing sensitivities and requirements for these drugs.

This problem isn't limited to this hospice physician. It is a problem across the country. In an effort to reassure physicians, in 1994 the Medical Board of California issued a statement explaining their position on narcotic drug utilization:

> Large doses [of narcotic pain medications] may be necessary to control pain if it is severe. Extended therapy may be necessary if the pain is chronic. . . . The Board believes that addiction should be placed into proper perspective. Physical dependence and tolerance are normal physiologic consequences of extended opioid therapy and are not the same as addiction. . . . Federal and California law clearly recognize that it is a legitimate medical practice for physicians to prescribe controlled substances for the treatment of pain, including intractable pain. . . . Concerns about regulatory scrutiny should not make physicians who follow appropriate guidelines reluctant to prescribe or administer controlled substances . . . for patients with a legitimate medical need for them.

Chronic pain syndromes and the intractable pain of cancer and other terrible diseases are a harsh reality of human existence. As it is, even with our medications we sometimes cannot do enough to provide full comfort to individuals with these disorders. If you are medication-sensitive and develop a disease that requires prolonged treatment with narcotic drugs, your tolerance will likely increase. However, the speed and degree of that tolerance may vary greatly from that seen with other individuals. Close cooperation between you and your physician is necessary to assure sufficient treatment without causing overmedication and its resultant side effects.

PART 6

Medications for Allergies and Motion Sickness

SIXTEEN

Antihistamine Medications

In-depth Analysis

Seldane (terfenadine)

Other Medications

Second-Generation Antihistamines

Claritin (loratadine)
Zyrtec (cetirizine)
Allegra (fexofenadine)
Hismanal (astemizole)

First-Generation Antihistamines

Benadryl (diphenhydramine) (also in Benylin
tablets and cough syrup, Bufferin Nite Time,
Excedrin PM, Nytol Tablets, Sleep-eze 3
Tablets, Sominex Caplets and Tablets, Tylenol
Cold Night Time, Tylenol PM, Unisom with
Pain Relief-Nighttime Sleep Aid, and others)

Brompheniramine (also in Alka Seltzer Plus
Sinus Allergy Medication, Dimetane and
Dimetapp products, Dristan Allergy Nasal
Caplets, and Drixoral Syrup)

First-Generation Antihistamines (Cont'd):

> Chlorpheniramine (also in Ornade, Teldrin, and
> some preparations of Comtrex, Contac,
> Coricidin, Dristan,
> 4-Way Cold Tablets, Sinarest, Sinutab, Tylenol
> Cold and Tylenol Flu remedies, Triaminic,
> Vicks, and others)
> Tavist (clemastine)
> Other First-Generation Antihistamines

About Antihistamine Medications

Histamine is a naturally occurring substance in the human system that is involved in a host of cellular and tissue actions and reactions. Best known are the allergic reactions—itchy skin or eyes, rashes, swelling, nasal congestion—in which histamine plays a key role. Allergies are common, ''the sixth most prevalent cause of chronic disease in the United States.''

The medications that inhibit histamine-mediated allergic reactions are therefore the ones commonly called antihistamines. This group includes the top-selling drugs Claritin, Seldane, Hismanal, Benadryl, and Tavist. Many popular nonprescription allergy and cold remedies contain antihistamines.

The antihistamines that block allergic phenomena actually represent only one of several antihistamine groups. This is because histamine is involved in other body functions, including the stimulation of stomach acid. The drugs that block allergic reactions, which we call antihistamines, are H1 blockers. These are the medications that are discussed in this chapter.

The medications that selectively block the stomach's production of hydrochloride acid, the H2 blockers, include Zantac, Tagamet, Axid, and Pepcid. These drugs are well known for their use in the treatment of ulcers and other gastrointestinal disorders. Most people don't think of them as antihistamines, but in fact they are. They are discussed in detail in Chapter 10.

THE SECOND-GENERATION ANTIHISTAMINES

The second-generation antihistamines are newer and generally more effective with fewer side effects than their older, first-generation counterparts. The prototype second-generation antihistamine is Seldane. Hismanal, Claritin, Zyrtec, and Allegra are more recent additions to the second-generation antihistamine group.

Available only by prescription in the United States, these drugs rarely cause the sedation frequently seen with first-generation antihistamines. They also are far less prone to producing blurred vision, incoordination, constipation, or mental confusion.

Dose flexibility was not a priority in the production of Seldane in 1985, or in that of its earliest rivals, Hismanal and Claritin, which were released in the early 1990s. All three come with manufacturer-recommended one-size-fits-all dosages. In the case of Seldane and possibly Hismanal, this limitation in dose flexibility has contributed to the occurrence of serious, occasionally fatal side effects in a small percentage of patients. The availability of lower doses, shown to be effective in pre-release studies of Seldane, may well have prevented or at least lessened these reactions.

FIRST-GENERATION ANTIHISTAMINE MEDICATIONS

The original antihistamines date back many decades. They still rank among the most utilized medications in the world.

The first-generation antihistamines are versatile drugs, and they continue to enjoy many applications. In addition to allergy symptoms, members of this group are used for motion sickness, nausea and vomiting, and nervous tension, as well as being the main ingredients in many cough and cold remedies (conditions for which antihistamines have yet to the proven effective).

First-generation antihistamines are also used to treat insomnia, a usage based on their most frequent side effect—sedation. Surprisingly, the dosages sometimes recommended for insomnia with one preparation are often identical to those recommended for allergies or other conditions with another.

For instance, Sominex is marketed in two sizes, 25-mg tablets and 50-mg caplets. Another manufacturer offers this same drug, diphenhydramine, at this same dosage *three or four times a day* for allergy symptoms. Is there a contradiction here? No wonder people get sedated.

All of the first-generation antihistamines are sedating, extremely so for some people. These drugs are also prone to produce dizziness, impaired coordination, stomach irritation, blurred vision, and other side effects, especially in the elderly. Their overall side effect rate is considered "very high, perhaps up to 50%" according to *Meyler's Side Effects of Drugs*. Most antihistamine side effects are dose-related. Lower dosages cause fewer problems.

CHOOSING THE CORRECT ANTIHISTAMINE

Antihistamines are effective medications when used properly. This is the key.

Antihistamines are very useful for allergic reactions. First-generation antihistamines are also employed for insomnia or motion sickness. There is little evidence that antihistamines provide effective relief from colds.

Side effects are far fewer with the second-generation antihistamines. Seldane and Hismanal can cause rare, sometimes fatal cardiac irregularities, especially when mixed with certain other drugs. Doses lower than those recommended by the manufacturers decrease the risk.

Because of the potential cardiac risks with Seldane and Hismanal, when Claritin was released in 1993, it became an instant success. By 1995, it surpassed Seldane, the perennial leader, in U.S. outpatient prescriptions. In 1996, Zyrtec and Allegra arrived on the scene. Allegra is similar to Seldane but without Seldane's potential for cardiac problems. Zyrtec appears to possess some additional efficacy beyond its competitors in controlling allergic conditions, especially skin diseases such as atopic dermatitis and eczema, and in preventing or treating the skin reactions to mosquito bites in bite-sensitive individuals.

First-generation antihistamines are contained in scores of non-prescription remedies. Drug manufacturers spend millions to advertise their nonprescription products, yet the difference between many of these remedies is slight. Because the competition is fierce and the rewards are great, advertisers constantly seek new ways of making products attractive to the public. A dermatologist at the University of California, San Diego, told me that as television and magazine advertising has increased for antihistamines (including second-generation drugs such as Claritin), he has been beset by an increased and unnecessary demand for these products. Don't be influenced by advertising. Select a specific product based on your symptoms and the product's cost and dose flexibility. Be aware of any side effects that develop.

Interindividual variation can be considerable with any antihistamine. Individualization of dosage is always recommended.

In-Depth Analysis: Seldane (Terfenadine)

For nearly a decade, Seldane was the most prescribed antihistamine by far in America. No other prescription antihistamine came close.

For example, in 1991, 15.3 million prescriptions were written for Seldane, somewhere between 500 million and 1 billion pills. This popularity made Seldane the No. 9 selling prescription drug in the world, and these numbers didn't include over-the-counter sales of Seldane in Canada, Great Britain, and several other countries.

Seldane's instant popularity stemmed from its ability to block allergic reactions without sedating people. Compared with the highly sedating first-generation antihistamines such as Benadryl, Seldane represented a new generation of non-sedating antihistamine—a huge improvement. But like all medications, Seldane has its side effects and its hidden dangers.

* * *

Chuck Kohler is aware that any medication can cause unexpected side effects, yet because of allergies he's been taking Seldane daily for years. His dosage? One pill daily—that's 60 mg a day, half the manufacturer's recommended dosage. Chuck isn't small. He's 5 feet 11 inches tall and weighs 170 pounds. He's 48 years old and healthy and takes no other medications on a regular basis. So why does he take only half the manufacturer's recommended dosage of Seldane?

"It works," he says. "When the pollen is really bad I take more, but most of the time one pill lasts all day and night. Besides, I know that everything I take runs through my liver and kidneys, and I don't want to mess them up."

Chuck is right about medications sometimes affecting people's livers or kidneys, but his low-dose approach with Seldane is especially wise for another reason—Seldane's effect on the heart.

SELDANE AND IRREGULAR HEARTBEATS, CARDIAC ARRHYTHMIAS, AND DEATH

In August 1990, in response to a growing number of reports about serious heart abnormalities associated with Seldane, the FDA ordered the manufacturer to add strongly worded warnings to Seldane's package insert and PDR write-up. It also prodded the manufacturer to send warning letters to practicing physicians. Nevertheless, as reported in *JAMA* two years later, "cases and fatalities continue to be reported to the FDA."

After the initial reports, it was discovered that Seldane affected the depolarization—i.e., the electrical discharge—of the heart. Notice that this very serious side effect wasn't discovered until nearly five years after Seldane was released for general usage.

The cause of the cardiac irregularity is related to the direct effect of Seldane on the heart. And the effect on the heart is directly related to dosage.

In most people, Seldane (terfenadine) is quickly metabolized to another molecule, terfenadine carboxylate, that retains an antihistaminic effect but doesn't alter the heart rhythm. It's Seldane itself that's the problem, so any factor that hinders Seldane's quick metabolism to terfenadine carboxylate may cause higher blood levels, which can result in an altered heart rhythm, extra or irregular heartbeats, and in a few cases, death.

When unmetabolized, Seldane acts on the heart like the potent heart drug quinidine. The danger depends directly on the level of Seldane in the blood—a function of the dose and the individual's ability to metabolize Seldane quickly. But as we've seen in previous chapters, there's a great deal of variation in different individuals' ability to metabolize medications. Seldane is no exception.

SELDANE AND INTERINDIVIDUAL VARIATION

Seldane is metabolized by a liver enzyme, the hepatic cytochrome P450 enzyme, CYP3A4. Research has shown that there's a 10-fold range of interindividual variation in the activity of this enzyme. In other words, some patients metabolize Seldane a tenth as quickly as others, which means that the Seldane molecule responsible for cardiac arrhythmias lingers far longer in the bloodstreams of some people than others. As *JAMA* put it, "It is possible that those 1% to 2% with the lowest enzyme activity are at risk of developing high concentrations of terfenadine. . . . Some normal individuals may have low enough levels of enzyme activity to accumulate potentially dangerous concentrations of the drug."

If approximately three million people use Seldane in the United States, 1% to 2% equals 30,000 to 60,000 people who may not metabolize Seldane quickly enough to prevent it from affecting their heart function. Across the world, the number would be many times higher.

WHY SELDANE'S CARDIAC EFFECT IS DIFFICULT TO PREDICT

Complicating the problem is the fact that so many factors predispose a patient to Seldane-induced arrhythmias. Already recognized are the Seldane interactions with the drugs erythromycin and ketoconazole (an antifungal agent), as well as liver disease and Seldane overdose. Physicians have also been warned about combining Seldane with other drugs such as itraconazole, fluconazole, metronidazole, clarithromycin, quinidine, procainamide, disopyramide, sotalol, haloperidol, thioridazine, probucol, pentamidine, and others.

Other recognized predisposing factors include coronary artery disease, hypothyroidism, and low potassium and magnesium levels in the blood. In addition, some people are born with abnormal cardiac electrical rhythms (technically speaking, congenital prolonged QT syndrome or secondary forms of delayed repolarization), which may also predispose to Seldane-provoked arrhythmias.

Prior to 1993, twenty-five cases of Seldane-related arrhythmias had been reported to the FDA. All twenty-five patients required hospitalization; two died.

Considering the millions of Seldane prescriptions written annually, twenty-five reported cases is a small fraction—as long as it's not you or someone you know. Moreover, not all Seldane-related arrhythmias are identified as such. And not all identified cases are reported to the FDA.

Thus, the actual incidence of this problem hasn't been accurately quantified. It's almost certainly far higher than the official numbers. Furthermore, predisposing factors continue to be identified. Studies revealed that the enzyme that metabolizes Seldane can be inhibited by the naturally occurring flavonoids in grapefruit juice. This interaction was confirmed by a 1996 study in which six known slow metabolizers of Seldane were given the drug at the standard dosage for seven days. Their blood levels of Seldane and their electrocardiograms were then measured. For another week they continued the Seldane and added grapefruit juice twice daily. At the end of the second week their blood levels of Seldane had increased and their electrocardiograms showed changes typical of the Seldane effect.

Does this mean that people who drink grapefruit juice and take Seldane are at risk? Or those taking vitamins containing grapefruit or other flavonoids and Seldane? Nobody knows. The point is that we don't know and may never know all of the factors that trigger Seldane's cardiac effect.

Because this adverse reaction is so severe, the FDA, the manufacturer, and the medical establishment have called upon doctors prescribing Seldane to anticipate predisposing conditions in order to, as *JAMA* put it, "thereby avoid this serious and potentially deadly complication." But how are physicians to anticipate so many drug interactions and other complicating factors? Are physicians to perform electrocardiograms on every patient before starting Seldane? And with new risk factors continually being discovered, the anticipation of predisposing conditions is impossible, especially since, as reported in the *American Hospital Formulary Service 1994*, "Serious cardiac effects also have been reported rarely during terfenadine [Seldane] therapy in apparently healthy individuals with no associated risk factors."

What then is the solution? Since Seldane's effects on the heart are directly related to dosage, using lower doses would greatly diminish the risk. Yet few if any have raised this possibility. Why? Because the manufacturer has always recommended a Seldane dosage of 120 mg a day (60 mg twice a day) for all patients, the FDA approved that dosage, and even though people have died at this dose, it hasn't been reduced.

Instead, in early 1997 the FDA proposed withdrawing its approval of Seldane. If Seldane's approval is revoked, it will be withdrawn from the market. Seldane's manufacturer announced it would fight the FDA proposal, claiming that Seldane's serious side effects were rare. Others called for an immediate, voluntary removal of all Seldane products from drugstores and distributors. While the battle ensued, Seldane continued to be recommended and prescribed (4.3 million U.S. prescriptions during January–November, 1996) at the standard dosage, and no one suggested otherwise.

ONE-SIZE-FITS-ALL VERSUS LOW-DOSE SELDANE

The literature is filled with studies at the recommended 120 mg a day and higher dosages of Seldane, but just a few that have studied lower, safer dosages. Their results were impressive but apparently ignored.

Seldane's 1996 PDR dosage guidelines are: "One tablet (60 mg) twice daily for adults and children 12 years and older."

That's it, except for a warning set in large capital letters about using higher doses of Seldane because it may cause cardiac side effects. There's not one word about using lower doses.

Nor do Seldane's dosage guidelines offer one word about individualizing the Seldane dosage according to patients' size, state of health, or medication sensitivities. Not one word about reducing the dosage, when possible, with patients taking Seldane on an ongoing basis. Not even a word about lower dosages for the elderly.

This is surprising, since five years before Seldane's release, several studies established Seldane's effectiveness at significantly lower doses, doses 50% less than the manufacturer's recommendation. For example, a 1980 study convincingly showed that 20 mg of Seldane taken three times per day (60 mg daily) was as effective as CPM (chlorpheniramine), the effective but sedating antihistamine already on the market. This study not only compared 20 mg of Seldane three times a day (60 mg a day) to CPM and placebo, but also 200 mg of Seldane three times a day (600 mg a day). The lower Seldane dosage was more effective than the dosage ten times higher, helping 77% of subjects versus 67%, respectively (Table 15.1).

Table 15.1. Lower Doses of Seldane Are Safer and Effective

This 1980 study, published five years before Seldane's release, demonstrated that at 20 mg three times a day, Seldane was highly effective. A dosage of 20 mg three times a day is 50% lower than the 60 mg twice a day (120 mg/day) dosage recommended in the PDR and prescribed by doctors. A 20-mg dose also subjects the body to a third as much medication at any given time, thereby markedly reducing the risk of adverse effects and drug interactions.

(Adapted from M.L. Brandon and M. Weiner, *Annals of Allergy*, 1980, and the same authors in *Arzneimittel-Forschung/Drug Research*, 1982)

	ANY IM-PROVEMENT (%)	MODERATE OR BETTER (%)
Seldane 20 mg TID (60 mg/day)	84	77
Seldane 200 mg TID (600 mg/day)	83	67
Chlorpheniramine 4 mg TID (12 mg/day)	85	71
Placebo	69	50

TID = three times a day

The authors concluded, "The data indicate that daily dosages of 60 mg terfenadine (20 mg three times a day) were as effective as 12 mg (4 mg three times a day) of chlorpheniramine maleate [CPM]. Larger doses of terfenadine [Seldane] were . . . no more effective."

Two years later, the same authors published another article involving low-dose Seldane. The results: 84% of subjects taking 60 mg a day of Seldane reported some improvement in their allergy symptoms. This is a very high percentage. By comparison Prozac, a most effective medication for depression, never yielded improvement in more than 65% of subjects in pre-release studies.

Because of Seldane's repeatedly impressive performance at the lower dosage, the authors once again concluded: "None of the terfenadine [Seldane] dosage schedules up to 200 mg 3 times a day [demonstrated] efficacy greater than seen with 20 mg 3 times a day." But even these convincing results were not enough for Seldane to be produced and recommended at a lower, safer dosage.

WHY SELDANE IS RECOMMENDED AT A HIGHER DOSAGE

Why was the higher dosage selected for recommendation by Seldane's manufacturer? Why were the impressive results at a 50% lower dosage dismissed? I submitted these questions to Seldane's manufacturer. The company wrote in reply: "Apparently, the minimum effective dose which allowed twice daily dosage was selected for marketing."

This rings true. The manufacturer wanted to market Seldane as a medication to be used twice a day, not three times. There are some advantages to a twice-a-day dose schedule. People frequently forget to take their medications, and studies have shown that the more often people have to take a drug, the more often they forget. A three-times-a-day medication is truly harder to remember than a twice-a-day drug.

But Seldane is an antihistamine. In most cases, Seldane is taken for symptomatic relief—congested noses, itchy eyes—not medical exigency. With medications such as blood thinners or heart drugs or insulin, missing a dose can be dangerous. This is rarely the case with Seldane.

So doubling the total daily dose of Seldane (from 20 mg three times a day to 60 mg twice a day) to be able to market a twice a day drug wasn't a matter of medical necessity. On the other hand, Seldane's strongest competitors were Benadryl and Chlortrimeton (chlorpheniramine), both drugs taken three or four times a day. Seldane, introduced as a twice-a-day remedy, would possess a definite marketing edge.

Well, no matter, Seldane's pre-release side effect profile seemed benign enough at 60 mg twice a day: headache, 15.8%; drowsiness, 8.5%; gastric problems (nausea, vomiting, stomachache), 7.6%; dry mouth or throat, 4.8%; fatigue, 4.5%. These numbers are actually pretty low compared with those of most drugs. So why not market Seldane at this dose?

There was no indication that Seldane caused serious cardiac effects. There was little indication that using 120 mg a day of Seldane might prove more risky than 60 mg a day. So why not go with the more marketable 60-mg twice-a-day dosage?

Just one reason—that no drug is well known until years after its release. That pre-release studies inevitably have their limitations; new side effects and unexpected problems always turn up later. Just one reason—caution.

A LOWER TWICE-A-DAY SELDANE DOSAGE?

The great irony about Seldane is that by making it a drug used twice a day instead of three times a day, the manufacturer actually increased the risks. And not just because the total daily dosage increased from 60 to 120 mg.

The cardiac arrhythmias caused by Seldane are directly related to the amount of medication *taken at any one given time*. Total daily dosage isn't as important as how much is taken at one time. It's obvious that taking 20 mg of Seldane each time is safer than 60 mg, so clearly the 20 mg taken three times a day is safer than 60 mg twice a day.

What's interesting is that a dosage of 40 mg three times a day is also less likely to cause cardiac irregularities than 60 mg twice a day. The total daily dose is the same, 120 mg a day. But with the 40-mg dose, the amount taken each time is 33% lower.

Indeed, a study published in 1977 suggested that 40 mg twice a day might be effective in treating some individuals. This study examined the effects of oral Seldane on allergic skin reactions. When given doses of 40 and 60 mg each three times a day, the 40-mg dose performed as well as the 60 mg. The 60-mg dose was also studied on a twice-a-day schedule; the 40-mg dose wasn't. However, the researchers observed that the 40-mg dose maintained its strength beyond ten hours, and some of its effect lasted for twelve hours.

This study was performed on healthy male volunteers with an average age of 29 years. In essence, the study group was younger, larger, and likely healthier than the general population—meaning that the Seldane requirements and tolerances of this study group would be higher than the average patient seen in doctors' offices. In the general population, 40 mg of Seldane twice a day might be plenty for some.

Why wasn't the 40-mg dose studied in more diverse and older populations? Why wasn't Seldane produced in both 40- and 60-mg pills, thereby providing patients and physicians some flexibility in dosing? We can only guess—time, money, the pressure to market a new, promising product.

So only the dosage of 60 mg twice a day was tendered to the FDA, which approved it. Only the 60-mg pill was marketed. Only a one-size-fits-all dosage of 60 mg twice a day was recommended. And as of February 1998, it was removed from the market.

SELDANE AND THE ELDERLY

The 1995 PDR offers no specific dosage guidelines for elderly individuals prescribed Seldane. Geriatric patients, like everyone else, are given the same 60 mg twice a day. As revealed in Seldane's pre-release research, this dosage is unnecessarily strong for many adult patients.

Remarkably few studies appear in the literature regarding Seldane and the elderly. The scant research that is present offers conflicting results. A 1992 study of healthy elderly and younger adults revealed similar rates of metabolism and low frequencies of side effects, but this provides no assurance for less able elderly patients. In contrast, a 1990 study found that 5 of 8 healthy elderly females (average age 68) became sedated with Seldane. And the article in *JAMA* stated: "Old age may also be a factor that could lead to toxic concentrations of terfenadine [Seldane] after usual dosages."

Although the research doesn't confirm whether elderly individuals require lower Seldane dosages than younger adults, it does reveal that the very lowest effective Seldane dosage for elderly patients, especially for those with other illnesses or taking other medications, was never defined. This places elderly patients in jeopardy because many older patients take cardiac drugs, and some cardiac drugs interact adversely with Seldane. Once again, dosage is key. Lower doses usually cause fewer problems.

INADEQUATE RESPONSES TO A SERIOUS PROBLEM

You'd think that with the discovery of Seldane's connection to life-endangering heart arrhythmias, the manufacturer's dosage recommendations would have been expanded to include guidelines for lower dosages. Since it had already been shown that doses of 20 mg as well as 40 mg three times a day are effective, and strongly suggested that 40 mg twice a day may be sufficient for some people, why not encourage physicians to start patients at these lower, safer dosages? For people who require higher dosages, the dose can readily be adjusted up to the standard 60 mg a day.

Why not provide lower, safer dosing schedules for mild conditions, or for small, sickly, or medication-sensitive persons, or for those taking other medications? Why not provide lower dosages for the elderly?

As of early 1997, none of these preventive measures has been implemented. True, in the years since the discovery of Seldane's association to cardiac abnormalities, some changes have been made in Seldane's package insert and PDR description. Bold-print, all-cap, or otherwise highlighted warnings about Seldane-induced cardiac arrythmias, cardiac arrest, and death are plastered all over Seldane's two-page description in the PDR. These warnings not only let doctors know about Seldane's dangers, but also caution them not to prescribe Seldane in dosages above the recommended 120 mg a day. This means that both Seldane's minimum recommended dosage *and* its maximum recommended dosage are 120 mg a day—i.e., the same. Not much flexibility for a medication shown to exhibit a 10-fold range of interindividual variation.

But guidelines for lower, safer doses? Not a one. Not even a word about the findings of the studies with Seldane at lower doses. In the meantime, the approved dosage guidelines for Seldane remain the same in 1997 as when Seldane was first released in 1985—and so do the risks.

RECOMMENDATIONS

Despite the problems discussed above, in 1995 Seldane remained America's No. 46 top-selling drug as measured by outpatient prescriptions—that's 7 million prescriptions purchased from U.S. pharmacies. In 1996, Seldane still ranked among the top 100 prescribed drugs, holding position No. 84.

In 1997 the FDA announced its intention to withdraw Seldane from the market. Seldane's manufacturer responded that it would fight this action because serious side effects with Seldane are very infrequent—indeed, far less frequent than with many other drugs that doctors prescribe. However, in the case of Seldane, newer, safer, and equally effective medications such as Claritin and Zyrtec are now available. Also, in 1996 Seldane's manufacturer released Allegra, a derivative of Seldane without the potential cardiac problems.

So as of this writing, no form of low-dose Seldane is available. Fortunately, the 60-mg Seldane pill is a tablet that, although not scored, can be easily split. Of course, not everyone will respond adequately to Seldane at lower doses, but the issue here is dose flexibility. Knowing about the rare but serious cardiac effects of Seldane and the demonstrated effectiveness of Seldane at lower doses, at least consider starting with a lower dose to determine your individual sensitivity to the drug. This is no different than the *Journal of the American Medical Association* suggests: ''Dosage restriction [of Seldane is] . . . essential for prevention of this serious reaction [cardiac arrhythmias].''

As stated previously, any adjustments in dosage should first be discussed with your physician. This is especially true with Seldane. Fewer physicians are prescribing this drug, but in 1996 Seldane remained among the top 100 most prescribed drugs in America. There is no reason for this—many alternatives exist. Allegra is almost chemically identical to Seldane with the same 60-mg twice-a-day, one-size-fits-all manufacturer-recommended dosage (despite studies that show the effectiveness of lower doses). Claritin and Zyrtec have already proven themselves to be as effective or more so than Seldane. If your physician intends to prescribe Seldane for you, ask about these alternatives.

Other Antihistamines

SECOND-GENERATION ANTIHISTAMINES

CLARITIN (LORATADINE)

Within a year of its release in 1993, Claritin advanced into the ranks of the top 200 drugs in U.S. outpatient prescriptions. The reason was that unlike Seldane and Hismanal, Claritin was the first second-generation antihistamine that was not associated with potentially dangerous effects on the heart. Consequently, many physicians, hospitals, and nursing homes switched to Claritin as their preferred antihistamine. The result was that in 1995, Claritin (No. 27) surpassed Seldane (No. 46) in U.S. outpatient prescriptions; in 1996, Claritin ranked No. 20.

Claritin's manufacturer recommends a dosage of 10 mg for all ages over 12 years. In fact the same dosage, 10 mg once daily (2 teaspoons of Claritin syrup), is recommended for children ages 6 to 11. The only exception is people with liver or kidney impairments, who are advised to take 10 mg every other day.

Were any studies done with Claritin at dosages below 10 mg? A review of the pre-release literature reveals none. Nor was Claritin's manufacturer able to locate any studies for me.

The limitations of a one-size-fits-all dosage have been discussed at length in this book. This problem is underscored by statements in Claritin's 1996 PDR description that in pre-release studies ''considerable variability'' was seen in Claritin's activity in test subjects. This variability resulted in ''a 25-fold range of distribution in healthy subjects.''

In other words, the range of interindividual variation with Claritin in healthy subjects was quite broad. In the elderly, the range of variation may be even greater. According to the 1997 PDR Supplement A, blood levels of Claritin were increased about 50% in elderly individuals as compared with younger adults. The risk of side effects likely mirrors the increased blood levels of Claritin in the elderly. Nonetheless, dose recommendations for elderly individuals are the same as younger adults.

Although Claritin's popularity is based in part on its lack of sedation, one physician I know who isn't sensitive to medications or sedation gets very drowsy with Claritin. This surprised him until he checked Claritin's side effect profile: headache, 12%; somnolence, 8%; fatigue, 4%.

Additional variation may be seen when Claritin is taken with other medications. Because Claritin is metabolized by the cytochrome P450 3A4 enzyme, its effects may be greatly increased by drugs that inhibit this enzyme such as Nizoral (ketoconazole) and possibly Sporanox (itraconazole), erythromycin antibiotics (erythromycin, Biaxin), Tagamet, and others.

Because the 10-mg dosage is recommended for all ages over six, it is unlikely that many physicians will think about prescribing any other dosage. Indeed, even for people with impaired liver or kidney functioning, the 10-mg dosage is still recommended— every other day. For these people or other medication-sensitive individuals, this isn't an ideal solution because there's no guarantee that Claritin will remain effective for two days. A better approach is probably 5 mg daily.

Why wasn't this dosage recommended instead? Possibly because it simply wasn't studied. Also, for children ages 6 to 11, it's difficult to believe that their dosage can be the same as adults many times their size (6-year-olds are small!) without some increased risk. Why not suggest 1 *or* 2 teaspoons (5 *or* 10 mg) once daily just to provide some flexibility? Actually, with small children, it may be wise to start even lower.

These criticisms notwithstanding, Claritin has proven to be an effective, well-accepted, and apparently generally safe antihistamine. Still, side effects do occur with Claritin, so if you are sensitive to medications or prone to side effects, especially sedation, you may want to start at a lower dosage until your specific dose requirement and tolerance is established.

Claritin is produced in breakable tablets and a syrup, making flexible dosing easy. It is also manufactured as a fast-acting Reditab that dissolves in the mouth and is then swallowed.

ZYRTEC (CETIRIZINE)

Approved by the FDA in late 1995, Zyrtec quickly climbed among the ranks of the top 200 prescribed drugs in America, ranking No. 159 in 1996. Zyrtec is chemically related to hydroxyzine (Atarax, Vistaril), a first-generation antihistamine that has been used for decades. But Zyrtec is chemically different enough from hydroxyzine to lack its high incidence of side effects. Still, Zyrtec does cause sedation in approximately 15% of people, and if you are sensitive to sedating drugs or alcohol, you should start with a low dose of this drug.

Recent reports suggest that Zyrtec may possess additional activity in comparison to other antihistamines. Specifically, Zyrtec not only blocks histamine, but may also reduce the production of eosinophils, a type of white blood cells that are usually increased in allergic disorders. This attribute seems to make Zyrtec quite effective in treating skin disorders such as atopic dermatitis, eczema, hives, and severe cases of congenital dry skin. It also may explain Zyrtec's apparent ability to reduce the severity of skin reactions in people sensitive to mosquito bites; in fact, Zyrtec taken before exposure has been reported to have a protective effect.

The manufacturer-recommended dosage of Zyrtec is 5 or 10 mg once daily; most clinical trials used 10 mg. There are no specific geriatric dosages. For people with impaired liver or kidney functioning, 5 mg daily is recommended. Unlike all other second-generation antihistamines, Zyrtec is offered in two pill sizes, 5 and 10 mg, both breakable tablets.

According to pre-release studies, the most common side effects are sedation (14%), fatigue (6%), and dry mouth (5%)—all dose-related. Zyrtec is not recommended in pregnancy or nursing mothers.

If you are sensitive to medications, prone to side effects, small, or elderly, or simply want to find the very lowest effective dosage of Zyrtec, start with 5 mg a day. This dosage was shown to be effective in several pre-release studies. In one study, all of the subjects were started at this dosage and immediate improvement in allergic symptoms was seen. The subjects were allowed to increase to higher doses, and the majority ultimately did. But 13.4% chose to remain at 5 mg a day. In another study, the authors concluded "the once daily 5-mg dose was found to be an effective minimum dose." These authors noted that with increased Zyrtec dosages, the incidence of side effects also increased.

The 1997 PDR includes some information about interindividual variation with Zyrtec. Several measures of Zyrtec in blood levels showed "a two- to four-fold variability in healthy subjects," so an increased effect can be expected in medication-sensitive or side-effect-prone individuals. And although the manufacturer claims that the blood level of Zyrtec doesn't build up with each 10-mg dosage, the drug effect does last for at least 24 hours, suggesting that some medication remains in the system when the next dose is taken.

In the elderly, the manufacturer notes that Zyrtec clearance from the blood is slowed on average by 40%, which explains why the half-life (the time required for the blood level of Zyrtec to drop by a half) was extended by 50%. This means that high blood levels of Zyrtec last much longer in elderly persons.

If you are highly sensitive to medications or specifically sensitive to sedating drugs, you can begin with Zyrtec 2.5 mg by splitting the 5 mg tablet. If 2.5 or 5 mg a day are ineffective, you can increase to 7.5 mg rather than doubling from 5 to 10 mg a day. Another way to reduce the tendency for sedation or other side effects is to split the total daily dosage into two doses twelve hours apart, such as 2.5 or 5 mg of Zyrtec twice a day. Zyrtec is also produced as a syrup (5 mg per teaspoon) with which different doses can be easily measured.

If Zyrtec is too sedating for you at any dosage, Claritin and Allegra are less likely to cause this side effect.

ALLEGRA (FEXOFENADINE)

The newest among the second-generation antihistamines, Allegra was released in late 1996. Chemically related to Seldane, Allegra provides the same results without Seldane's dangerous drug interactions or cardiac risks.

The manufacturer-recommended dosage of Allegra is 60 mg twice a day for everyone 12 years and older. The recommendation for dosage for the elderly is the same. The only exception is for those with reduced kidney function, for whom 60 mg a day is recommended. Allegra is produced in only one size, a 60-mg capsule, making flexible dosing difficult (at least Seldane is produced as a breakable tablet).

In pre-release studies, side effects with Allegra were infrequent. The most common were nausea, stomach upset, and drowsiness—all reportedly occurring in less than 2% of subjects. Interestingly, although Allegra is chemically very similar to Seldane, its most frequent side effects don't include headaches, a fairly common event with Seldane. Allegra is not recommended in pregnancy or nursing mothers.

In early studies, low doses of Allegra demonstrated substantial antihistamine effect. Doses of 20 and 40 mg reduced allergic reactions for up to twelve hours in some studies. In one study comparing doses of 40, 60, and 120 mg a day of Allegra, all doses provided significant relief of allergy symptoms during the 14 days of the trial. Thus, 40 mg twice a day may be quite sufficient for many people, not only those who are sensitive to medications, and 20 mg twice or three times a day may be enough for some who are medication-sensitive. You may recall that similar findings were demonstrated with Seldane more than fifteen years ago (20 mg three times a day was very effective), but like the latter medication, Allegra is not offered at these lower doses.

In the elderly, 60 mg of Allegra produced markedly increased medication blood levels. In a study using only 20 mg of Allegra four times a day, a group of elderly subjects demonstrated peak levels and total amounts of medication in the blood that were about 70% higher, and a rate of drug clearance that took about 30% longer, as compared with a matched group of younger adults. These results suggest a more potent effect of Allegra in the elderly. With greater potency usually comes a greater propensity for side effects. Yet despite these very significant findings, elderly individuals are prescribed the same Allegra dosage as younger folks. Moreover, these findings were obtained with healthy elderly individuals; medication effects, and therefore side effects, are likely to be even greater in elderly persons with other illnesses or taking other medications.

If healthy elderly individuals developed such high blood levels of Allegra, other people who are sensitive to medications may likely encounter similar heightened responses to the manufacturer-recommended dosage of Allegra.

Allegra is one of the most recently marketed drugs reviewed in this book, but once again we are confronted with a virtually one-size-fits-all dosage, compounded by the availability of only one dose size, a 60-mg capsule. This greatly restricts dose flexibility. Although Allegra does demonstrate a low incidence of side effects in pre-release studies, this was also true of Seldane and many other drugs that later, years after their release for general usage, were found to cause more problems than anticipated.

In the meantime, Allegra may be most useful for transferring people from standard doses of Seldane to the identical dose regimen with Allegra. For those who are sensitive to medications or otherwise at risk for drug side effects, ask your pharmacist about preparing low-dose capsules of Allegra for you. By simply spreading the contents of a single 60-mg Allegra capsule between two or three empty capsules, doses of 20 or 30 mg, respectively, can be fashioned. Initiating treatment with a low dose of Allegra will allow you to determine the lowest effective dose required for your system and allergies.

An easier alternative is to start with an antihistamine that offers greater dose flexibility. Both Claritin and Zyrtec come as breakable tablets and syrups.

HISMANAL (ASTEMIZOLE)

In 1995 Hismanal ranked No. 174 among the 200 most prescribed drugs in America; in 1996, it disappeared from the list. Yet in 1993 Hismanal ranked No. 81. Its decline coincides with Claritin's (and more recently Zyrtec's) gaining favor.

Hismanal's slide is warranted. Like Seldane, Hismanal can cause rare yet very serious cardiac problems, especially when used in combination with certain drugs. Like Seldane and Claritin, Hismanal is recommended in a one-size-fits-all dosage. The manufacturer-suggested dose is one 10-mg tablet daily for all ages over twelve years.

The deficiencies of a one-size-fits-all dosage has been discussed previously in this book. However, Hismanal is produced as a scored tablet. It is easily breakable, affording dose flexibility for people who are small, elderly, sensitive to medications, or prone to side effects, or those who simply prefer to start treatment at a low dosage.

Among the physicians I've asked, Hismanal rarely ranks as a favorite antihistamine. The most common complaint about it is that it starts working slowly. Zyrtec, Claritin, Seldane, and Allegra work faster, an advantage if your allergy is acute or severe. In addition, as mentioned above, Hismanal shares the same potential drug interactions and cardiac reactions as Seldane.

FIRST-GENERATION ANTIHISTAMINES

BENADRYL (DIPHENHYDRAMINE)

A health professional I know has dermographia, a skin condition that makes his skin extremely sensitive to injury, no matter how slight. The mildest scratch or abrasion creates immediate intense redness and itching lasting 15 minutes. His doctor prescribed Benadryl at the high dose of 100 mg three times a day. Incredibly, the man developed no side effects, not even sedation. He laughed when he told me this because he has friends who get very sleepy with 25 mg.

The Benadryl controlled his condition, but although he wasn't medication-sensitive, he was concerned about taking so much medication, particularly because dermographia is permanent and requires daily treatment. On his own, this man reduced his dosage to 50 mg three times a day, then 50 mg only at bedtime without any loss of effectiveness. Now, twelve years later, he takes 25 mg of Benadryl at night, and it continues to do the job. In this case, side effects weren't the reason using a lower dosage. Instead, as the man put it, "I have to take the medication daily. I was concerned about taking more medication than I needed year after year."

Benadryl is available in both prescription and nonprescription strengths. Its generic form, diphenhydramine, can be found in a myriad of other prescription and nonprescription products: Benylin tablets and cough syrup, Bufferin Nite Time, Excedrin PM, Nytol Tablets, Sleep-eze 3 Tablets, Sominex Caplets and Tablets, Tylenol Cold Night Time, Tylenol PM, Unisom with Pain Relief-Nighttime Sleep Aid, and others.

The PDR-recommended dosage for adults taking Benadryl is 25 to 50 mg three or four times daily. For insomnia, 50 mg at bedtime. Benadryl's dosage recommendations also come with a warning in capital letters: "DOSAGE SHOULD BE INDIVIDUALIZED ACCORDING TO THE NEEDS AND THE RESPONSE OF THE PATIENT." Good idea, but Benadryl is produced in only two sizes, 25- and 50-mg capsules, so flexible dosing is limited. Even at the lower 25-mg dose, many people experience substantial sedation.

The PDR provides no dosage guidelines for elderly patients;

seemingly, the recommended dosage is the same as for younger adults. Yet the manufacturer does acknowledge that elderly patients are more likely to encounter problems with antihistamines, including dizziness, sedation, and a drop in blood pressure. For this reason, many physicians don't prescribe Benadryl or other first-generation antihistamines to the elderly. No matter your age, if you are medication-sensitive, starting with lower doses is suggested until your sensitivity can be determined.

BROMPHENIRAMINE

Brompheniramine is found in prescription Dimetane products, as well as in many nonprescription remedies such as Alka Seltzer Plus Sinus Allergy Medication, Dimetane and Dimetapp products, Dristan Allergy Nasal Caplets, and Drixoral Syrup. The usual recommended dosage (Dimetane-DC Cough Syrup) is 4 mg every 4 to 6 hours. Dosages for the elderly are usually the same.

The uses and problems of this entire class of drugs apply to brompheniramine. Sedation is the most frequent adverse effect. Individual tolerance to brompheniramine varies considerably. The recommended dosage of Dimetane, a prescription cough syrup, will sedate many adults and elderly persons. Half or quarter dosages may be preferable until your individual sensitivity can be ascertained.

CHLORPHENIRAMINE (CPM)

Even more omnipresent than Benadryl, CPM is an ingredient in a dazzling array of top-selling nonprescription products: Ornade, Teldrin, and some preparations of Comtrex, Contac, Coricidin, Dristan, 4-Way Cold Tablets, Sinarest, Sinutab, Tylenol Cold and Tylenol Flu remedies, Triaminic, Vicks, and many drugstore brands. The list in the 1994 nonprescription PDR of remedies containing CPM is two columns long.

The usual recommended dosage for CPM is 4 mg every 4 to 6 hours. CPM possesses the same general side effect tendencies of other first-generation antihistamines, including sedation.

Individual tolerance to chlorpheniramine varies considerably. A local physician told me, "I weigh 220 pounds, but if I take 2 mg of CPM [that's half the usual dose], I walk around all day long shaking my head. 'Thick' is the best way I can describe it.''

CPM is supposed to wear off in four to six hours, but in the elderly and others sensitive to CPM's sedating properties, the effect can linger. Many CPM preparations don't contain lower-dose recommendations for elderly individuals. Nevertheless this age group, as well as other medication-sensitive persons, should consider initiating treatment with CPM at lower than recommended dosages.

TAVIST

Like other first-generation antihistamines, drowsiness is the most common side effect with Tavist. Hence Tavist comes with a highly visible recommendation to individualize dosage. Fortunately, unlike Benadryl, Tavist makes this possible with breakable tablets.

The 1994 PDR dosage recommendations for Tavist offer some dosage flexibility. The starting dose is 1.34 mg twice a day, which can be increased to a maximum dose of 2.68 mg three times a day. Patients with known sensitivity to the sedating properties of antihistamine drugs may want to begin at even lower dosages. This is possible because Tavist is produced as a scored, easily breakable tablet.

Tavist's manufacturer offers no dosage provisions for the elderly, although it does mention the dizziness, sedation, and low blood pressure that antihistamines can cause in this age group. Whether you are elderly, taking other medications, or medication-sensitive, starting with a lower dose may be wise until your individual sensitivity can be determined.

OTHER FIRST-GENERATION ANTIHISTAMINES

The first-generation antihistamines comprise a broad group of drugs. Other members of this group include Actifed (triprolidine), Phenergan (promethazine), Midol and Pamprin (pyrilamine), Dramamine (dimenhydrinate), and Bonine (meclizine).

Different first-generation antihistamines are marketed for different purposes. For example, Dramamine, Bonine, and Phenergan are best known for treating motion sickness (see Chapter 17), Phenergan also for nausea and vomiting, and Midol for menstrual distress.

No matter the usage, first generation antihistamines share similar properties and side effects. If you experience sedation with one member of this group, you are likely to be sedated by the others, although the degree of sedation may vary. Sedation and most other side effects with first-generation antihistamines are dose-related. Starting at lower doses may cause you fewer or milder side effects.

SEVENTEEN

Motion Sickness Medications

Transderm-Scop (scopolamine patch)
Dramamine (dimenhydrinate)
Meclizine—Antivert, Bonine, Dramamine II
Phenergan (promethazine)

About Motion Sickness

Motion sickness can occur with any vehicular movement, whether on land or sea, in the air or in space. Most of us think of cars, boats, or airplanes in relation to motion sickness, but many experience a moment of it in a fast elevator in a skyscraper. The most frequent symptom of motion sickness is nausea. Others include vomiting, chills, pallor, and sweating.

The most commonly used medications to prevent and treat motion sickness are scopolamine (Transderm-Scop) and prescription and nonprescription first-generation antihistamines. Among the latter group is Dramamine, Bonine, and Antivert. Atarax and Vistaril may also be used, but these are more often employed for their anti-anxiety effects and are listed in Chapter 7. Benadryl is sometimes used for motion sickness, but more often for allergy symptoms, insomnia, and as an ingredient in nonprescription remedies for colds and coughs.

Among the antihistamines, the *AMA Drug Evaluations Annual 1994* states that Phenergan (promethazine) is the most effective for motion sickness and is used by astronauts in the space program. However, Phenergan can be highly sedating. Second-generation antihistamines (Seldane, Hismanal, Claritin) are ineffective for motion sickness because these drugs do not appreciably enter the brain.

HIGHER INCIDENCE OF SEDATION (ANTIHISTAMINES)

Dramamine (dimenhydrinate)
Meclizine—Antivert, Bonine, Dramamine II
Phenergan (promethazine)
Other Antihistamines: Marezine, Benadryl

LOWER INCIDENCE OF SEDATION

Transderm-Scop

Medications Used for Motion Sickness

The Transderm-Scop patch is considered the most effective medication for motion sickness. However, for individuals not sensitive to sedating medications, antihistamines offer greater dose flexibility and the generic nonprescription preparations are less expensive.

Transderm-Scop and the first generation antihistamines are more effective when used prior to travel rather than after symptoms have developed. Among these remedies, there is considerable variation in effects and side effects. Some are short-acting (Dramamine), while others may persist for one (meclizine) to three days (Transderm-Scop).

The first-generation antihistamines cause drowsiness in a large proportion of people, while Transderm-Scop reportedly causes sedation in about 16%. Thus, people known to be sensitive to the sedating effects of medications might consider Transderm-Scop as their first choice. On the other hand, for those who are insensitive to the sedating properties of first-generation antihistamines, this group offers greater dose flexibility and less cost. Most side effects with motion-sickness medications are dose-related.

Is it important to use the lowest effective dosage of motion-sickness medications? We don't usually consider these drugs dangerous, yet in August 1996, Derek Smith died from respiratory failure related to motion-sickness medication. Smith, 34, was an excellent professional basketball player until injuries curtailed his career. At the time of his death, he was an assistant coach with the Washington Wizards and was on a cruise with other team members and families, including his wife and two children. The accounts didn't mention which medication Smith had taken or if there were complicating factors such as other illnesses, medications, or alcohol. Either way, respiratory depression is usually related to dosage. Smith was young and well over six feet tall, but whichever motion sickness medication he took, the dosage was too much for his system.

Transderm-Scop
(Scopolamine Patch)

It has long been known that scopolamine, the active ingredient of Transderm-Scop, is very effective in preventing and treating the dizziness, nausea, and vomiting of motion sickness. Some authorities consider it the most effective of all motion sickness medications. For decades, however, scopolamine's use was limited because of a high incidence of side effects that made the drug intolerable for many people.

Transderm-Scop, a patch fixed to the skin behind the ear, was developed to provide a convenient means of providing a continual, low-dose infusion of scopolamine through the skin and directly into the bloodstream. The overall dosage by this method is substantially less than when scopolamine is administered by mouth, thereby reducing the risks of side effects, yet the effectiveness of Transderm-Scop remains high. In one study exposing subjects to rough seas for seven hours, 76% on placebo became sick, 45% on dimenhydrinate (regular Dramamine), and only 25% on Transderm-Scop.

The Transderm-Scop patch comes in only one size, containing 1.5 mg of scopolamine; only a third of this amount gets through the skin and into the bloodstream. The manufacturer recommends placing the patch behind the ear about four hours before exposure to motion. However, one study suggested that placement eight to twelve hours before traveling may be more effective.

One patch lasts seventy-two hours in most people, but less in some individuals. For briefer exposures, the patch can be removed sooner. For exposures beyond seventy-two hours, the old patch should be removed and a new patch applied behind the other ear.

MOST COMMON SIDE EFFECTS

Dryness of the mouth occurs in about 67%, drowsiness 16% (substantially less than with antihistamines for motion sickness), blurred vision. The manufacturer recommends caution for those driving or operating machinery. Use with caution with intestinal or urinary obstructions, or liver or kidney disorders. Transderm-Scop shouldn't be used in when the patient has glaucoma or is pregnant. Use with caution in the elderly. Withdrawal reactions—nausea, dizziness, incoordination—have occurred with this drug.

LOW-DOSE TRANSDERM-SCOP

Transderm-Scop is produced as an adhesive patch in only one size, which limits dose flexibility. Interestingly, different areas of the body of the same individual produce different rates of absorption. Studies have demonstrated a wide variation in skin permeability with Transderm-Scop. In cadavers, the variation was five- to ten-fold. Limited tests in healthy individuals demonstrated similar variation. In cadavers, absorption was greatest when the patch was applied to the skin behind the ear, followed in order by the skin of the back, chest, stomach, forearm, thigh. The skin behind the ear was ten times more permeable than the thigh.

RECOMMENDATIONS

Transderm-Scop is the most effective medication therapy currently available for motion sickness. Produced as a three-day patch, it's most useful for longer periods of motion exposure such as a cruise or an all-day fishing trip. Because it is available in only one size, dose flexibility is limited. However, theoretically speaking, applying Transderm-Scop to less permeable skin areas lowers the amount of medication that enters the body. Theoretically speaking, if you develop intolerable side effects with Transderm-Scop placed as recommended behind the ear, you may be able to obtain benefit with fewer side effects by applying the patch to a less permeable part of the body. No studies exist testing this hypothesis, so it cannot be recommended. However, if you are medication-sensitive, prone to motion sickness, and intolerant of Dramamine, meclizine, and other medications, you and your physician may want to consider some adaptation of the Transderm-Scop patch approach. Be aware that once you attach the patch to one area, if you then move it to another, it won't work.

Dramamine (Dimenhydrinate)

Dramamine is perhaps the antihistamine best known for motion sickness. Dramamine works like other antihistamines by reducing the sensitivity of the balance mechanism in the inner ear and by reducing symptoms of nausea. Some authorities believe that scopolamine (Transderm-Scop patches), promethazine (Phenergan), and meclizine (Bonine) may be more effective than Dramamine. However, Dramamine is shorter acting than Bonine and can be taken for brief exposures. Dramamine is less prone to cause side effects than Phenergan in many people. Thus, Dramamine remains a useful, short-acting motion sickness medication, particularly for people who develop side effects to Transderm-Scop patches.

For greatest effectiveness, Dramamine should be taken at least thirty minutes before exposure to motion. The manufacturer-recommended dosage is 50 to 100 mg every four to six hours; maximum total dosage is 400 mg a day. Note that regular Dramamine (dimenhydrinate) differs from Dramamine II, which contains long-acting meclizine (see below).

MOST COMMON SIDE EFFECTS

Dramamine often causes sedation, drowsiness, and sleepiness. Other common side effects include stomach irritation, dry mouth, headache, blurred vision, impaired coordination.

RECOMMENDATIONS

As with all antihistamines, considerable individual variation occurs in response to Dramamine. Medication-sensitive individuals and those known to be sensitive to sedation may want to start with lower doses of Dramamine. Some authorities suggest that antihistamines should not be used in the elderly.

Dramamine is produced by the Upjohn Company; generic dimenhydrinate is made by many manufacturers. Usually available as tablets or capsules; tablets are preferable for flexible dosing. Some tablets are chewable, which increases the speed of absorption. Also available as a liquid (12.5 mg a teaspoon), the most flexible dose form. Liquid dimenhydrinate is also absorbed quickly. Generic dimenhydrinate is usually less expensive than brand-name Dramamine.

Meclizine—Antivert, Bonine, and Dramamine II

Nonprescription Bonine, Dramamine II, and prescription-only Antivert are brand names for meclizine, a long-acting antihistamine frequently used for motion sickness. In 1995, meclizine ranked No. 32 among the generic medications in outpatient prescriptions written by physicians. In that year, nearly 1,200,000 outpatient prescriptions were written for meclizine, and this number doesn't include the millions of times that people purchased it in a nonprescription form.

Meclizine works by reducing the sensitivity of the balance mechanism in the inner ear and thereby reducing symptoms of nausea. Some authorities believe that scopolamine (Transderm-Scop patches) and possibly promethazine (Phenergan) are more effective in preventing or treating motion sickness. An advantage of meclizine products over Dramamine (dimenhydrinate) is their prolonged effect, requiring only one dose per day. For the best results, meclizine should be taken at least an hour before traveling.

The manufacturer-recommended dosage of meclizine is 1 to 2 25-mg pills per day.

MOST COMMON SIDE EFFECTS

Meclizine often causes sedation, drowsiness, dry mouth, fatigue, blurred vision, impaired coordination.

RECOMMENDATIONS

As with all antihistamines, considerable individual variation occurs in response to meclizine. Meant as a twenty-four-hour medication, meclizine's duration of action lasts eight to twenty-four hours, meaning that for some people one dose may last far less than a day. On the other hand, medication-sensitive individuals may be particularly prone to sedation or other side effects with this medication and may want to start with lower doses. Some authorities caution against the use of antihistamines in the elderly.

Meclizine can be purchased as Bonine, Dramamine II, Antivert, and several kinds of generic preparations. It is available as tablets and capsules in various sizes: 12.5, 25, and 50 mg. Tablets are preferable for flexible dosing. Chewable tablets are the most flexible and, when chewed instead of swallowed, work more quickly. Meclizine is not available in liquid form.

Prescription Antivert and generic meclizine preparations are available at half dosage, 12.5 mg, and Bonine (25 mg) is breakable. The nonprescription forms of meclizine generally cost less.

Phenergan (Promethazine)

Chemically a member of the phenothiazine group (Thorazine, Mellaril, Stelazine, Haldol), Phenergan's effects are more like those of antihistamines. One of Phenergan's effects is to prevent or reduce the symptoms of motion sickness. Some authorities consider Phenergan more effective than Dramamine or Bonine. Phenergan reportedly has been used in the space program for motion sickness.

Phenergan is also employed in other areas including the treatment of nausea and vomiting resulting from illness and cancer chemotherapy. A very sedating medication, Phenergan can also be used for insomnia, anxiety, and allergic reactions.

Phenergan dosages vary according to its usage. For motion sickness, the manufacturer-recommended dosage is 25 mg twice a day. For nausea and vomiting, 25 mg every four to six hours orally; if vomiting prevents oral usage, 12.5- or 25-mg rectal suppositories can be used every four to six hours. For allergic reactions, 25 mg at bedtime, or 12.5 mg four times a day. For sedation, 25 to 50 mg.

Phenergan is produced in 12.5-, 25-, and 50-mg tablets. Suppositories in same dosages. Phenergan liquid available in a concentration of 6.25 mg a teaspoon. Also available as generic promethazine.

MOST FREQUENT SIDE EFFECTS

Phenergan frequently causes sedation, sleepiness, drowsiness, blurred vision, dry mouth, dizziness. The manufacturer cautions against driving or operating dangerous machinery until Phenergan's effect in the individual is known. It must also be used with caution in patients with seizure disorders, glaucoma, peptic ulcer.

COMMENTS ON RECOMMENDED DOSES

Because Phenergan is known to be highly sedating in many people, doses lower than 25 mg should be considered in people with histories of sedation with other medications, especially with first-generation antihistamines.

Phenergan's effects are usually apparent within twenty minutes of oral ingestion. Considerable interindividual variation may be seen; the effects of Phenergan generally last four to six hours, yet may persist up to twelve hours in some individuals. Phenergan should be taken half an hour to an hour before travel and repeated eight to twelve hours later. May be used every four to six hours if nausea develops.

For medication-sensitive individuals requiring Phenergan at doses below 25 mg, a breakable 12.5-mg tablet or the 6.25 mg/teaspoon Phenergan liquid offer the greatest dose flexibility. For those whose nausea makes all intake impossible, Phenergan suppositories can be used; these can also be split with a knife to reduce the dose. If you are using prescription Phenergan, be sure to discuss any changes in your dosage with your physician.

PART 7

Other Medications

EIGHTEEN

Other Medications

Antibiotics
Antifungal medications and a new, low-dose
treatment for fungal nails
Digoxin
Haldol (haloperidol)
Zofran

Antibiotics

You go to your physician for an infection in some part of your body. In most cases, your doctor takes a culture and prescribes an antibiotic. The infection goes away. This is medical practice in its classic, most basic form.

But it doesn't always work this well. A 30-year-old woman developed bronchitis. She was prescribed an antibiotic that made her so dizzy she could hardly stand; as a result, she missed several days of work. She tried to stick it out. "I just thought it was me," she told me. That's what most people think when a side effect occurs. Finally she called her physician, who told her to break the tablets in half, reducing her dosage by 50%. The dizziness went away. So did the infection. Obviously, the lower dose was sufficient. "It never occurred to me that it could be the dosage," she said. But it was—not surprising when you consider that she weighs 100 pounds, yet her initial dose was the same used for people twice her size.

Antibiotics comprise the most prescribed group of drugs in America. In 1995, five antibiotics ranked within the top 20 most prescribed outpatient medications in the United States. In 1996, seven antibiotics ranked within the top 30. Among generic drugs in 1996, six of the top 11 were antibiotics.

Antibiotic dosages are usually standard. Most are prescribed in one or two dosages. Amoxicillin, perhaps the most prescribed drug in the United States, is usually prescribed at 250 or 500 mg every eight hours, although the dose may be modified with small children and the very old. For everyone else, dosage decisions are usually based on the nature and severity of the infection, as opposed to the potential medication sensitivity of the patient.

Some antibiotics are produced in only one size. These include Zithromax (azithromycin, ranking No. 49 in sales), Maxaquin (lomefloxacin), and Noroxin (norfloxacin). This may sometimes be a problem for people at risk for medication side effects. For example, with Zithromax the PDR tells us that elderly women develop peak blood levels that are 30% to 50% higher than other groups, yet no dose alterations are suggested. Also, a 1993 study found that some patients with cirrhosis developed peak blood levels of Zithromax that were 70% higher than in healthy subjects, and elimination rates were prolonged by about 25%, but the manufacturer doesn't recommend lower doses for this group either. However, the 1996 *American Hospital Formulary Service* drug reference makes note of these discrepancies: "While the manufacturer makes no specific recommendations for azithromycin [Zithromax] dosage adjustment in patients with hepatic impairment, caution should be exercised in such patients since the drug is eliminated primarily via the liver."

ANTIBIOTIC DOSAGES: A COMPLICATED ISSUE

If you are sensitive to medications, the dosage of antibiotics sometimes can be adjusted according to your tolerance and need, but this is a more tricky procedure than with most other medications. Unlike the other medications reviewed in this book, the effect of antibiotics isn't actually directed at you or some organ or system within your body. Instead, antibiotics are targeted toward an interloper—the living and propagating bacteria that have invaded your system, causing an infection.

Using lower doses may be more tolerable for your system, but will it be enough to eradicate the bacteria? Underdosing with antibiotics has dangers. Sometimes it may worsen the infection by allowing the most resistant bacteria to survive and thrive, and possibly spread further. For this reason, if you are prone to medication side effects, using antibiotics presents a delicate balance between a dosage that is low enough for you to tolerate, yet potent enough to ward off the infection.

Complicating the picture even further is the fact that different infections may require different dosages and durations of antibiotic treatment. For example, in the majority of women with cystitis, a common bladder infection, the infection can be treated with just a one-day course of antibiotics. But for 10% to 15% of women, that's not enough to fully extinguish the infection. Thus, most physicians prescribe three to five days of treatment to all women with cystitis in order to be sure to adequately treat everyone. Perhaps someday we will possess the technology to determine exactly when the infection is gone, and then we will be able to individualize the duration of treatment with antibiotics to your exact need.

DISCREPANCIES BETWEEN DRUG REFERENCES AND CLINICAL PRACTICE

Genital infections offer a different kind of dilemma. The world's most common causative agent of sexually acquired infection is chlamydia trachomatis, which can cause urethritis (infection of be urethra), prostatitis in men, and pelvic infection in women.

Chlamydia is treatable with several types of antibiotics. The problem is that chlamydia can be stubborn organisms, and even when the infection seems gone, the chlamydia can persist within human cells, making them undetectable. When this occurs, it is called a subclinical infection, and in some cases may silently do considerable damage, leading to chronic prostatitis or reactive arthritis in men, and infertility and ectopic pregnancy in women.

Many drug references, including the PDR and *The Pill Book*, recommend antibiotic therapy of seven to ten days. However, the research literature and clinical physicians maintain that this is inadequate for many people to fully eradicate a chlamydial infection. Instead, twenty-one to thirty days of treatment, including treatment of the sexual partner who may also harbor the chlamydia, is often essential. The only exception is with the antibiotic Zithromax (azithromycin), which is usually taken for six days because it saturates the tissues and maintains its effect much longer.

Even if your symptoms disappear within seven to ten days of antibiotic therapy, this doesn't mean that all of the chlamydia (or other causative organisms such as mycoplasmas or ureaplasmas) have been destroyed. Neither can cultures always be relied upon.

"In my male patients with urethritis," a urologist told me, "even those with obvious infection-related discharges from their penises, we still aren't able to culture the causative organism in about half of the cases."

Unfortunately, if your physician does prescribe a proper three- to four-week course of antibiotics, some insurers will approve only enough pills for ten days, claiming that this is all that is necessary based on the manufacturer's recommendations in the package inserts and PDR. In these instances, your physician has to give you a prescription with several renewals, which means extra trips to the pharmacy and additional copayments—disincentives that reduce the proportion of people who actually finish the necessary three to four weeks of treatment.

Despite these potential problems, I want to emphasize the importance of completing a full course of antibiotic therapy for genital infections. Full treatment is highly successful, whereas inadequate treatment that leads to subclinical infection can be very difficult to detect and very harmful to the individual in the long run.

LOW-DOSE ANTIBIOTICS

You and your physician do have some flexibility in choosing antibiotics and dosages. Recently, a woman I know was prescribed Biaxin (ranked No. 16 in 1996), a new and highly effective type of erythromycin. For her infection, as well as her size (small) and age (48), 250 mg twice or three times a day would have been adequate, but her physician prescribed 500 mg twice a day. At the higher dose the woman experienced an extremely dry mouth and insomnia. The physician reduced the dose, the side effects disappeared, and within a few days so did the infection.

If you are small or elderly or you frequently encounter side effects with medications, ask your physician if using lower antibiotic dosages are possible for your specific infection. If the infection is mild, often a lower dose will suffice.

If you are prescribed an antibiotic and it causes problematic side effects, it may mean that you are taking more medication than necessary. Ask your physician about lowering the dosage or switching to another antibiotic.

A physician I know began taking Levaquin (levofloxacin), a new antibiotic, for an infection caused by mycoplasma, and organism similar to chlamydia. While he was not usually sensitive to medications, the Levaquin caused ringing in his ears so loud that his hearing was impaired. He reduced his dosage by 50% and has done much better.

Another instance in which less antibiotic may be sufficient involves women who've had recurrent urinary tract infections. Typically, women with this problem are placed on a low dose of daily antibiotic. In the March 1997 issue of the *Journal of Urology*, a study was done in which one group of such women received 125 mg a day of Cipro (ciprofloxacin), which is the usual approach. The other group took the same dose of the same drug, but only after intercourse (average, twice a week). During the year of the study, both groups obtained similar results; only two women in each group of 67 developed urinary infections. Nine women in the daily Cipro group encountered side effects; four in the after-intercourse group.

Unfortunately, the PDR and most other drug references provide little information about the range of variation seen with a given dose of antibiotic. Without this information, physicians aren't alerted to the variations in drug absorption and metabolism between individuals. These variations can produce very different levels and durations of antibiotics. In one instance I called the manufacturer of an antibiotic and learned that with their drug, a 2.5-fold range of variation in peak blood levels was seen in subjects during research studies. Such variation would provide guidance for adjusting antibiotics according to individual sensitivity or a patient's reaction to the medication during treatment, as well as to the nature and severity of the infection.

OTHER THINGS YOU CAN DO TO MINIMIZE ANTIBIOTIC PROBLEMS

Of course, the best way to minimize antibiotic side effects is to use antibiotics only when they are truly needed. It is generally agreed that antibiotics are overprescribed. This results in increased medical expenditures and adverse reactions that shouldn't have happened in the first place, and it further abets the emergence of antibiotic-resistant bacteria.

When antibiotics are required, there are things you can do to minimize the impact on your system. Diarrhea and vaginal infections are common consequences of antibiotic treatment, because the antibiotic kills off not only the invasive bacteria but also friendly, protective bacteria in the gastrointestinal and vaginal tracts.

Eating yogurt or taking lactobacillus supplements during and after antibiotic treatment can help maintain and restore the natural flora of the gastrointestinal tract. In addition to these, yogurt and other types of douches can help maintain the normal bacterial balance of the vagina and prevent yeast overgrowth and other antibiotic-induced superinfections.

Antifungal Medications and a New, Low-Dose Treatment for Fungal Nails

Athlete's foot is a common fungal infection of the skin between the toes that is easily treated with antifungal lotions or creams. But when the fingernails or toenails develop a fungal infection, they become unsightly and difficult to cure. Toenail infections are particularly recalcitrant.

Fungal nails are not harmful or dangerous. The fungus is not highly invasive and usually doesn't spread to other tissues in healthy people. Treatment is initiated mainly for cosmetic reasons. Treatment usually involves from six weeks to four months of oral medication therapy. Success rates with oral antifungal drugs are about 50% to 75%, but 10% to 20% of people experience recurrences of the fungal infection after medication is discontinued. Furthermore, all current oral antifungal drugs cause side effects, some serious.

SPORANOX (ITRACONAZOLE)

The most widely advertised drug for treating fungal infections of the nails is Sporanox. Sporanox is effective in about 50% to 60% of cases, but some practitioners prescribe it reluctantly because of rare reports of hepatitis and even rarer instances of liver failure, causing death, with this drug. Sporanox is an inhibitor of the liver metabolic enzyme cytochrome P450 3A4, which causes it to interact with many other drugs. The manufacturer-recommended dosage is 200 mg a day for twelve weeks. A new, low-dose regimen is 200 mg twice a day for one week each month for four months.

DIFLUCAN (FLUCONAZOLE)

Diflucan is chemically related to Sporanox and Nizoral, another antifungal agent. However, Diflucan is considered by many physicians to be safer and more effective, which explains its No. 83 ranking among the top 200 drugs in 1996 U.S. outpatient prescriptions.

Diflucan is primarily excreted by the kidneys and therefore causes far fewer drug interactions via liver enzymes. Nevertheless, rare instances of liver toxicity have been reported.

For fungal nails, Diflucan has been used in doses of 100 mg every other day for three to six months, or 150 mg once weekly for the same duration. Diflucan is not FDA approved for treating fungal nails, which simply means that the manufacturer decided to study its effectiveness for other fungal diseases in developing the drug. Nevertheless, Diflucan is considered equally effective as other related drugs in treating fungal nails.

However, because Diflucan isn't FDA approved for this usage, some insurers use this as an excuse for refusing to pay for Diflucan for treating fungal nails—despite the fact that Diflucan is preferred by many physicians and is generally considered safer than the FDA-approved treatment, Sporanox.

LAMISIL (TERBINAFINE)

Oral Lamisil is a new antifungal drug that is specifically approved for fungal nails (topical Lamisil has been used for years for athlete's foot). Oral Lamisil was approved for usage in the United State in 1996; it has been used in Europe since 1992. The recommended dosage is 250 mg a day for twelve weeks, and cure is seen in 60% to 80% of toenail cases, 90% in fingernail cases. An alternate dosage regimen of 250 mg twice a day for one week each month for four months has also been used successfully. Often the full effects of Lamisil aren't seen until well after treatment has been discontinued, because it takes many months for new, healthy nails to fully appear. Lamisil is about half as costly as Sporanox.

A SAFER, LOW-DOSE ALTERNATIVE

Among the standard treatments for fungal nails listed above, Lamisil may be the safest and most effective (and least expensive) medication, but because it is the newest oral antifungal agent, its long-term side effects aren't as well known. Diflucan is considered by many physicians to be the safest of its group, which includes Sporanox and Nizoral (ketoconazole).

However, when you think about it, doesn't it seem like overkill to take an oral medication, have it course through all of your tissues and be metabolized by your liver or excreted by your kidneys, just to get a small amount of it to your fingernails or toenails? Fungal nails are not harmful or dangerous. This is why some physicians hesitate to prescribe oral antifungal drugs, which have known, sometimes serious side effects, for what is mainly a cosmetic problem..

Now, perhaps, there may be a more direct and vastly safer solution. Most sensible would be a treatment that you could apply directly to your nails and the skin surrounding them. Presently available lotions and creams aren't able to penetrate the nail, cuticle, and skin well enough to eradicate the fungus that infects the nail beds and leads to distorted nail formation. According to *Conn's Current Therapy 1995*, several topical agents that can penetrate into the nail beds are under investigation, but these agents aren't available yet.

Over recent years, pharmacies known as compounding pharmacies have appeared in most major cities. These pharmacies operate like apothecary shops of old, producing custom-designed medications that are overlooked by or unprofitable for major pharmaceutical companies. One such medication is a combination of Diflucan diluted in a skin-penetrating vehicle.

One type of vehicle is a transdermal cream, similar to the ones used in medication patches for cardiac drugs or the nicotine patches used in smoking cessation. Anti-inflammatory drugs administered via transdermal creams have been shown to be effective. For fungal nails, a transdermal cream containing 2% to 5% of Diflucan can be applied once or twice daily to the skin and cuticle surrounding each fungal nail.

Another type of vehicle that also may be mixed with Diflucan is DMSO, a solvent that readily penetrates through the nails themselves as well as the surrounding skin. According to my local compounding pharmacist, a preparation of 1% Diflucan in 99% DMSO applied once daily has been used successfully by many physicians. DMSO is a controversial but well-known chemical with purported anti-inflammatory properties for arthritis and muscle pain. Although not FDA approved for usage in humans, DMSO is approved for such usage in several states and is widely used in Europe. DMSO is also used extensively by veterinarians in animals for tendon, joint, and other problems. DMSO can cause irritation to the skin; if this occurs, less concentrated solutions of 50% or 30% DMSO with 1% Diflucan can be made.

The data on these new, topical treatments of fungal nails is sparse. Anecdotal testimonials are all that support their usage at this time. However, I can state that I witnessed the use of these preparations in a man who developed fungal fingernails and toenails while taking a prolonged course of antibiotics. Both the transdermal- and DMSO-Diflucan combinations worked.

Most surprising was the effect of the DMSO-Diflucan preparation on the nails themselves. Already an opaque white-gray from the fungus, the DMSO turned the nails back to a normal shade of pink. The effect occurred gradually over several weeks, and it was fascinating to see the healthy pink regions gradually overtake the sickly-looking gray ones like an army pushing back another.

And this occurred while the man continued on his antibiotics. I was amazed. I'd been taught that once a nail turned fungal, it was permanent. Only by the growth of new, healthy nails from the nail beds would the old, disfigured nails be pushed away. Apparently this is incorrect, for the DMSO/Diflucan penetrated straight through the nail, killing the fungus and restoring the infected nail to its original healthy-looking state.

These direct, transdermal methods not only appear to be much safer, but seem to work faster because of their direct effects on infected nails. Furthermore, the price of topical therapy is substantially less than oral antifungal drugs. Some insurers cover topical antifungal treatments produced by compounding pharmacies, but others don't. Because these topical preparations contain a prescription drug, Diflucan, they require a physician's prescription. You can locate the compounding pharmacy nearest to you by calling the Professional Compounding Centers of America, at 800-331-2498.

Digoxin

Cardiac medications such as digoxin are usually prescribed flexibly, starting with lower doses that are increased according to the patient's response. However, even with these methods, some people are unusually sensitive and encounter substantial side effects at the lowest standard doses.

One expert told me, "I have found that with quinidine, digoxin, and other cardiac medications, the 'normal range' is really talking about the optimal therapeutic dose for the average patient, but some people just need a whisper of the stuff to really have it work. Other doctors give up on these drugs if patients develop side effects at the lower end of the therapeutic range rather than seeing if a 'subtherapeutic' dose can be effective without the side effects."

A highly experienced internist agreed. For people with a history of medication sensitivity, "I use less of everything," he told me. With the very elderly, he frequently begins at extremely low, "homeopathic" doses with considerable success and far fewer side effects.

A 1997 article in the *Journal of the American College of Cardiology* supports these low-dose approaches. In a study of people with mild to moderate heart failure, a very low dose of 0.125 mg a day of digoxin was compared with a more typical dose of 0.25 mg a day. The results: "We conclude that moderate dose digoxin [0.25 mg/day] provides no additional hemodynamic or autonomic benefit for patients with mild to moderate heart failure over low dose digoxin [0.125 mg/day]. Because higher doses of digoxin may predispose to arrhythmias, lower dose digoxin should be considered in patients with mild to moderate heart failure."

If you are medication-sensitive, depending upon the acuteness and severity of your condition, ask your physician about the possibility of initiating treatment with cardiac drugs such as digoxin at a very low dose that can be increased, if necessary, according to your response and tolerance.

Haldol (Haloperidol)

Haldol is frequently used in the treatment of schizophrenia, manic-depressive disorder, the confusional or belligerent episodes that sometimes occur with Alzheimer's disease and other types of dementia, other psychotic disorders, severe agitation, explosive behavioral syndromes, Tourette's disorder, and other conditions.

Haldol is a neuroleptic, a group that includes Thorazine and Mellaril. Relatively nonsedating compared with these latter drugs, Haldol can cause serious side effects including parkinsonian-like muscle rigidity, seizures, menstrual irregularities, dry mouth, sedation, and seizures, nearly all of which aren't are directly related to dosage.

Over the years, many drug references and physicians have gravitated toward lower Haldol dosages. Although some patients do require high dosages, multiple studies have shown that lower doses can be effective and are less prone to side effects. In a 1994 article in *Clinical Psychiatry News* it stated "there is good evidence that 'minidoses' [of Haldol] that were unthinkable a decade ago may be as effective, at least for some patients, as far greater amounts." The article quoted Dr. D. L. Garver of the University of Texas Southwestern Medical School. "A minidose of haloperidol appears to be an effective initial dosage strategy for most psychotic patients with illness of less than 5 years."

A report given by Dr. Robert Zipursky at the 1997 annual meeting of the American Psychiatric Association supported this approach. The report announced the results of a clinical trial in which Haldol was given in a low-dose, stepwise manner until the desired results were attained. According to the report, "Optimal dosage was far lower than had been anticipated." Nearly 70% of subjects responded to doses of just 2 to 5 mg a day, suggesting that patients in the early stages of schizophrenia may be highly sensitive to Haldol and other neuroleptic drugs.

Low Haldol doses are not only effective, but less likely to cause side effects such as muscle rigidity or spasms that often cause patients to quit treatment. In Dr. Zipursky's study, if patients continued to experience agitation, an anti-anxiety benzodiazepine medication was added rather than increasing the Haldol dosage.

Side effects with benzodiazepines are less frequent and much less severe than higher doses of Haldol.

Dr. Zipursky stressed that since many cases of schizophrenia, Tourette's syndrome, Alzheimer's and other dementias require prolonged or ongoing medication therapy, the long-term prognosis depends on the patient's ability to maintain medication treatment as long as necessary. Therefore, as in treating other conditions such as hypertension, diabetes, depression, or elevated cholesterol, the early experience of people requiring medication is key. Keeping doses of side-effect-prone neuroleptic medications such as Haldol as low as possible is instrumental in the ultimate success of treatment.

Interindividual variation with Haldol is also seen between ethnic groups. Several studies have demonstrated that Asian patients develop higher blood levels of Haldol and more Haldol-related side effects at equivalent doses than Caucasian patients. Thus, Asian patients may require lower Haldol doses to obtain the same medication effects while avoiding side effects than other ethnic groups.

The 1997 PDR offers clear guidelines for flexible dosaging with Haldol for moderate or severe symptomatology, geriatric or debilitated individuals, or chronic or resistant cases. Even within these groups, a range of recommended doses is offered. These manufacturer-dosage recommendations reflect the wide range of interindividual variation seen in response to Haldol. The clear, concise manner in which the manufacturer offers these dosages could serve as a model for many other drug dosage recommendations.

Although it is not well known, Haldol may also be very useful in treating severe nausea or vomiting. Haldol in very low doses, sometimes as little as 0.5 to 1 mg, can be very effective in stopping nausea. Although related drugs such as Phenergan and Compazine are better known for this effect, Haldol is sometimes equally or even more effective. For people whose nausea or vomiting prevents them from taking Haldol orally, it can be used in suppository form. Another, often preferred method is to use liquid Haldol and have the individual merely swish it around his mouth. The oral mucosa readily absorbs the Haldol, which reaches the bloodstream much more rapidly that when swallowed. The nausea and vomiting may begin to diminish within a few minutes.

Zofran

Zofran is an extremely important medication in treating the sometimes severe nausea and vomiting caused by cancer treatment. "Zofran works when nothing else does," a hospice nurse told me. "It's been a major advancement over previous anti-nausea drugs and usually causes fewer side effects."

The nausea and vomiting following cancer chemotherapy are not only extremely unpleasant but also potentially dangerous. Maintaining adequate nutrition is imperative, and Zofran improves the ability of cancer patients undergoing treatment to do so. Zofran is also used in some types of radiation therapy that cause nausea and vomiting.

Zofran is given both after treatment and prior to a course of therapy, thereby preventing or reducing nausea and vomiting. Zofran can be administered by injection for those unable to keep oral medication down. This analysis relates to oral Zofran dosages only.

MANUFACTURER-RECOMMENDED DOSAGE

The manufacturer-recommended dosage of oral Zofran is 8 mg twice a day when used for the nausea and vomiting associated with cancer chemotherapy; three times a day for usage in radiation therapy. The dosage for the elderly is the same. The first pill may be taken thirty minutes before chemotherapy or radiation treatment to prevent or reduce treatment-related nausea and vomiting. Zofran treatment is usually continued one or two days after completion of a course of treatment. With liver impairment, the total daily dosage should not exceed 8 mg a day.

Zofran is produced in 4- and 8-mg tablets that are unscored but can be split with a pill cutter.

MOST FREQUENT SIDE EFFECTS

The reported incidence of side effects to Zofran exceeds 30%, but many are mild. Most common are headaches (24%), malaise or fatigue (13%), constipation (9%), abdominal pain (5%), dry mouth (2%); also dizziness, light-headedness, diarrhea. Occasionally, an increase in liver enzymes occurs, possibly indicating liver irritation. The safety of Zofran in pregnancy and nursing mothers is not established; its usage should be decided by you and your physician depending on the circumstances of your case.

LOW-DOSE ZOFRAN

According to the 1997 PDR, the current, manufacturer-recommended Zofran dosage is 8 mg twice a day if you are undergoing cancer chemotherapy. Interestingly, in the 1995 PDR, the recommended dosage was 8 mg three times a day. In essence, after a few years of usage in the general population, the recommended dosage for cancer chemotherapy has been reduced by 33%.

This is not surprising. Prior to the release of Zofran for general usage, several studies indicated the effectiveness of significantly lower dosages. In these studies, 4 mg three times a day produced very similar results as the recommended dosages. In fact, 1 mg three times a day also proved effective for a substantial proportion of patients.

Indeed, in the 1995 PDR, in a footnote to a complicated chart, the substantial effectiveness of the 4-mg dose three times a day is quantified. In one study, three times a day dosing with 8 mg prevented any vomiting episodes in 66%, with 4 mg, 65%; with 8 mg, 16% of patients experienced more than five vomiting episodes (indicating limited medication effect); with 4 mg, 23%. In the second study, three-times-a-day dosing with 8 mg prevented any vomiting episodes in 66%, with 4 mg, 64%; with 8 mg, 15% had more than five episodes; with 4 mg, 19%.

Clinical experience supports these findings. "We cut Zofran tablets in halves and quarters and start many patients, especially those who are frail, very old, or with liver disease, at 2 mg," the hospice nurse said. "These lower doses help a lot of them."

The data from the studies with Zofran 1 mg (three times a day) is not mentioned in the 1997 package insert or PDR. The footnote about the effectiveness of the 4-mg dose three times a day dose in the 1995 PDR has been eliminated from the 1997 PDR. On the other hand, in those two years the manufacturer-recommended dosage for cancer chemotherapy has been reduced 33%, from 8 mg three times a day to twice a day.

If you are medication-sensitive or you are experiencing significant side effects with standard doses of Zofran, using the 4 mg tablet twice or three times a day may be worth discussing with your physician. If even these reduced doses are too much for you, doses of 2 or even 1 mg twice or three times a day should be considered.

PART 8

How to Improve the System

NINETEEN

Slow Responses to Serious Side Effects: The Coumadin Story

This book has asserted the proposition that most, if not all, medications should be used in the very lowest effective doses for a given individual. It has also stated that in regard to drugs and dosages, you cannot always rely on the knowledge of your physician or the recommendations of drug references, including and especially the *Physician's Desk Reference*.

For many of these medications, the problem has been the failure of the manufacturer to define the very lowest effective dosage (Mevacor, Halcion, Restoril, Zantac), or to include known low-dose information in the package insert and PDR description (Prozac, Motrin, Voltaren), or to provide a range of doses and pill sizes that allow flexible dosing for medication-sensitive individuals (Prilosec, Dalmane, Redux, Prozac initially). Contributing to these problems, of course, is the FDA's failure to require such steps.

This chapter focuses on the fact that even with medications that are supposedly well known, that have been used for years or decades, the dosages that physicians prescribe may be too high—with disastrous effects. Yet even when the problem comes to light, it may take many years for the system to correct itself, and you or others may suffer unnecessarily.

This isn't a problem of some bygone era, but of today. As discussed in Chapter 16, the occurrence of dose-related, severe cardiac reactions to Seldane was recognized prior to 1990, yet the manufacturer-recommended (one-size-fits-all) dosage remained unchanged. The actual number of victims of Seldane reactions isn't known, but at least a hundred or more people have been hospitalized and several killed. This was enough for the FDA to finally, in 1997, call for Seldane's withdrawal from the market.

This chapter chronicles another, even more unsettling story about a medication that has been used for over sixty years, a medication that when used properly has helped millions, but when used improperly from the 1970s into the 1990s has unnecessarily harmed hundreds of thousands and killed thousands. The issue once again has been one of dosage, and it underscores the importance for you to insist on the very lowest effective dose of any medication, prescription or nonprescription, that you may take. Until we create a system that is committed to developing the very lowest, safest, effective drug dosages and to immediately correcting newly discovered errors, your own vigilance remains your best and sometimes your only defense.

COUMADIN: A MEDICATION WITH A DELICATE BALANCE

Anticoagulants are substances that thin the blood. Coumadin and its generic, warfarin, are our most prescribed anticoagulants. In 1996, Coumadin ranked No. 10 in U.S. outpatient prescriptions, three spots behind Prozac and ahead of Mevacor, Prilosec, Pepcid, Zoloft, Paxil, and every antihistamine, sleep remedy, anti-anxiety and anti-inflammatory drug.

Coumadin is a very important medication. For a number of conditions, thinning the blood is a vital aspect of treatment, extending both the quality and duration of people's lives. Unfortunately, the treatment isn't without risk. Anticoagulant therapy has the highest rate of morbidity and mortality of any outpatient prescription treatment. If the dosage of Coumadin is too high, the blood becomes too thin and people bleed. They hemorrhage, as the PDR states, "from any tissue or organ. This is a consequence of the anticoagulant effect."

Bleeding episodes aren't the only side effects of anticoagulant treatment. Other adverse effects include gastrointestinal disturbances, dermatitis, fever, reduced white cell count, allergic reactions, loss of hair, elevation of liver enzymes, and priapism (a constantly erect penis). In addition, many drugs affect Coumadin's activity or breakdown and must be avoided.

Because of the seriousness of its side effects, Coumadin isn't prescribed like other drugs. With most drugs, physicians prescribe what they consider appropriate dosages and hope that side effects don't occur—in essence, a trial-and-error approach. With Coumadin, as with insulin, trial and error won't do because the gap between effectiveness and side effects is very narrow, and an adverse reaction can be catastrophic. Therefore, beginning in the late 1930s, doctors have employed blood tests to closely monitor the effect of anticoagulant drugs.

TWENTY-FIVE YEARS OF EXCESS DOSAGING?

When treatment with Coumadin or generic warfarin is begun, the standard approach is to test the patient's blood very frequently, sometimes daily, for about two weeks, then weekly for several months. As long as an individual remains on Coumadin, the blood is checked regularly, and with any variation in the person's condition or any sign of an adverse reaction, the blood is retested immediately.

The blood test utilized to measure the degree of Coumadin-induced anticoagulation is called the prothrombin time (PT) determination. It measures the time required for Coumadin anticoagulated blood to form a clot in comparison to normal blood. The PT with Coumadin anticoagulated blood should fall within a therapeutic range. A PT falling below or above the therapeutic range indicates inadequate or excessive anticoagulation, respectively. These in turn indicate inadequate treatment or increased risk of spontaneous bleeding—both dangerous circumstances.

A lot depends on the PT test—its reliability, its consistency, its accuracy. PT determinations that are consistent and accurate will facilitate a proper degree of anticoagulation—that is, a proper dosage of Coumadin. PT determinations that are inconsistent or inaccurate cause physicians to prescribe incorrect amounts of Coumadin, increasing the risks of an already risky treatment.

Studies published over the last decade have shown that since the late 1960s, the results from performing the PT test in North America often have been unreliable and inconsistent. "As a result," a 1989 article stated, "many clinicians have unknowingly increased the dose of warfarin to treat patients." This means that for about twenty-five years Coumadin dosages frequently were unnecessarily high—and the frequency of side effects, including hemorrhage, had been unnecessarily high as well.

HOW A VITAL TEST WENT AWRY—
AND UNNOTICED

The PT determination requires a reagent, thromboplastin, an organic chemical derived from living tissue. In the 1940s, hospital laboratories prepared their own thromboplastins. Based on the methodology at that time, in 1948 the American Heart Association recommended a targeted PT therapeutic range for Coumadin anticoagulation of 2.0–2.5, meaning that the anticoagulated patient's blood should require 2–2.5 times as long to clot as normal blood.

In the late 1960s and early 1970s, clinical laboratories stopped producing their own thromboplastins and turned to national producers for these supplies. These commercially produced thromboplastins were less sensitive than those locally produced, and they required more anticoagulation (i.e., more medication) to obtain the same targeted PT ratio of 2.0–2.5.

As these changes took place, the recommended PT ratios should have been adjusted to compensate for the less sensitive commercial reagents. They weren't. As the 1989 article described: "This change in responsiveness of thromboplastins, which was unsuspected by most clinicians, led to an increase in the dose of warfarin used to treat patients." In other words, the change in reagents caused a shift in PT results, which in turn led to higher Coumadin dosages. Yet the patients didn't actually need more Coumadin, and the result was an increased incidence of bleeding episodes.

Compounding the problem was the fact that commercially prepared reagents displayed substantial variability between producers and lots. This added another layer of inaccuracy to the PT determination. For example, patients transferred from hospital to home usually had to switch labs. If the new lab obtained a lower PT result, doctors increased the patient's Coumadin dosage; yet the change in the PT result may only have been a reflection of the difference in sensitivities of the PT reagents used by the two different laboratories.

Utilizing the same laboratory reduced the variability but didn't negate it. Even if the lab always purchased its reagent from the same source, which wasn't always the case, significant variations sometimes existed between different lots of thromboplastins from the same supplier. Consequently, even under the most ideal circumstances—a stable patient, a competent physician, and a reliable lab—the PT results utilized to guide Coumadin treatment were subject to unrecognized and uncorrected variability.

This variability affected more than a small number of people. "The more than half a million Americans receiving long-term anticoagulant therapy," stated an article in a 1993 issue of the *New England Journal of Medicine*, "face unnecessary risks of bleeding or thromboembolism [blood clots] because of variability in the commercial thromboplastins used by clinical laboratories to determine prothrombin times." This article also contained an eye-opening chart that underscored the difference in the standard method of anticoagulant dosing then prevalent in North America versus lower doses: in four separate studies, the annual rate of bleeding episodes was 200% to 650% higher with the standard dosing.

A DANGEROUS OVERSIGHT

Bleeding is the main complication of anticoagulant therapy. Bleeding episodes are categorized as major or minor depending on the site and degree of bleeding. Most Coumadin-related bleeding episodes are, fortunately, minor, causing limited discomfort and/or discoloration of the skin. Major bleeding, however, can be incapacitating, if not lethal, especially if it occurs in the brain.

A survey of studies in which anticoagulation was performed at the higher dosages common to the 1970s to the mid-1990s revealed a risk of bleeding episodes between 11.8% and 39.7%. Episodes of major bleeding were reported in several studies as occurring in more than 7%. Fatal hemorrhage occurred at rates of 2% to 4%, but at higher rates in some specific categories. For example, in people with prosthetic heart valves require lifelong anticoagulation, approximately 7% of their major bleeding episodes proved fatal. These are very high rates of severe adverse effects. In contrast, known cardiac fatalities attributed to Seldane have occurred in probably fewer than one in one million Seldane users.

On the other hand, it must be remembered that anticoagulation treatment is employed in conditions which themselves have high rates of major complications and death. Overall, it's been shown that when performed properly, anticoagulant therapy, though not without risk, enhances and extends the lives of people whose conditions require it.

THE PROBLEM EMERGES, SLOWLY

As the dosages of Coumadin crept up, didn't anyone notice? In fact, a few physicians did question the altered level of dosing. From the late 1950s into the early 1980s, a sprinkling of articles showed up in various journals challenging the higher Coumadin dosages and questioning the reliability and sensitivity of the commercially produced PT thromboplastins. A few of these articles in fact demonstrated the efficacy and enhanced safety of lower dosages. These findings were largely ignored.

Finally, in 1982 a study appeared in the *New England Journal of Medicine* comparing different intensities of anticoagulation in the long-term treatment of venous thrombosis (clotted veins). The study reported that by reducing the dosages of anticoagulants, the rate of clinically important bleeding was reduced from 22% to 4%—a huge improvement.

Based on these findings, the study estimated that by utilizing lower dosages of anticoagulants for only one disorder, venous thrombosis, 43,000 incidents of clinically important bleeding could be averted *per year*. Extrapolating these statistics to all conditions requiring anticoagulation, it was estimated that over 100,000 cases of important bleeding (and several thousand deaths) could be averted annually. And these numbers didn't include the reduction in "unimportant" bleeding—incidents of minor medical significance, perhaps, but nonetheless unpleasant and unnerving to patients.

In the same year, a British study was published reporting the marked differences in Coumadin dosages among countries. The cause? Differences in the types of thromboplastins utilized to determine the PT. This led to the following statement in an American publication: "If the therapeutic ratio used by most British hospitals is correct, patients in North America . . . are being treated with unnecessarily high doses of oral anticoagulants and are being exposed to an unnecessary risk of bleeding."

Finally, by late 1993, American medicine was beginning to take notice. In contrast, by 1983, after nearly two decades of examining the problem, European investigators adopted an international standard for thromboplastin reagents utilized in PT determinations. Actually, anticoagulant dosing had gone less awry in Europe than America because the Europeans had stuck with high sensitivity thromboplastins while North American laboratories switched to low sensitivity ones. Nevertheless, the Europeans felt there remained too much variability from laboratory to laboratory, and in 1983 they established an international standard, thereby creating an additional level of safety.

The Europeans called their new standard the INR, the International Normalized Ratio, based on a World Health Organization reference preparation of thromboplastin. Thereafter, all European thromboplastins were tested against this international reference standard, and all PT results were calibrated accordingly, thus correcting any inaccuracies in PT results due to variability among European reagents. Even before this standardization, European PT methodology was more accurate than the American method, and still the Europeans worked to further improve their techniques— and save lives.

In the wake of these developments, in 1984 the Committee on Antithrombotic Therapy of the American College of Chest Physicians (ACCP) and the National Heart, Lung and Blood Institute (NHLBI) convened. Two years later its recommendations were reported in *Chest*. Noting that the international system had been accepted by most Western countries but not in North America, the committee called for all PT results in North America to be standardized using the INR, the new international system of calibration. They added that such standardization shouldn't be left to the discretion of commercial thromboplastin producers and laboratories, but instead should be required, and they debated whether the FDA should be asked to insist upon such standardization.

It would be reassuring to report that the response throughout the medical community was instantaneous, but in fact it was imperceptible. For years the situation remained unchanged. Despite repeated articles on the subject, North American thromboplastins remained unstandardized, PT results remained uncalibrated, and anticoagulant dosages and bleeding complications remained unnecessarily high.

In 1988, an article in *Thrombosis and Haemostasis* reiterated the discrepancies in anticoagulant dosages in different countries. Again it suggested "that manufacturers calibrate their thromboplastin reagent against the WHO reference standard and provide the user with an [accurately calibrated] value. If this was done, individual hospital laboratories could report the results in a standard way based on the INR." After describing the benefits of these reforms, the authors acknowledged that "to date, however, this recommendation has been adopted by only a very small percentage of laboratories throughout North America."

In the six years since the first major American article on the subject, published in the *New England Journal of Medicine* in 1982—with its estimate that 100,000 cases of major bleeding could be averted *annually*—hardly anything had changed. In the five years since Europe had adopted the INR, no systematic improvements in American PT methodology had been put into use.

Three years later, in 1991, Dr. Jack Hirsh, one of the leading proponents for PT standardization, wrote in *Drug Therapy*: "For reasons that are difficult to explain on scientific grounds, the INR system of reporting has not been adopted by the vast majority of institutions in North America."

Equally discouraging, the first-line medical journals continued to publish studies on oral anticoagulation without requiring any standardization of the PT results, rendering their conclusions not only meaningless, but misleading. About which Dr. Hirsh warned:

"The present system . . . has the potential to compromise patient care and makes clinically meaningful comparisons of efficacy and safety of oral anticoagulant therapy between studies difficult. The situation could be corrected by introducing the INR system and using more sensitive thromboplastins."

In 1993, an article entitled "Effect of Laboratory Variation in the Prothrombin-Time Ratio on the Results of Oral Anticoagulant Therapy" appeared in the *New England Journal of Medicine*. It stated that because of the variability in U.S. PT determinations, the resultant higher anticoagulant dosages in patients with atrial fibrillation (ineffective contractions of the heart's atria) produced higher rates of complications, which was no surprise. The surprise was the scope of the problem, which the authors quantified as a 50% lessening of the beneficial effects of anticoagulant therapy and a 500% increase in the cost-effectiveness ratio of anticoagulant treatment.

The authors also restated previously reported disparities in the thromboplastins of fifty-three laboratories: "This means that although two laboratories may report the same prothrombin-time ratio, the intensity of anticoagulation may differ substantially." Indeed, the very same blood sample, when tested at different labs, obtained different results. Thus, as the authors pointed out, anticoagulant therapy, even when medically necessary, could in the United States actually have a poorer prognosis than no anticoagulation at all.

MOVING TOWARD MORE RELIABLE, LOWER DOSE ANTICOAGULATION

Though the laboratories didn't get the message, physicians gradually did, as finally reflected by the lowering of the recommended Coumadin dosages in drug references around 1994. Previously, it was believed that a large, initial "loading dose" of Coumadin was necessary to expedite anticoagulation, but this practice fell into disfavor, as reflected in the *AMA Drug Evaluations Annual 1994*: "The former custom of giving a large loading dose . . . is no longer recommended. . . . Avoiding a loading dose minimizes the danger of hemorrhage in patients with diminished tolerance or unusual sensitivity to the anticoagulant."

Even earlier, Coumadin's manufacturer had updated the information in the package insert and PDR. Coumadin's 1990 PDR description contained many of the recommendations of the Committee on Antithrombotic Therapy for improving PT testing methods. The 1990 PDR informed physicians about the new international system of PT standardization and explained the importance of calibrating all PT results in order to reduce variability. This is one instance in which a pharmaceutical company was way ahead of physicians.

Still, the 1990 PDR dosage recommendations, though reduced, remained high in comparison to present standards. In 1990, 10 mg a day of Coumadin was the recommended initial dosage. By 1994, it was to 2 to 5 mg a day, a reduction of 50% to 80%.

Reductions in the recommended Coumadin dosages in the PDR and other references were a welcome step, but this didn't guarantee immediate changes in how physicians prescribed Coumadin. They still had to rely on PT tests to monitor Coumadin treatment, and it took time for laboratories and hospitals to change their methods. For example, it wasn't until 1993 that one local hospital instituted the use of the international standard, which it announced with a memo to its medical staff: "Because of the long-standing problem of variable sensitivity of thromboplastins producing widely variable PT results, we started reporting the PT using the international normalized ratio (INR). . . . The main advantage is to allow a lower dose of Coumadin and therefore less bleeding complications."

This hospital may have been in the forefront. A year later in 1994, twelve years after the issue first gained national prominence via the article in the *New England Journal of Medicine*, a pathologist told me, "I'm lecturing at a well-known Los Angeles hospital next week. It's going to be a shock to the clinicians. They're going to be amazed when they switch over [to the international standard in PT testing], how it's going to reduce the dosages of warfarin they use."

WHY DID IT TAKE SO LONG?

Reduced Coumadin doses are important, but they still depended on reliable PT determinations. By 1994, many hospitals had begun adjusting their PT methods to international standards.

I asked one laboratory physician why it had taken so long. He replied, "Frankly, I didn't think it was a big deal when I first heard about it. I didn't realize the impact. In the lab, we are always altering and fine tuning our laboratory methods. But after going back and reading the 1982 studies, I thought, Geez, this is obvious. Why didn't people flock to this system?"

Part of the problem was the high degree of specialization that has become part of our medical system. Pathologists usually run hospital laboratories, overseeing hundreds of tests and procedures. But pathologists don't treat patients, so they don't observe first-hand the dosing and side effect problems with any particular group of drugs. On the other hand, the clinicians who prescribe Coumadin and follow patients don't involve themselves in the laboratory aspects. They generally assume that the best and most accurate methods are being applied. Clearly this gap played a role in the unnoticed escalation of Coumadin dosages beginning in the late 1960s and early 1970s.

The gap finally has been closed. According to one expert, in 1992 most labs didn't calibrate their PT results to the international standards; by 1994, most did. And with each year, the dose recommendations in the PDR became more specific about using lower doses, using them flexibly according to individual response, and judging dose effectiveness upon PT results that were calibrated to the international standard (INR). Coumadin tablets come in seven sizes (1, 2, 2.5, 4, 5, 7.5, and 10 mg), and all are scored tablets.

LESSONS FROM THE COUMADIN EXPERIENCE

One of the themes of this book is that once a drug is released by a manufacturer at specific recommended dosages, and once physicians learn them, subsequent changes in dosing are slow to be adopted—even when lower doses are proven to be safer and effective. This has been the story of many medications in this book: Dalmane, Prozac, Mevacor, Seldane, Zantac, Zoloft, Prilosec, Voltaren, Halcion, to name just a prominent few. In many of these instances, lower dosages have yet to be adopted by the general medical community.

In the case of Coumadin, the necessity for lower dosages arose from an unexpected source, a change in laboratory techniques during the late 1960s and early 1970s. Yet despite the fact that tens or, more likely, hundreds of thousands of patients were adversely affected annually, despite repeated warnings in the medical literature and in the 1980s calls from a prestigious task force and major medical associations, it was well into the 1990s before the necessary changes were generally adopted.

You and I have to wonder if somehow the process couldn't have moved more quickly. We have to wonder why after the Europeans adopted the INR in 1983, the FDA or some empowered agency didn't seize the moment to initiate immediate action.

We understand that it is the nature of institutions to change slowly. This includes the medical establishment, the pharmaceutical industry, and the FDA. Sometimes the conservatism of these institutions works for the better. No one wants to repeat the thalidomide experience of the 1950s, when a supposedly safe medication caused severe birth defects in children. But when a well-known, top-selling medication is causing unnecessary and serious harm because the dosage is too high, it seems that it shouldn't take an act of Congress, or a decade, to rapidly impose a newer, safer standard.

Unfortunately, for now that's the way the system sometimes works—very slowly. This may be why the issues of medication sensitivities and interindividual variation in dosage between people taking the same medications have not received their due recognition. But solutions are possible and long overdue, and I will suggest plenty of them in Chapter 20.

TWENTY

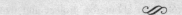

Solutions

EVERYONE HAS A STORY

In the years I've contemplated, researched, and written this book, it seems that just about everyone I've spoken to about this project has volunteered a story about themselves, a family member, a friend or coworker.

I was taking a class on nutrition where a nurse I met asked about my work. I told her about this project. She volunteered, "I have cystic breast disease, and if I drink a cup of coffee, my cysts flare up overnight. The condition is that sensitive to caffeine—at least in me."

The mother of one of my son's friends understood the issue of medication sensitivities. One-quarter of a Xanax is all she needs to calm her irritability when she's premenstrual. Her doctor didn't believe her, claiming that such a small dose couldn't possibly work. Yet I knew she was right—I'd seen similar small doses work in some of my patients.

One day I called a pharmacy. The pharmacist, who knew about my project, said, "By the way, I've got a young woman working for me now who's sensitive to everything. A cup of coffee makes her hyper. Antihistamines zonk her. It's amazing."

I replied, "Unfortunately physicians and drug manufacturers hardly pay attention to them."

"From what I see," the pharmacist countered, "they don't pay *any* attention to them."

At my son's birthday party, I got into a conversation with Lee Kaplan, a dermatologist. I told him about the project and that everyone I've mentioned it to has a story. "It's true," he agreed. "I have stories. My patients have stories. My family has stories."

Dr. Kaplan volunteered to read my section on Seldane, a drug that had been recommended at the same dosage for everyone and a drug he used to prescribe frequently. He suggested a few minor changes in the text but overall concluded, "When you think about it, it's ridiculous to think that everyone would respond to the same dosage of medication, but that's exactly what we do."

A MEDICATION-ORIENTED SOCIETY

We are a medication-oriented culture. When a symptom arises or a condition strikes, our first instinct is often to take something to rid ourselves of the symptom. That's one of the reasons that the pharmaceutical industry is one of the largest in the world: in 1996, sales of prescription drugs to pharmacies amounted to over $85 billion. That's why drug companies spend hundreds of millions of dollars introducing new nonprescription products such as Aleve or Pepcid AC or Zantac 75. That's why perhaps as many as one hundred million Americans take medications regularly. And that's why iatrogenic (that is, treatment-related) illness, particularly medication side effects, is itself a major medical problem.

There's nothing wrong with taking a couple of Tylenol or other products for a headache. The discovery of drugs such as antibiotics, insulin, hormones, anti-seizure medications, ulcer remedies, and a host of others have contributed to medical advancements in the twentieth century that dwarf those of all the previous centuries combined. Yet success may foster excess. When, for example, people with hypertension or medical obesity can control or reduce their disease by modifying their diets, stopping smoking, and exercising regularly, yet many prefer to simply take a pill, perhaps we've become too enamored of using medications to solve problems that may originate in our lifestyles. Antihypertensive and weight-reducing drugs aren't benign; all have potential, sometimes serious, occasionally lethal side effects. Drug therapy should be the last resort, not the first.

If you are medication-sensitive, you've already learned the lesson. Your experiences with medications, the side effects you've encountered with standard doses, have taught you that medications are powerful substances—foreign chemicals that can be helpful or toxic.

If you are medication-sensitive, you have probably already learned to use medications only when absolutely necessary. You might have learned to use lower doses—or you might not have. Most people I've met haven't considered the possibility of using lower doses. Either a drug works or it's discontinued. My wife, Barbara, represents a health-care organization at a local health club. A new enrollee explained how a medication she was taking for a rapid heart rate made her feel sleepy all morning, although she took the pill at night. Her solution was to drink a cup of coffee with breakfast. Barbara suggested that maybe the medication dosage was too high. "That's a good idea," the woman said. "I didn't think of that."

People don't think about dosage, about adjusting what's given. Many physicians don't either. Drug companies and drug references often don't suggest it or even study it. The FDA doesn't demand it. These are all part of the problem. They can also be part of the solution.

DRUG MANUFACTURERS

Effexor is one of the newer antidepressants, yet this caveat can be found among Effexor's four pages of information in the PDR: "The effectiveness of Effexor in long-term use, that is, for more than 4 to 6 weeks, has not been systematically evaluated in controlled trials." Effexor was released just a couple of years ago, yet we knew little about its effects beyond six weeks despite the fact that most people taking it will do so for months, years, or perhaps decades. Nor was Effexor's very lowest effective dose ever defined, despite high side effect rates exceeding 20% to 30% in each of several categories, and despite a dropout rate of almost 20% due to drug side effects in pre-release studies.

Did the manufacturer study Effexor in clinical trials as thoroughly as possible to test its effectiveness at enough different dosages to ensure its safety when released for general usage? Did the FDA demand it? The side effect and dropout statistics make us wonder.

Effexor isn't unique. Its research and development are similar to many drugs. Being a new drug, the research methods and dosage decisions with Effexor represent the current state of the art. That's the problem.

Here is a list of measures that manufacturers can undertake to improve our knowledge of medications before they are released and thereby reduce the risks of drug-related side effects:

1. Define the very lowest effective dosage. This dosage may not be effective for as many people as are higher dosages, but it is likely to cause fewer side effects. If only 40% respond to this low dosage, that's still a very large number of people. Besides, as we have seen, study subjects often may not be representative of the general patient population; a dosage that helps 40% in pre-release studies may be beneficial to an even greater percentage in the hands of general physicians or gerontologists (specialists in treating the elderly).

The manufacturer doesn't have to recommend this low dosage for everyone; it merely should inform us of the possibilities. A statement such as "Drug X was significantly effective at doses starting at 5 mg" would be sufficient; this statement should appear in the dosage guidelines. Better yet would be a chart that defines dosages and their resultant rates of effectiveness.

This recommendation seems simple enough, but there are barriers. Dose research is mainly performed Phase 2, early in the process of drug development. A relatively small number of subjects and a brief period of time are committed to this most important effort. As an article in the *Journal of Clinical Pharmacology* explained: "Often, a commercial sponsor does not want the Phase 2 to be prolonged, and hence, the extra time needed to explore the full dose range and various dose intervals to obtain good dose and concentration information may not be committed."

In addition, competitive pressures can encourage the development of higher dosages that yield more "impressive" responses— i.e., effective for more people, even if such dosages produce more side effects. As we have seen, this certainly has been the story with Prozac, Seldane, Mevacor, Halcion, Prilosec, Axid, and some antihypertensive, anti-inflammatory, and other drugs.

The emergence of many prescription drugs in new, nonprescription doses underscores the fact that lower doses can be effective for mild conditions as well as for medication-sensitive individuals. Here is an example: for decades, physicians have been giving prescription-strength Tagamet, Zantac, Axid, and Pepcid to patients complaining of heartburn or gastric irritation, including even mild cases because prescription dosages were the only ones available. Yet, during this time data were available on the effectiveness of lower dosages (Chapter 10). Now, finally, we have nonprescription preparations of all of these drugs. Why did it take up to twenty years for these lower, safer doses to be available? Is there some reason that they were not available at the same time as the higher, riskier dosages of these drugs?

Small people, medication-sensitive individuals, the elderly, people taking several other drugs—these have always been part of medical practice. Lower doses that may be safer yet effective for these populations should be the first available, not the last.

Providing data on the very lowest effective dosages is particularly important for elderly individuals. As we have seen, this population demonstrates even more variability than younger individuals. Furthermore, it's virtually impossible to conduct large-scale clinical studies on the very old, very frail, or very sick—the people that most often require the smallest dosages, dosages called "almost homeopathic" by one insightful internist. Perhaps there is a correlation between the fact that about 80% of medication side effects are dose-related, and the elderly exhibit the highest rate of medication side effects.

Medication side effects sometimes aren't discovered until after years or decades of usage. We know that when a drug is released for general usage, there's often much yet to be learned. For example, a recent report stated: "A thyroid hormone medication taken by millions of Americans when over age 50 causes bones to weaken, says a UCSD [University of California, San Diego] study published today." The report went on to suggest using the very lowest possible doses of this thyroid hormone. Yet it shouldn't take this kind of discovery to motivate us. We know problems will develop with many drugs. Defining and utilizing the very lowest effective dosages is, therefore, preventive medicine at its best.

2. Avoid one-size-fits-all dosages. Provide a range of effective drug dosages that provide dose flexibility for physicians and patients. One-size-fits-all drug dosages are irrational. Interindividual variation is a constant in all clinical situations. Different people will respond differently to the same dosage of the same drug. This is basic scientific fact.

We know that some people are slow metabolizers. We know that the enzymes responsible for drug metabolism may exhibit many variations in form and activity from person to person, thereby affecting the rate of drug metabolism. We know that as people age, their ability to metabolize drugs decreases. Medications must be provided in a range of flexible dosages to reflect these individual differences.

Yet new drugs continue to be released with one-size-fits-all dosages. The antihistamine Allegra, the appetite suppressant Redux, and the smoking cessation drug Zyban are the most recent examples.

Medications are potent substances that usually have multiple actions within the human system. If we are to reduce the high incidence of medication side effects, we must be able to tailor our medication dosages to the individual.

3. Provide all drugs as breakable tablets in multiple dose sizes, thereby allowing for flexible dosing. Only when chemically necessary, such as with extended-release preparations, should capsules be permitted, and the capsules should be produced in multiple sizes that facilitate flexible, gradual dosing. Because of the importance of flexible, precise dosing, the anticoagulant Coumadin is produced in seven scored-tablet sizes. Several preparations of thyroid hormone are made in twelve sizes, all scored tablets. But as repeatedly discussed in this book, many medications are produced in only one or two dose sizes. Also, dosage increases are often recommended in jumps of 50% to 100%. Medical authorities advise physicians to pay special attention to dosage and side effects, especially when prescribing new drugs, but this isn't possible when a drug is produced as capsules or unbreakable tablets in only one or two sizes.

With medications produced only as capsules, your pharmacist can fashion lower-dose capsules for you. Some people buy empty gelatin capsules (available at pharmacies and many health food stores) and make their own low-dose pills. However, medical authorities discourage this because of the possibility of dosage errors or getting powder in the eyes.

4. Medication studies should simulate clinical situations. Drug studies should serve as a model for clinical usage, not an impediment. Drug studies are indeed costly, but brief studies may produce potentially harmful biases, in part because some side effects may emerge only from longer periods of drug usage. In addition, brief studies sometimes necessitate the rapid increase of dosages. This not only may bias the results toward higher dosages and miss long-term side effects, but also may leave the impression that such rapid upward dosaging is the sanctioned method. In the real world, starting low and going slow is much less likely to provoke side effects and more likely to result in a satisfactory outcome.

Many drug studies are geared toward proving that a new drug is superior to an already established competitor. Doing so may tend to bias studies toward the use of higher dosages that yield higher rates of efficacy, but also would be likely to show a higher incidence of side effects. A 1990 journal article cited this problem and offered a suggestion:

> *In the future, there will perhaps be more clinical trials that do not address the traditional goal of detecting significant differences between two treatments. Perhaps more trials will be directed toward validating that a more conservative treatment is equivalent in efficacy to a standard but more toxic treatment.*

In other words, an effective but safer treatment.

Historically, aspects of drug studies have been done with subjects who may have little resemblance to "typical" patients. Studies that have utilized subjects who are predominantly male, young, white, or healthy may produce findings that aren't accurately applicable to patients in everyday medical practice. For example, younger and healthier male subjects often require and tolerate dosages that may be higher than necessary in typical patients. The

FDA has attempted to correct these biases, but studies still are not always ideally balanced or sometimes exclude important subgroups such as people with major illnesses that are common in the general population and that influence drug response.

The 1990 article quoted above defined what drug studies should accomplish: "When the study is completed, there ought to be clear guidelines for the clinician to design initial, individualized, optimal dosage regimens or for subsequent adjustment of the regimen." Optimal dosages, individualized treatment—these are what drug studies should but sometimes don't produce.

5. Update drug information annually. Most of all, include new uses and dosages for medications, and newly revealed side effect information. Prozac has been on the market almost ten years. Multiple studies and physician reports have proven its effectiveness for a wide variety of conditions, often at dosages below those recommended in the package insert and PDR. For instance, Prozac is often prescribed for panic disorders and agoraphobia (Chapter 7). Because of the tendency for insomnia or agitation with Prozac in these individuals, authorities recommend dosages as low as 2.5 or 5 mg a day. Most of the information on this usage is published in psychiatry journals that few other practitioners tend to read. This information has been known for many years, but it's not reflected in the sources that doctors use most, the package inserts, manufacturer's advertising, and Prozac's PDR description. Instead, physicians relying on these sources will likely prescribe the usual recommended initial dosage, 20 mg a day.

A substantial proportion of side effects with a new drug are often discovered after its release in the general population. Also, higher rates of already known side effects are sometimes found. Except with extremely serious side effects, this information does not necessarily show up in the medication's package insert or PDR description. It should—and promptly.

6. Use once-a-day dosing judiciously. Studies have repeatedly shown that the simpler the dosing, the better people remember to take their medication. Once-a-day pills are easier to remember than those taken four times a day.

Once-a-day drugs also may provide a more even, continuous medication effect than the peaks and valleys in blood levels sometimes seen with drugs that require multiple daily dosing.

But once-a-day dosing may have a downside. Longer-acting once-a-day drugs may tend to accumulate in the bodies of slow metabolizers more readily than shorter-acting drugs.

Once-a-day and even twice-a-day medications may require larger amounts of medication to be taken at one time—and side effects sometimes are directly related to how much medication is introduced into the body at a given time. A good example is Seldane, a twice-a-day medication that has produced serious cardiac problems in some people. The cardiac reactions were in large part related to the amount of Seldane (60 mg) taken at one time. Meanwhile, pre-release studies showed that 20 mg three times a day was highly effective in treating allergy symptoms, but this dosage was never released or recommended. Although it is harder to remember to take Seldane three times a day instead of twice a day, it would likely cause substantially fewer cardiac and other Seldane adverse reactions.

All of these issues should be weighed carefully by manufacturers in developing and by the FDA in approving new medications. Ease of usage and a continuous level of drug activity, as accomplished with once-a-day medications, are important factors in providing effective treatment. But it also must be remembered that spreading the daily dosage of a drug across multiple doses also has its advantages, such as providing greater opportunity for dose adjustment and the sometimes safer effect of introducing smaller amounts of medication into the human body at one time.

And if a manufacturer decides to produce a once-daily drug, it should offer it in several pill sizes to allow dose flexibility. When Prozac was first released, it came in only one size, a 20-mg capsule—an amount that was excessive for about half of my patients. (Prozac now is also produced in a 10-mg capsule and a liquid.) Prilosec is available only as a 20-mg capsule, despite findings that lower doses are effective. On the other hand, Oruvail is made in 100-, 150-, and 200-mg capsules, and Relafen is produced in 500- and 750-mg breakable tablets.

THE *PHYSICIANS' DESK REFERENCE* (PDR)

Although the PDR may be a less than objective vehicle for the pharmaceutical industry to promote their products, an overwhelming majority of physicians rely upon it for drug information. In addition, approximately half a million PDRs are sold to the public each year. The PDR may be our most used drug reference, but the information it provides is far from comprehensive or current. These shortcomings affect the way medications are prescribed and utilized, and thus play a role in the high rate of iatrogenic illness.

In July 1996, the *Archives of Internal Medicine* published a special article by Dr. Paul Insel and me listing many of the shortcomings of the PDR. In response to our criticisms, a spokesman for the PDR stated that criticizing the book was like criticizing the messenger. He was partially correct, because the PDR is essentially a collection of package inserts of various medications arranged in a reference format. Shortcomings of the PDR represent shortcomings in the data provided by drug manufacturers in package inserts. Thus, the PDR is a conduit for getting manufacturer-selected drug information to physicians. Or, as some have said, the PDR is a form of advertising.

The FDA also plays a key role in the contents of the PDR. The information in package inserts must be approved by the FDA; information that is included (or omitted) is done so with the FDA's explicit (or implicit) consent.

The PDR could be a superb resource if the larger medical community determined to make it so. The drug industry, the FDA, and medical establishment should work together to develop mechanisms for accomplishing this very attainable and important goal. Here are three suggestions.

1. Most important, the PDR should be regularly updated, preferably on an annual basis. Because a new edition of the PDR is published annually, it may seem that the contents are regularly updated. This isn't the case. Many medication descriptions in the PDR are ancient, in some cases ten or twenty or more years old. In many instances, important new uses of a drug, or newly discovered side effects or drug interactions, or a revised frequency of known side effects, are not added to PDR descriptions. As a primary source of drug information, the information contained in the PDR must be comprehensive and current.

2. Every medication description in the PDR should offer data on the very lowest effective dosages of drugs. As new data accumulates after a drug is released, new uses of the drug should be listed and the lowest effective dosages defined. To obtain FDA approval for new drug, a drug company must demonstrate its effectiveness in treating one disease. However, manufacturers know that after the drug is released, physicians may use it for many other disorders. These new uses may or may not require different dosages. Often, as information accumulates about new uses of the drug in post-release studies and by usage in the general population, little of this information is added to the PDR.

Drug manufacturers aren't the only source of the problem. According to drug company representatives, adding new information to package inserts or PDR descriptions isn't an easy task. The FDA may require extensive and expensive new studies, and submitting an application to the FDA is costly and time-consuming. On the other hand, since drug manufacturers are not required to provide this new information after a drug has been approved, it's easier for the manufacturer not to do so. For example, according to a representative of Zeneca Pharmaceuticals, the company would like to include all of the new uses (e.g., pain control) in its PDR description of Elavil. However, the process isn't simple or cost-effective.

The FDA should develop a means by which manufacturers are required to add information about new uses and newly recognized side effects involving their products, and it should create a process for doing so in an efficient, quick, and low-cost manner.

3. Explain the relevance of placebo data that is provided with side effect data. If placebo data is provided with side effects, should it also be provided with the beneficial effects of drugs? When listing the side effect data on many new drugs, manufacturers offer lists or charts comparing these results with placebo. For example, with the antidepressant Wellbutrin, the PDR lists an incidence of headaches 25.7% in study subjects; with placebo, 22.2%. While it's helpful to know the placebo numbers, there is a danger that the comparison may cause physicians to assume that the "true" drug-related incidence is the difference between these two numbers—in the case of Wellbutrin and headaches, 3.5%— and then dismiss this side effect as a minor problem. Yet the fact is that among subjects given Wellbutrin in pre-release trials, headaches did occur in 25%—one in four, a substantial proportion— and physicians can expect to encounter this problem with similar frequency in their patients.

The placebo effect is a real phenomenon that researchers continue to try to decipher. Interpreting placebo data can be tricky. In pre-release studies with the tricyclic Anafranil, the PDR states that headaches occurred in 52% of subjects given Anafranil and in 41% given placebo. Does this mean that only 10% of the headaches were "really" caused by the medication? If 52% of people prescribed Anafranil develop headaches, what should their physicians do? Assume it's mainly a placebo reaction and do nothing, or assume it's the medication and take appropriate steps, such as perhaps reducing the dosage?

On the other hand, placebo comparisons are generally omitted when the PDR states the effectiveness of many drugs. In the 5-mg Prozac study completed before Prozac's release, 54% of subjects improved on 5 mg, 64% on 20 mg—and 33% on placebo. Should readers of the PDR know this? On the other hand, the data might lead people to think that Prozac "really helps" only 20% to 30% beyond what is observed with placebo, but clinical experience indicates that Prozac helps far more.

The main question is: why are the placebo numbers listed for side effects but not for beneficial effects? What is gained by providing the placebo percentages for side effects? What is lost by omitting them for beneficial effects? Does the current method enlighten or confuse? If placebo data is being provided regarding side effects, should they also be provided regarding drug effectiveness?

These questions aren't easily answered. I raise them because in researching this book, I have found the placebo data included in package inserts and PDR descriptions informative yet confusing, and I suspect that it may have a similar effect on other readers of these sources of drug information.

THE FOOD AND DRUG ADMINISTRATION (FDA)

The FDA is the agency that oversees drug development and usage. All new drugs, prescription and nonprescription, must be approved by the FDA.

There's no medication that won't harm someone. The FDA performs an important and difficult service—a sort of balancing act in deciding how much medication-prompted harm (i.e., side effects) is acceptable in exchange for the benefits of a drug. I believe that such decisions would be made easier if the very lowest effective dosages were identified and made available. Dosages that are only slightly (but significantly) more effective than placebo may nevertheless be useful in a sizable proportion of the general population. I believe that the birth of new drugs should not commence with higher dosages that are lowered years later, as is often the case—but instead with the very lowest, safest, effective dosages.

1. Require drug companies to determine the lowest and safest effective drug dosages. Current FDA regulations require a new drug to be proven "safe and effective." These regulations leave a lot of latitude. How do we define "effective," and even more subjective, what is "safe"? This is a thorny philosophical and practical issue, since some would contend that no risk is the goal, while others would argue that risk (i.e., adverse effects) is an unavoidable consequence with any foreign substance administered to a large number of people.

However, we do know that the safest dosage is most likely to be the very lowest effective amount of a drug, but the regulations don't require that a new drug be "safest." They don't require that it be shown whether doses lower than those tested by a manufacturer and submitted for FDA approval might be "safer" or equally effective. For example, when Prozac was approved by the FDA at a recommended initial dosage of 20 mg a day for everyone, data already existed showing 5 mg a day to be quite effective in some settings. The FDA approved Prozac at the submitted dosage; not a word about the lower, safer dosage of a 5 mg a day appeared in the package insert or PDR. It still doesn't.

A researcher who knows the system wrote to me: "One of the major reasons for the lack of availability of low-dose medications is the FDA requirement that the medication must be shown to be both safe and efficacious. This is a requirement written into law and interpreted quite rigidly by the FDA. Once a medication has been demonstrated to be efficacious in high dose, low-dose testing can be quite expensive, particularly since testing for low-dose efficacy often requires a larger number of test subjects. The FDA's rigid interpretation of the requirement for efficacy is thus an important factor in the limited availability of low-dose drugs."

This is a crucial issue. FDA regulations and methods play an integral role in the manufacturer-recommended dosages. As this book has demonstrated, too often these dosages are not the lowest effective dosages, and the range of recommended dosages is too narrow to account for interindividual variation. These shortcomings are directly related to the high incidence of medication side effects. A wide range of flexible drug dosages is fundamental to a system in which physicians individualize treatment for you and me.

2. Require manufacturers to include pertinent data on all effective dosages of a drug in the package insert and PDR. As shown with Motrin, Voltaren, Halcion, Prozac, and many others, manufacturers often fail to provide important low-dose data that was determined before these drugs were released. Consequently, physicians and the public are not aware of the effectiveness of significantly lower and safer dosages—and a higher than necessary rate of side effects may be the result.

3. Require manufacturers to provide a range of recommended drug dosages in order to accommodate for interindividual variation. Allegra (fexofenadine), a new antihistamine, is one of the newest drugs reviewed in this book. Allergra was developed and FDA approved at 60 mg twice a day *for everyone*. It is a one-size-fits-all drug. Considering what is known about interindividual variation, one-size-fits-all dosing is irrational.

Pre-release studies with Allergra demonstrated a relatively low incidence of side effects, but that has been true with many drugs that subsequently caused serious adverse effects, many of which were dose-related. Seldane, the top-selling antihistamine for a decade, is a classic example. In pre-release studies, low doses of Allegra were found effective for a significant number of people, but these doses were not developed.

When a one-size-fits-all medication is developed and approved, it tells me that the pharmaceutical industry and FDA are dismissing one of the basic realities of medical practice: patients come in many different sizes, ages, states of health, medication and drug (e.g., alcohol, caffeine, smoking) usages, and medication sensitivities. To me, dismissing such consequential variables is fraught with risk.

One-size-fits-all dosing will mean undermedication for some and overmedication for others. For the latter group, the medication-sensitive group, an unnecessarily higher incidence of drug-related side effects may be the result.

4. Require manufacturers to provide annual updates of their package inserts and PDR descriptions reflecting new information on usages and side effects. Some PDR descriptions are very outdated. The FDA should provide guidelines that facilitate a simple and efficient method for drug manufacturers to make yearly updates of new usages, dosages, side effect data, and overdose measures for all medications.

5. Require manufacturers to produce drugs in multiple dose sizes and breakable tablets, except when medical concerns dictate otherwise. Capsules, which reduce dose flexibility, are often produced for marketing, not medical, purposes. In most instances, capsules serve no useful medical purpose. The price we pay for colorful, bullet-shaped capsules is a steep one—dose flexibility.

As mentioned earlier, Coumadin and some hormones are made in seven to twelve different doses, all as scored tablets. Thus, dose flexibility is possible with most medications, if drug manufacturers and the FDA decide it is a priority.

6. Require manufacturers to publish all relevant studies, especially dosage studies, before approving any new drug. In 1997, Zyban was approved for usage for smoking cessation. Yet none of the manufacturer's research had been published in the medical literature. In other words, the data upon which the FDA approved Zyban wasn't available for independent review of the design and conclusions of the manufacturer's research. Doctors had to depend on information from a nonobjective source, the drug company, at the very same time that the manufacturer initiated a huge advertising campaign encouraging people to ask their doctors for Zyban. The little information that was contained in the package insert was hardly convincing that Zyban's effectiveness was worth the risk (see Chapter 9), or that its usage had any substantial impact on the long-term ability for people to remain off cigarettes. Nor was there any information about individual subjects' response to various doses of Zyban.

In essence, the FDA approved a new drug with virtually no prerelease research unequivocally demonstrating its effectiveness in smoking cessation. The manufacturer's data wasn't particularly impressive, nor had it been published and therefore subjected to independent, objective review—the cornerstone of the scientific process.

Zyban isn't alone. When Allegra was released in 1996, no studies could be found in the medical literature, including data suggesting that a dosage of 40 mg twice a day, 33% lower than the manufacturer-recommended 60 mg twice a day, was effective. Nor, of course, is this information provided in the Allegra package insert or PDR description.

7. Revise the regulations on nonprescription drugs. Nonprescription Motrin IB, Advil, Aleve, Orudis, and other forms of anti-inflammatory drugs have proven to be very useful and effective for many people with arthritis, tendinitis, and similar ailments. Yet for many years, only the prescription forms of these drugs were available, meaning that some people may have had to use dosages higher than they needed.

Anti-inflammatory drugs prompt more adverse-reaction reports to the FDA than any other drug group. The medical establishment and medication references repeatedly stress the importance of using the very lowest effective dosages of these drugs. But if nonprescription anti-inflammatory drugs work, then the very lowest effective dosages weren't originally defined, produced, or released. Only with the advent of the nonprescription preparations did lower-dose and more flexible dosing become possible.

Is the current model of higher prescription doses first, lower nonprescription doses later, the best approach? What will happen when a new generation of anti-inflammatory drugs that don't cause serious gastrointestinal irritation, ulcers, and hemorrhage arrives? Will these new drugs be reserved for prescription-only usage, leaving the nonprescription market to the older, more side-effect-prone drugs we have today?

Perhaps it is time to reevaluate when lower, potentially safer, "nonprescription" drug doses should be developed and released.

8. Provide the population with better information about interindividual variation in drug response and the fact that some people are sensitive to the usual recommended dosages of many medications. The FDA publishes a pamphlet that you can obtain upon request. It is titled "FDA's Tips for Taking Medicines: How to Get the Most Benefits with the Fewest Risks." It contains a lot of advice about using medications properly, keeping a chart if you are taking several medications at a time, and warnings about mixing prescription and nonprescription drugs.

Unfortunately, it doesn't contain one word about the fact that the range of interindividual variation with any given drug is four- to forty-fold. It doesn't state that about 85% of medication side effects are dose-related. It doesn't mention anything about people who may be sensitive to medications. It doesn't suggest informing your physician about your experience with prior medications and side effects. It doesn't hint that doses lower than those recommended by the manufacturer may be safe and effective for many individuals.

In other words, it doesn't discuss any of the information or suggestions provided in this book.

PHYSICIANS

When I discuss the issues in this book with nonprofessionals, the most frequent question they ask is "Why don't doctors know about the effectiveness of low-dose of medications?" This is the quintessential question, because if doctors were informed about interindividual variation, medication sensitivities, and the low-dose data in the medical literature, our epidemic of iatrogenic illness wouldn't exist and this book wouldn't be necessary.

I must admit that for many years I was completely unaware of the scope of the problem. I did, however, believe my patients when they reported unusual side effects or side effects at so-called standard dosages. Perhaps I was open to their input because I've always been sensitive to sedating drugs and alcohol. Tiny doses of antihistamines or Valium put me out. So complaints of other side effects at seemingly proper doses wasn't a concept foreign to my own experience.

Nevertheless, even I sometimes was skeptical, tending to trust my medications more than my patient. Medications are, after all, the heart of the profession we call medicine. Sometimes it's psychologically difficult and frustrating to have to face the fact that our best weapons have failed. That we have caused harm when we only intended good. Perhaps this explains why, when a cardiac technician tried to tell physicians that she was seeing an unusual number of abnormal heart valves in patients taking fen-phen, it was received with considerable skepticism. "There was a lot of debate among the doctors about if this meant anything or not," according to one physician. Such skepticism is a sign of overconfidence in our medications. A report of a severe side effect, especially a series of such incidents reported by a competent professional, should without hesitation be taken seriously until proven otherwise.

Similarly, physicians aren't taught to question the dosage guidelines they are given. Not once in my medical training did a professor ever raise the issue that the dosages provided by the PDR and other drug references might be wrong, too high, or lacking in thorough study and reporting. The methods of the pharmaceutical industry in researching and marketing drugs dosages was never raised. We were never told how brief and limited prerelease drug research can be. Our professors probably didn't know.

In the succeeding years, it seems that things haven't changed. In my recent work with medical students, I've never heard anyone except me raise these issues.

Nor are most physicians trained to individualize medication treatment, to take careful medication histories and to prescribe accordingly. We are taught a lot about how medications work, their interactions in the body, and the specifics of their metabolism and elimination by the liver and kidneys. But rarely are medication dosages—how they were determined and if they are ideal—issues of serious scrutiny.

The result is that by default, physicians learn to rely upon the information provided by the pharmaceutical industry via the new PDRs they receive each year, and to accept this information without critical appraisal. This leads to a major blind spot in medical practice: the well-entrenched assumption that the manufacturer-recommended dosages are the correct dosages.

Thus, if you complain of a side effect not listed in the PDR, the odds of your physician believing you may be low. That's why, even when low-dose information is presented, physicians often fail to act on it. How else to explain, for example, the prescribing of Zantac at 150 mg for over a decade when the PDR states that 100 mg is just as effective. Or if you are prescribed "nonsedating" Claritin and get drowsy, or Motrin and develop anxiety—both rare but documented side effects—your physician may not heed your complaint.

To hopefully improve this situation, here are a few humbly offered recommendations for physicians (and for you to remind your physician):

1. Remember the concept of interindividual variation with every patient, with every prescription. Use medications flexibly. Just because manufacturers recommend one-size-fits-all initial dosaging for medications such as Allegra, Claritin, or Prilosec, that doesn't mean this is the ideal dosage for every person. Just because the PDR doesn't offer information about lower doses of drugs such as Prozac or Ambien, that doesn't mean data on lower, effective dosages don't exist. Just because many people respond to 400 mg of Motrin, that doesn't mean that others won't do just as well at nonprescription 200 mg, as studies dating back to 1966 confirm.

Cardiac drugs are no different. One physician told me: "I have found that with quinidine, digoxin, and Pronestyl, the 'normal range' is just the therapeutic dose for the average patient, but some people just need a whisper of the stuff to really have it work." Other doctors, he said, give up too quickly when people develop side effects; they don't try lower than recommended dosages, although these in fact work with some individuals. Studies concur with his perspective.

Using drugs flexibly implies an understanding that drug company guidelines aren't biological truths or federal laws; the recommended dosages are only approximations, not irrefutable facts. Physicians should be skeptical of all drugs that are recommended at an one-size-fits-all initial dosage. As one textbook emphasizes, "Clinical trials by physician-scientists are done on groups of patients. . . . Clinicians, however, do not treat groups of patients. Rather, they treat individuals." The goal of any prescription is to help someone—if a dose lower than the manufacturer recommends works, so much the better.

Speaking as a physician, I find that using medications flexibly and creatively is challenging and fun, and the rewards are great. Flexible dosing heightens the level of my prescribing skills and improves results. Patients recognize the difference, the attention to details such as obtaining a thorough medication history and fully discussing dosing issues, and are appreciative. The time expenditure is minimal; indeed, flexible, careful dosing that reduces the risks of side effects ultimately saves time.

2. Obtaining a history of medication experiences and drug sensitivities, past and present, is mandatory before initiating or adjusting medication treatment. Recognize that many people are sensitive to medications. Often they are sensitive to alcohol or coffee, which can be clues. As one internist put it, "The ones who say they're very sensitive are very sensitive, and the ones who say they have an iron stomach have an iron stomach."

3. Physicians have an obligation to inform patients of potential side effects with medications. According to a 1992 report in the *British Medical Journal* entitled "Adverse drug reactions and secrecy": "Traditionally, doctors have told their patients little about possible unwanted effects of prescribed medicines. Two British studies have shown that only a quarter of patients knew what side effects their medicines could cause, and half of these 'informed' patients became aware of problems only when they themselves were affected."

From my experience, this is not an exaggeration. To me, it signifies that physicians are not fully involving patients in the decision-making process about drugs and dosages. And it means that patients aren't asking enough questions.

4. Physicians must listen closely and believe their patients, especially regarding complaints about drug side effects. When I first went into practice, I didn't know that Tofranil could cause memory deficits at a dose of 30 mg. My training had taught me otherwise, but the patient was credible and her description of the subtle memory deficits was convincing. We lowered the dosage to 25 mg, a seemingly small (yet 17%) reduction. The side effect disappeared, the antidepressant effect remained.

Subsequent situations reaffirmed this experience, and learning to use lower and more carefully graduated doses served me well. Thus, when Prozac was released, I knew how to direct patients to make small dose adjustments after many of them encountered unpleasant side effects at the manufacturer-recommended initial 20-mg dosage.

Some physicians are very willing to listen to what patients tell them. Others, more skeptical, are nevertheless willing to learn. One internist told me I was dispensing "placebo treatment" when I started his patient on 25 mg of Elavil. His opinion changed when he jumped the dosage to 50 mg and side effects nearly landed the man in the hospital.

Still others, perhaps perceiving their prestige or credibility at stake, are too quick to dismiss complaints of side effects with which they are not familiar.

Many physicians (and science in general) have a difficult time dealing with ambiguity—for example, treatments that work sometimes, or doses that work for some patients. As scientists, physicians rightly feel most comfortable with methods that are scientifically proven, which is why the random, controlled, double-blind study has become the gold standard for validating the effectiveness of a medication. Although this type of study may be the most reliable, many fruitful avenues of scientific investigation have been prompted by an unusual finding, response, or reaction. Examples include the discovery of penicillin, the association of *Helicobacter pylori* with ulcers and gastritis, the unexpected side effects such as anterograde amnesia with Halcion and cardiac reactions to Seldane.

Physicians must be careful to keep their minds open to things patients tell them that may not have yet been scientifically reported, studied, or fully clarified.

If your doctor has difficulty understanding your medication sensitivities, try to educate him; give him your filled-out medication-sensitivity form (see pages 27–29); give him this book; go to the medical library and obtain copies of the relevant studies listed in the reference section of this book. You will not only be helping yourself and him, but performing a service that may benefit many of his patients. If all of these attempts fail, find a physician who is more open to you.

5. Physicians who listen and acknowledge their patients' concerns are greatly appreciated and rarely sued. Most people don't like taking medication. When they have to do so, it's not without some trepidation. Such people appreciate physicians who take care to minimize the risk.

People who feel that their physician has made every effort to use medications carefully are more accepting when problems occur. It has been repeatedly reported that the more people like their physician, the less they are likely to sue. Considering that drug-related side effects are the leading cause of iatrogenic illness, and iatrogenic illness is what often prompts malpractice suits, it further behooves physicians to employ every means possible to minimize medication risks.

Some physicians may feel awkward about occasionally suggesting a nonprescription dose of a medication, believing that patients expect a prescription. Sometimes this is indeed the case. Physicians can handle this situation by including the patient in the decision process, pointing out the pros and cons of lower and higher dosages. Most people, when told that one nonprescription Advil or Aleve or Pepcid AC may suffice, but if not, they can double the dose, will agree with this more flexible, initial approach.

A disincentive, however, may be that most insurers don't pay for nonprescription drugs. Perhaps in time they'll realize that by avoiding side effects and extra doctor visits and hospitalizations, money may be saved by honoring a physician's recommendation for a nonprescription drug.

People also appreciate physicians who try to minimize their discomfort. My dermatologist adds a buffering agent to lidocaine so it doesn't sting when she injects it. My orthopedist uses the smallest size needle necessary for injecting an inflamed tendon.

Because of their desire to spare me unnecessary pain, I appreciate and am loyal to them—and give others their names.

6. Physicians, remember the principle best expressed by medicine's most respected drug reference, *Goodman and Gilman's Pharmacological Basis of Therapeutics*:

> *Therapy as a science does not apply simply to the evaluation and testing of new, investigational drugs in animals and man. It applies with equal importance to the treatment of each patient as an individual.*

When I've spoken to physicians individually, most of them readily understand the point I make, that the wide range of interindividual variation makes one-size-fits-all dosaging irrational. Given the proper tools such as comprehensive low-dose data and flexible pill sizes, I believe that many physicians would adopt the methods required for individualization of medication therapy. Indeed, we already do this with insulin, digoxin, and hormones. As I've said previously, the process of careful individualization of drug therapy isn't new—it's just not been applied to most medications.

Unfortunately, low-dose data is generally not readily available for physicians' usage. It's not in the PDR and infrequently in the other most used drug references. Finding the low-dose data means digging it out of the medical literature, and even then it is often a difficult and time-consuming process. Journal abstracts often omit the various doses used in a study and rarely mention individual responses. Physicians who today are given as little as eight minutes for each patient hardly have time to obtain a decent medication history, let alone spend hours at the medical library delving into the literature. It is my hope that this book may help to fill this information gap.

MOST IMPORTANT—YOU, THE PATIENT

"Both my mother and sister are very sensitive to medications," a woman told me. "Of course their doctors don't believe them, but they're very persistent and always demand the very lowest doses. Usually they get what they want."

The interaction between you and your physician constitutes a relationship. Previously, this relationship usually consisted of a paternalistic physician dispensing treatment and advice to the recipient. In recent times, as people have become more interested in and knowledgeable about health issues, the relationship has become more equal, at least with some physicians. But in the realm of medications and dosages, physicians have generally continued to be the font of all knowledge. The goal of this book is to allow you to become an active participant in the process. There are many steps you can take to accomplish this.

1. If you are medication-sensitive, tell your physician. Provide specific examples of adverse drug reactions and/or responses at lower doses. Fill out the medication-sensitivity form in Chapter 1 (pages 27–29) and ask that a copy be placed on your chart.

2. Be clear with your physician about your preference to avoid medications whenever possible. Many physicians believe that most patients want and expect a prescription. Physicians quickly learn that a recommendation against medications or for lower-dose nonprescription remedies is often met with disappointment or outright hostility. As a hypertension specialist explained, most patients would rather take a pill than follow his advice about losing weight, stopping smoking, and reducing salt. Your physician may mistakenly assume that you're like everyone else; let him know otherwise.

3. If you require medication therapy, involve yourself in the choice of drug and dosage. Ask questions! Ask about the side effects with any medication that your physician may prescribe to you. Ask specifically about data on lower, potentially effective dosages. Ask your physician the source of his information. If you are medication-sensitive or elderly and your condition isn't acute, ask about starting with a lower, safer dosage, and together form a strategy for gradually increasing the dosage if necessary.

Be persistent, or you may not get the information you want. As the article "Adverse drug reactions and secrecy" stated: "Traditionally, doctors have told their patients little about possible unwanted effects of prescribed medicines. Two British studies have shown that only a quarter of patients knew what side effects their medicines could cause, and half of these 'informed' patients became aware of problems only when they themselves were affected.''

4. If you are taking medication on an ongoing basis, ask about reducing the dosage to a lower maintenance level. Once a condition is controlled, medications can often be reduced to lower, maintenance levels. Sometimes this possibility is overlooked. Other times, the data on the effectiveness of lower dosages isn't well known. Obtaining the data and presenting it to your physician should facilitate discussion about the benefits and risks, if any, of reducing your medication.

5. Do not rely on the PDR or medication package inserts, *The Pill Book,* or other medical references for low-dose information. Most PDR descriptions provide no data on doses below those recommended by the manufacturer, but a small percentage do. Check the ''Clinical Pharmacology'' section. This section may also provide other hints such as data on the range of individual variation of medication blood levels. Sometimes the ''Dosage Guidelines'' section may suggest, if not define, lower dosages. If you are sensitive to medications, elderly dosages may sometimes be helpful even if you're not over sixty. Overall, however, most PDR descriptions offer no low-dose data.

The Pill Book and standard medical references such as the *AMA Drug Evaluations Annual* series, the *American Hospital Formulary Service, Drug Information* series, and the *Conn's Current Therapy* series contain a lot of good information, but not in regard to low-dose medication therapy. The best source of information about lower dosages and interindividual variation is the medical literature. Medical libraries contain computers that access Medline, the database on the medical literature. Reference experts at medical libraries will assist you in learning the system and finding the journal articles. Many hospitals contain reference libraries.

If you're hooked up to the Internet, you can access Medline and other sources of medical information. Medline itself can provide a lot of leads, but the brief summaries or abstracts it offers often omit the dosages used in drug studies. You still may need to obtain the full journal articles at a medical library to learn about specific dosages and results.

Locating and interpreting medical articles is a time-consuming process. Hopefully, this book has provided you with the information you need to discuss your medication with your physician. I hope to provide future editions of this book with the latest information on current and newly released drugs.

6. Do not make medication decisions on your own. If your physician is skeptical about your history of side effects or dismissive of your requests for initiating treatment at lower, safer drug dosages, get another opinion. Ask friends and family about their physicians. Find one with a reputation for listening and taking patients' concerns seriously.

7. Practice prevention. The best way to avoid drug-related side effects is to avoid getting sick. Prevention is simple—take care of yourself. Exercise regularly. Eat a healthy diet. Use alcohol moderately. Don't smoke. Always buckle up. Keep stress down by seeking good work situations, developing good relationships, and keeping financial liabilities down. If you find yourself addicted to self-destructive behaviors or relationships, get counseling or seek support groups.

THE INFLUENCE OF ECONOMIC FACTORS ON DRUG DOSAGES

The marketplace is a powerful force in all venues of human endeavor, including the medical system. The marketplace generally operates without a moral compass, often with both positive and negative consequences.

The drive to develop newer and better drugs is anchored and underwritten by the vast profits that are reaped. Prozac, Mevacor, Motrin, Tagamet, Prilosec, Claritin, Redux: virtually all of the medications discussed in this book have proved highly useful as therapeutic agents and, in turn, have each generated millions or billions in profit for their manufacturers.

However, part of the success of these drugs involved being the first of their kind to reach the marketplace. Brief studies take less time and cost less money than prolonged ones, but they are less likely to uncover important side effects and may produce results skewed in favor of higher dosages.

It also saves time and money to study a limited range of dosages. Currently, drug manufacturers only have to find a dosage that's effective without causing an unacceptable rate of side effects in order to seek approval from the FDA. "Acceptable risk" is the operative—and unsettling—term. Manufacturers are not required to test lower dosages that may also be effective and would be likely cause fewer side effects.

Nor does the pull of the marketplace and the potential development of competing drugs encourage them to do so. Indeed, the marketplace virtually demands that a new drug must be more effective than already established competitors if physicians are to prescribe it. This again favors higher rather than lower dosages, because in pre-release studies a manufacturer will likely achieve higher rates of efficacy by using higher drug dosages in comparison to competing medications.

Of course, cost control is the lifeblood of every business and corporation. Drug companies are no exception. Funding the study of a broader range of dosages costs more money and reduces the amount available for the study of other drugs. No company can afford to waste precious funds. Research is expensive; marketing is expensive (nonprescription Aleve was released onto the market with a reported $100 million ad campaign). Perhaps the only way that drug companies will expand the study of drug dosages is if the FDA were to even the field, i.e., require it of all new drugs.

Similarly, once a drug is released, there's even less incentive for a manufacturer to undertake studies testing the effectiveness and safety of lower doses. Other researchers may do so, if clinical experience—i.e., side effects at standard dosages—suggests it, but it may take years for the new data to percolate through the system, reaching physicians and drug references. Such data may never be included in the PDR.

When a manufacturer's patent expires and the medication becomes available generically, further study is even less likely. As one researcher wrote to me about hydrochlorthiazide (HCTZ), an antihypertensive drug: "If one extrapolates the results of clinical trials with low-dose versus high-dose diuretic [HCTZ] on mortality and morbidity, one is left with the conclusion that increasing the dose of a diuretic in standard preparations may be responsible for thousands of unnecessary deaths and heart attacks. Unfortunately, there is no incentive for anyone to make lower-dose hydrochlorthiazide tablets, since it potentially costs millions of dollars to convince the FDA to permit these tablets to be marketed, and once marketed the tablet would not be under patent and could be copied by any competitor.''

Other promising methods also wither for lack of economic incentives. From 1987 through 1990, five papers were published involving the heightened effectiveness of Voltaren when combined with B-vitamins in treating pain syndromes. The study results demonstrated that not only was this combination effective, but it permitted the use of lower doses of Voltaren and shorter durations of drug treatment—and the risks of side effects were greatly reduced. Considering that anti-inflammatory drug side effects can cause serious side effects, was this approach studied further? Was it tried with other anti-inflammatory drugs or in treating other disorders such as arthritis or bursitis? As of 1995, no further articles appeared in the literature. And no mention of this method is noted in drug references or the PDR.

THE INFLUENCE OF ECONOMIC FACTORS ON PHYSICIANS' METHODS AND DRUG SELECTION

The economics of the medical system also affect physicians' practices. With the traditional fee-for-service system, the more patients a physician sees, the more money he makes. This encourages seeing more people and spending less time with each. An individual practitioner can do as he pleases, and many give each patient as much time as is needed, but those who work in groups may feel pressured by their peers to see a predetermined numbers of patients. For example, a friend of mine works with an emergency room group; indeed, he initiated the group and is its senior member. But he's extremely thorough and methodical, taking the time required to do a good job—and he gets a lot of flak from his partners because his numbers are less.

Under newer systems such as HMOs, in which physicians are salaried, the pressure to see a large number of patients is very strong. The economics of most HMOs require physicians to see a predetermined number of people per hour. With general physicians, the requirement may be as many as eight. Considering that physicians must also dictate notes, answer messages, give orders to nurses, and perform other ancillary duties, that leaves about five to six minutes per patient at best. For example, in Chapter 12 a hypertension specialist discussed how primary physicians often don't have the time to obtain medication-sensitivity histories or to individualize antihypertensive drugs.

More and more, one hears complaints about the impact of time pressures on medical practice. In a 1994 news article Dr. Robert Kane of the University of Minnesota School of Public Health stated: "As physicians feel under pressure to spend less and less time with their patients, they often don't spend the time needed to a take a thorough drug history." The result is side effects that might otherwise have been avoided, and many people drop out of treatment.

You'd think that there must be a system that encourages doctors to spend as much time as needed with every patient. One wonders if in the long run, by being more thorough and perhaps causing fewer side effects and other miscues, such an approach might actually be cost-effective. It would be interesting for someone to conduct a study that examines this issue.

In the meantime, you have to do what you can to obtain and keep your doctor's attention. Some physicians are impatient, but many will spend as much time as they can. Hopefully your physician is one of the latter, but if not, find one who is. If you are medication-sensitive, you need a physician who takes the time to listen because your medication tendencies require thoroughness.

MANAGED CARE AND MEDICATION CHOICE

Managed care, which includes most insurance plans as well as HMOs, has also begun to greatly influence medication treatment. Many managed care groups limit the quantity or types of medications they'll pay for. If you want to use the more flexible but more expensive liquid form of Prozac, your plan may refuse to pay for it. Or it may require your physician to submit a report explaining the need for the more expensive preparation. Such reports take time, frustrate physicians who believe they should possess the right to make medication decisions, and ultimately act as a disincentive for physicians to prescribe freely.

Some managed care systems have tried to reduce costs by narrowing their formulary (list of approved drugs), requiring physician members to choose among those the system offers. For example, Zoloft is a top-selling antidepressant that many psychiatrists prefer over Prozac, yet the 1997 formulary of Blue Shield of California didn't include it.

Soon some systems may start controlling physicians' choice even more directly. One managed care executive raised the possibility that his company might require the old, side-effect-prone but much less expensive tricyclic antidepressants be used first in treating depressed patients. The far better drugs such as Prozac, Zoloft, Serzone, Paxil, Wellbutrin, and others would be reserved for those who failed—i.e. encountered intolerable adverse effects with the side-effect-prone tricyclics. In other words, you'll first be required to take an older, far inferior, more side-effect-prone drug. You'll get the preferred medications only after reacting to the inferior drugs, while running the risk that while you're being put through this, your depression may continue and possibly worsen. Such requirements are inhumane.

Such economics-driven medicine also create tremendous moral dilemmas for physicians, whose first obligation is to "Do No Harm." Prescribing medications that they know cause more side effects directly conflicts with this ethic.

For patients, the dilemma is more concrete. They're the ones who will sustain the increased side effects and lower rates of success.

Adding to the confusion, drug companies have begun acquiring managed care programs. Will they pressure physicians to favor their products, even those that may be inferior to other brands?

Clearly the medical system is in flux. Disarray, some would call it. Where it will lead and the quality of care it will deliver— these remain to be seen. However things develop, our current, limited-dosage methods of developing and prescribing medications will not improve unless incentives are created. The marketplace may work well enough with clothing and automobiles, but I am concerned about its effect on the usage of medications. The FDA was created to safeguard the quality, effectiveness, and safety of medicinal products. But even if the pharmaceutical industry and the FDA were to fashion protocols for the development of the very lowest and safest effective drug dosages and the production of breakable tablets in multiple dose sizes, how much benefit will result if insurers and HMOs impede utilization of these products?

Perhaps the mandate of the FDA should be extended, or a new agency created, to ensure that new medical systems do not compromise the quality of medication treatment, to guarantee you and your physician the freedom to choose the best medications and dosages for your condition.

ECONOMIC FACTORS AND NONPRESCRIPTION DRUGS

"Don't take over-the-counter painkillers like candy, experts warn," was the title of a 1995 article published in a major newspaper. It's still good advice. Unfortunately, that's not the message we receive from television and newsprint advertisements extolling the virtues of one product or another. "We shouldn't think that just because these are over-the-counter drugs that they're the same as candy," the article quoted Dr. Paul K. Whelton of the Johns Hopkins School of Public Health. "Almost any drug that has a beneficial effect has some potential for an adverse effect." Other health professionals voiced similar concerns: "Prompted by TV pain-reliever pitches, Americans are swallowing over-the-counter analgesics for everything from headaches and bad backs to arthritis and routine athletic aches," the article stated. "Consumers need to take over-the-counter drugs seriously—and properly."

In 1995–1996, Axid AR, Pepcid AC, Tagamet HB, and Zantac 75 emerged as nonprescription preparations for mild heartburn and indigestion. Watching the intense, expensive advertising war between these very similar products has been enough to give one, well, heartburn. Equally stunning are the huge amounts spent perennially trying to convince you to use Advil or Nuprin or Motrin IB—all ibuprofen 200 mg.

Perhaps the worst effect is how this unrelenting advertising influences our attitudes about nonprescription drugs. "I think people are taking over-the-counter drugs way too casually," the same newspaper article quoted Peter Koo, a pharmacist and director of the pain consultation and management service at the University of California, San Francisco, as saying. Based on the vast amounts spent on these products, many people apparently do consider these drugs harmless. They aren't. As mentioned in Chapter 13, Tylenol (acetaminophen) and especially aspirin, when used frequently, are associated with increased incidences of serious side effects.

The availability of nonprescription drugs does provide us with the opportunity for using lower, safer doses of many drugs. But even at these dosages, no drug is entirely safe. Side effects can occur. Allergic reactions can develop. And frequent usage increases the risks.

It's discouraging to see manufacturers push the use of drugs such as Zantac 75 or Tagamet HB for heartburn when one or two Tums or Riopan tablets usually are effective, work faster, and produce fewer risks than a systemic medication. It's discouraging to see products containing ibuprofen being pushed for fever in children when ibuprofen may be more likely to cause stomach irritation than Tylenol or other forms of acetaminophen.

As with prescription drugs, nonprescription medications can be of great use, but they also must be used flexibly, cautiously, and only when necessary.

NEW AND BETTER METHODS OF MEDICATION THERAPY

Taking medications orally is a simple process: insert the pill into the mouth, drink some water, swallow. When you think about it, this method hasn't changed since ancient times. The drugs may be different, but the delivery system remains the same. That's another part of the problem. Whether you receive drug therapy by mouth or injection, the drug circulates throughout your entire body and affects most, if not all, of your cells.

New methods of medication delivery are slowly gaining interest. Already, skin-permeable (transdermal) delivery systems have been developed such as Transderm-Scop for motion sickness and nicotine patches to assist in smoking cessation. Transdermal patches are also used with cardiac medications, and specialty pharmacies can prepare transdermal creams containing hormones, anti-inflammatory medications, and other drugs. The advantages of the transdermal method are that it bypasses the effects of digestion and may deliver more consistent blood levels of medication. Some drugs, such as natural progesterone, are destroyed by the digestive process and are therefore ineffective when taken orally, but can be used via the transdermal method.

Similarly, some medications are now made as nasal sprays. The nostrils contain a rich supply of blood vessels and drug absorption can be very quick. Allergy medications already are available utilizing nasal inhalation, and other drugs such as hormones have been studied. Just like the sublingual (under the tongue) use for nitroglycerin, nasal inhalation provides a quick-acting method of getting medication into the system while bypassing the slower and less efficient oral route.

Just beyond the horizon is, I believe, a renaissance in medication specificity. Already, medical science has produced drugs that can more effectively target intended cells and evoke more precise responses. Prozac, Claritin, and Prilosec are examples of drugs that were intentionally designed to work more specifically and effectively than earlier, more side-effect-prone predecessors. Soon, perhaps, drugs will be introduced that are tagged in such a way they will target only the desired cells to produce responses without affecting other cells in the body. And it may be possible to engineer antibiotics that attack specific invasive bacteria without affecting human cells or other bacteria that compose the normal, benign intestinal, skin, and vaginal flora, thereby avoiding many side effects as well as the yeast or fungal overgrowths that sometimes occur with current antibiotic treatment.

Someday, our burgeoning knowledge of genetics may permit us to diagnose disease tendencies before they fully develop and to custom-design medications to prevent cancer, heart disease, diabetes and arthritis before they begin, perhaps even before we emerge from the womb. When illnesses do occur, simple tests may help us determine the specific genetic factors or boosters necessary to allow our systems to overcome the disease.

With these new technologies, side effects may still occur—interindividual variation will still be a factor—but the incidence and severity of side effects should plummet.

The future is bright, but what about the present? What can we do now? A lot. Most of all, we can perfect the usage of the tools

we already possess, specifically medications. The medical establishment recognizes that the rate of side effects is too high. What
can be done? We can prescribe and use our medications cautiously
and thoughtfully, paying heed to the fact that there's much we
don't know about the medications we use and that new side effects
and adverse drug reactions are discovered every day.

For example, in November 1996, it was reported that the effect
of Xanax, which has been available since 1981, is enhanced by
grapefruit juice, causing increased drowsiness. A few years back,
we learned that grapefruit juice increased the levels of Seldane in
the blood, possibly increasing the risk of serious cardiac arrhythmias. Now we know that grapefruit juice increases the blood levels of many drugs because of interactions with metabolic enzymes
in the liver. The medications that grapefruit juice, fresh or frozen,
may affect include Procardia XL, Calan and other forms of verapamil, cyclosporin (used in organ transplant therapy), estrogens,
caffeine, and possibly the asthma drug theophylline. In some instances, grapefruit juice causes an increase in the blood levels of
some drugs of over 100%.

The number of potential interactions between prescription
drugs, nonprescription preparations, and various foods is immense. The drug interactions we know about today probably represent just a fraction of what actually occurs. No one knew about
the interactions of Seldane with some antibiotic and antifungal
drugs until people began collapsing.

We can also improve our current methods by applying what we
already know about the broad range of interindividual variation
to medications. By paying heed to the fact that many people are
medication sensitive. And by maintaining a healthy, open attitude
to complaints of side effects even it they are not listed in the PDR.

The irony is that we spend billions on developing new technologies, new equipment, and new drugs. How much could we
save by perfecting what we already possess? And how much could
we save by reducing the costs of iatrogenic illness: pain, missed
work, office visits, hospitalizations, death?

Studies show that in regard to medications, people are most
concerned about effectiveness and safety, and they're willing to
pay for them. For a few cents extra per pill, much could be accomplished in developing lower, safer drug dosages?

As we have seen, the medical system changes slowly. New

drugs still arrive with limited information and minimal dose flexibility. New data about safer, lower doses often filter through the system slowly, if at all. We speak a lot about prevention. What could be more preventive than developing and utilizing the very lowest, safest, effective dosages of any medication? Or by ensuring that new data gets communicated to physicians and the public quickly?

TOWARD A GLOWING FUTURE

I hope I've made it clear that the suggestions and criticisms contained in this book are directed at one issue: how we can develop and utilize medications more effectively and safely. About Western medicine as a whole, I am very optimistic. We are on the verge of an era of unparalleled progress. Suddenly, possibilities unimagined just twenty years ago now beckon: genetic engineering, laser techniques, transdermal medications and injections without needles, artificial organs and tissues, artificial blood, cell-targeted medications, and perhaps most of all, an understanding of the human system on a biochemical basis that may eventually lead to diagnoses before diseases occur and treatments that are targeted to the molecular level.

Individually and collectively, we are and always will be a work in evolution. That's why we are here. The future is bright if we are willing to continually reassess our methods and improve them. That is the machinery of progress. That is what this book is all about.

Notes

Chapter 1. Side Effects—Why They Occur and How to Prevent Them

3: "Many adverse reactions probably arise from failure . . ." W. G. Clark et al., p. 48.

5: "It soon became apparent that many patients found the 20-mg dose . . ." N. Sussman and G. Stimmel, p. 25.

6: "According to the AMA . . ." American Medical Association, 1993, p. 33.

6: "It's because of this same wide range . . ." E. W. Martin, p. 202.

7: "As a 1996 journal article put it . . ." D. V. Sheehan and K. Hartnett-Sheehan, p. 51.

8: "As Goodman and Gilman's . . ." A. G. Gilman et al., p. 77.

8: "An adverse drug reaction is defined . . ." K. L. Melmon et al., p. 30.

9: "It is estimated that half of adverse drug reactions . . ." P. L. Price, p. 133.

9: "Considering that the sales of prescription drugs to pharmacies . . ." B. Buckley, p. 27.

10: "This may explain why, of about 37,000 adverse drug reactions . . ." G. A. Faich et al., p. 2068.

12: "Often, a commercial sponsor . . ." C. Peck, p. 117.

13: "It would disappoint the patients . . ." K. L. Melmon et al., p. 920.

15: "We found serious discrepancies in overdose treatment . . ."
W. H. Mullen et al., p. 255.

16: "But *The Pill Book* defines . . ." H. M. Silverman, p. 721.

18: "The regimen used . . ." *United States Pharmacopeia, Drug
Information* (USP DI), Monograph on colchicine, p. 18.

23: "Biologic variation in drug effect . . ." W. G. Clark et al.,
p. 19.

24: "Over the years she had considerable difficulties . . ." F.
Sjoqvist and L. Bertilsson, p. 369.

24: "Diclofenac [Voltaren], like other NSAIDS . . ." 1997 *PDR*,
p. 834.

Chapter 2. The Scope of the Side Effect Problem

30: "Patients, to a greater extent . . ." A. G. Gilman, et al., p. 77.

30: "Various studies have reported that from less than 10% to
more than 40% . . ." D. W. Bates et al., pp. 29–34. T. A.
Hutchinson et al., pp. 533–42. F. E. Karch and L. Lasagna,
pp. 247–54. C. R. Martys, pp. 1194–97. K. L. Melmon, et al.
A. G. Recchia and N. H. Shear, pp. 68–79.

30: "about 80 million people use medications regularly . . ." H.
Jick, pp. 555–57. K. L. Melmon et al.

30: "Serious medication side effects aren't rare . . ." T. Gibian,
pp. 1755–60. A. G. Recchia and N. H. Shear, pp. 68–79. K. L.
Melmon et al. S. M. Wolfe and R. E. Hope.

31: "Bad effects from prescriptions . . ." *Fort Lauderdale Sun-
Sentinel*, p. A–6.

31: "In the United States, hospitalized adults . . ." H. Jick,
pp. 555–57. K. Steel et al., pp. 638–42.

31: "Three percent experience side effects . . ." H. Jick,
pp. 555–57. K. L. Melmon et al.

31: "If the numbers from New York . . ." D. W. Bates et al.,
p. 29.

31: "The estimated medical expenditure for handling side effects . . ." P. L. Price, pp. 258–62.

31: "It is likely that only a fraction of the ADRs . . ." K. L.
Melmon et al., p. 44.

33: "Letters to the editors of medical journals . . ." F. M. Jacobsen, pp. 119–22.

33: "Years after Prozac's release . . ." 1997 PDR.

33: "A 1997 study showed that when determined by spontaneous reports of patients . . ." Dutch study attempts to qualify sexual dysfunction profiles among SSRIs, pp. 22–23.

33: "I think all the published figures are underestimates . . ." B. Jancin, p. 17.

35: "It would seem that with all these safeguards . . ." W. G. Clark et al., p. 42.

36: "The full range of adverse reactions . . ." *AMA Drug Evaluations 1993*, p. 41.

37: "Prozac, for example, has been available . . ." L. Orange, p. 20.

38: "A 1994 study found that a thyroid hormone . . ." C. Clark, p. B-3.

38: "We conclude that moderate dose digoxin . . ." M. L. Slatton et al., p. 1206.

39: "When prescribing newly released drugs . . ." American Medical Association, 1993, p. 43.

Chapter 3. Why People Respond Differently to Medications and What to Do About It

42: "The ultimate hazard is variability . . ." E. W. Martin, p. 202.

42: "The frequency at which adverse reactions occur . . ." W. G. Clark et al., p. 48.

44: "For example, the PDR tells us that with the antidepressant Norpramin (desipramine) . . ." 1995 PDR, p. 1417.

48: "Genetic polymorphisms [variations from the usual pattern] in enzymes . . ." K. L. Melmon et al., p. 878.

48: "With Xanax, the data shows that Asians . . ." K. M. Lin et al., pp. 365–69.

49: "Whereas most Caucasians respond well . . ." L. Abrams, p. 528.

50: "A 1972 study showed that while alcohol . . ." P. H. Wolff, pp. 449–50.

52: "For example, the 1997 PDR description of the anti-inflammatory drug Orudis . . ." p. 2875.

52: "A 1997 study in *Nature Medicine* . . ." Gender gap for pain, pp. 123–24.

53: "Women are also twice as likely as men to develop a biochemical depression..." K. Pajer, pp. 30–37.

53: "A 1996 study in *JAMA*..." C. B. Ambrosone et al., pp. 1494–1501.

56: "Hardly any people realize..." Correspondence, February 7, 1995, p. 3.

58: "Doctors may soon be able to tailor treatments..." K. Jegalian, p. 17.

59: "Many physicians are not aware..." K. L. Melmon et al., p. 800.

Chapter 4. Medication Sensitivities and Side Effects in the Elderly

60: "The normal aging process makes people..." Associated Press, p. 1.

61: "Illness caused by medications is arguably the most significant treatable geriatric health problem." T. Gibian, p. 1755.

62: "Mismedication of the elderly..." K. L. Melmon et al., p. 19.

62: "The risk of an adverse drug reaction..." S. M. Wolfe and R. E. Hope, p. vii.

63: "That is why, for example, the *United States Pharmacopeia* warns that with the anti-inflammatory drug colchicine..." *United States Pharmacopeia, Drug Information* (USP DI), Monograph on colchicine, p. 8.

64: "And although people over 65 years of age constitute about 12% of the population..." K. L. Melmon et al. N. Curzen and H. Purcell, p. 154.

65: "She was a vocal woman...." J. Van, p. D-3.

65: "Elderly patients often have multiple medical problems..." p. B-1.

65: "Indeed, a 1990 study found 9% of hospital admissions..." W. D. Smucker and J. R. Kontak, p. 105.

66: "According to the Public Citizen Health Research Group, a 1985 survey of 425..." S. M. Wolfe and R. E. Hope.

66: "For example, the 1997 PDR description of the anti-inflammatory drug Orudis and extended-release Oruvail (ketoprofen)..." 1997 PDR, p. 2875.

67: "A 1994 study found that elderly patients are most concerned about drug effectiveness and safety." R. P. Ferguson et al., p. 56–62.

67: "Recently approved drugs usually have not been given . . ." K. L. Melmon et al., p. 22.

68: "There are things that older people can do to help themselves . . ." G. Kolata, p. A-20.

Chapter 5. The Uses and Limitations of Low-Dose Medication Therapy

69: "Clinical trials by physician-scientists are done on groups of patients. . . ." K. L. Melmon et al., p. 942.

74: "The stepped-care approach does have one important attribute . . ." R. E. Rakel, p. 291.

74: "The thrust of this book is to reemphasize . . ." K. L. Melmon et al., pp. 942–43.

Chapter 6. Antidepressants

81: "Treatment should be initiated with very low dosages . . ." R. B. Lydiard and J. C. Ballenger, p. 164.

84: "With antidepressants, this variability can be enormous, up to 40-fold . . ." S. Dawling, pp. 56–61. D. J. Greenblatt, pp. 8–13. R. McCue, pp. 323–34. S. Preskorn, 1993, pp. 14–34. M. Rudorfer, pp. 50–54. U. Tacke et al., pp. 262–67.

84: "Treating all patients with standard dosing regimens can result in either undermedication or toxicity for many." M. Rudorfer, p. 54.

85: "Dosage is an art form . . ." Dr. Edmund Settle, as quoted in K. J. Bender, p. 2.

85: "But most guidelines fail to mention . . ." J. W. Cain, pp. 272–77. A. K. Louie, pp. 435–38. A. F. Schatzberg, pp. 14–20. F. Schneier et al., pp. 119–21.

86: "It's [dysthymic disorder], the most common form of medical depression . . ." D. L. Dunner, pp. 48–58.

86: "The problem was underscored in a 1988 study comparing Zoloft and Elavil . . ." F. W. Reimherr et al., pp. 200–205.

87: "the lowest effective antidepressant dose for a given individual . . ." S. L. McElroy et al., p. 50.

87: "For example, in a 1996 study, 58% of patients . . ." A. N. Bhandary et al., pp. 59–63.

87: "A 1997 report from the respected *Medical Letter on Drugs and Therapeutics* . . ." Drugs for psychiatric disorders, p. 34.

88: "A 1997 study has shown that when based on spontaneous reports . . ." Dutch study attempts to qualify sexual dysfunction profiles among SSRIs, p. 22.

89: "Dr. Alan J. Cohen reported . . ." E. L. Goldman, p. 5.

94: "This is why 1 million prescriptions for Prozac . . ." S. LaFee, p. C-3.

94: "Released for general usage in the United States in 1988 . . ." 1990 PDR.

95: "Of the 27 patients with both depression and panic disorder . . ." A. K. Louie et al., p. 437.

95: "Today, 20 mg a day remains the manufacturer-recommended initial Prozac dose . . ." 1997 PDR, p. 939.

96: "Nor do the manufacturer's dosage guidelines . . ." 1997 PDR, p. 937.

96: "When adverse reactions developed . . ." A. K. Louie et al., p. 436.

97: "From 1988 through 1995, while tens of millions . . ." 1990–1995 PDR.

97: "Meanwhile, studies began to reveal rates as high as 34% . . ." F. M. Jacobsen, pp. 119–22.

97: "Finally, in the 1996 PDR . . ." 1996 PDR.

99: "Typical is a case study in the renowned British journal *The Lancet* . . ." C. G. Fichter et al., pp. 520–21.

99: "A 1992 journal article recommended starting Prozac . . ." J. W. Stewart et al., pp. 23–36.

99: "The results of three dose-effect studies . . ." A. J. Wood, p. 1355.

100: "No lower limit for an effective dose . . ." J. Wernicke et al., pp. 186–87.

101: "Another article addressing lower, safer dosages . . ." A. C. Altamura et al., pp. 109–12.

101: "The 5 mg dose appears to have been effective in the treatment of depression . . ." A. C. Altamura et al., p. 111.

102: "Having noticed that patients responded . . ." S. M. Wolfe, p. 3.

104: "And, if Prozac isn't already popular enough . . ." M. Anchors, p. 1270.

105: "Soon after Prozac's release, a 1988 study . . ." J. Feighner et al., pp. 105–108.

105: "Some drug references recommend starting all elderly . . ." S. M. Wolfe and R. E. Hope, p. 235.

105: "At present, fluoxetine [Prozac] is available in the United States only as a 20-mg capsule . . ." C. Salzman, p. 41.

106: "Indeed, the February 1995 *Journal of Clinical Psychiatry* . . ." M. Fava et al., pp. 52–55.

107: "Many consultants to *The Medical Letter* . . ." S. M. Wolfe and R. E. Hope, p. 235.

107: "The dangers of Prozac accumulation were underscored . . ." J. W. Cain, pp. 272–77.

108: "Paxil is also used for conditions . . ." N. S. Kaye and C. Dancu, p. 1523. A. R. Lillywhite et al., pp. 551–54. A. L. Ringold, pp. 363–64. M. D. Waldinger et al., pp. 1377–79.

109: "The overall dropout rate in pre-release studies . . ." D. L. Dunner and G. C. Dunbar, 1992, p. 25.

110: "Although studies with Paxil and alcohol . . ." J. S. Kerr et al., pp. 101–108.

110: "In a study involving people with highly differing rates . . ." S. H. Sindrup et al., pp. 288–95.

110: "In the elderly group, maximum plasma paroxetine . . ." D. L. Dunner, p. 51.

112: "A good idea, but according to reports . . ." N. Sussman and G. Stimmel, p. 26.

113: "Indeed, in one study, the subjects were started . . ." E. W. Freeman et al., pp. 181–82.

113: "Two studies have shown that Serzone . . ." Nefazodone for depression, pp. 33–34. K. Rickels, pp. 802–805. R. Fontaine et al., pp. 234–41.

114: "effectiveness of Serzone in long-term use . . ." 1996 PDR, p. 772.

114: "For example, it has been shown that Serzone . . ." R. L. Elliott and S. D. Shillcutt, pp. 42–56.

116: "Before decreasing an otherwise effective dosage..."
M. D. Kline and S. Koppes, pp. 1521–22.

116: "In a study in which subjects were started..." D. P. Doogan, pp. 45–56.

117: "The stuttering was severe and involved virtually every word spoken." W. V. McCall, p. 316.

117: "A 28-year-old patient developed panic attacks..." S. H. Zinner, pp. 147–48.

117: "Reports and studies have suggested that in non-acute situations, waiting 2–4 weeks before increasing dosages may be preferable." M. D. Kline and S. Koppes, pp. 1521–22. S. Preskorn, 1994, pp. 13–19.

117: "In one study of severe depression..." D. P. Doogan and C. J. Langdon, pp. 95–100.

117: "Indeed, articles and anecdotal reports suggest..." S. Preskorn, 1994, pp. 13–19. S. H. Zinner, pp. 147–48.

120: "Articles and anecdotal reports suggest that lower doses [of Effexor] are useful..." S. L. McElroy et al., pp. 49–55. J. Mendels et al., pp. 169–74. S. Preskorn, 1995, pp. 12–21.

120: "According to my discussions with the manufacturer..." J. Mendels et al., pp. 169–74.

120: "A 1995 article described the complete cessation of panic episodes..." T. D. Geracioti, Jr., pp. 408–10.

121: "For example, in one study, 58% of subjects..." 1997 PDR, p. 2829.

123: "Also, studies before and after Wellbutrin's release..." R. L. Elliott et al., pp. 42–56. D. F. Kirksey and N. Harto-Truax, pp. 143–47. W. C. Stern et al., pp. 148–52.

123: "the wide variability among individuals and their capacity to metabolize and eliminate drugs...." 1994 PDR, p. 763.

123: "The PDR states that the variation seen..." 1997 PDR, p. 1178.

123: "A 1983 study found a 10-fold range of variation..." S. Preskorn, 1983, pp. 137–39.

123: "For years, anecdotal reports and a small study have suggested that Wellbutrin..." F. J. Ayd, p. 21.

124: "Wellbutrin [had] not been systematically evaluated in older patients." 1997 PDR, p. 1178.

125: "Luvox exhibits typical SSRI side effect tendencies..." 1997 PDR, page 2725.

125: "One journal article suggests . . ." W. K. Goodman et al., p. 32. D. Ginsburg, pp. 17–20.

126: "It [Desyrel] is also frequently prescribed . . ." M. J. Daamen and W. A. Brown, pp. 210–11. T. B. Pearlstein and A. B. Stone, pp. 332–35.

126: "Data from studies on trazodone . . ." A. F. Schatzberg et al., page 44S. G. Maletta et al., pp. 40–47.

127: "the more newly approved Anafranil . . ." 1995 PDR, pp. 598–99.

128: "Indeed, studies utilizing Anafranil . . ." R. G. Regalado, pp. 54–55. F. Rouillon, pp. 371–78.

128: "In one study with panic and agoraphobic subjects, 8 of 13 subjects . . ." S. Gloger et al., pp. 28–32.

128: "The literature contains a number of case reports of patients developing very high . . ." D. Roy and S. Dawling, p. 307.

133: "The manufacturer recommends that the 'dosage should be initiated at a low level and increased gradually.' " 1997 PDR, p. 1821.

95: Table 6.1. 1996 PDR, pp. 922–23.

101: Table 6.2. Adapted from J. F. Wernicke, p. 186.

102: New Possibilities, New Problems with Prozac. *Premenstrual Disorders (PMS)*: M. J. Daamen and W. A. Brown, p. 210. R. W. Pies, p. 348. *Prozac/Dilantin Toxicity*: U.S. Government Food and Drug Administration (FDA). *Prozac Risks During Pregnancy*: S. Duerksen, p. B–10.

109: Table 6.3. 1996 PDR, p. 2507.

Chapter 7. Anti-Anxiety and Anti-Panic Medications

145: "The benzodiazepines are often the drugs of choice . . ." *AMA Drug Evaluations, Annual 1994*, p. 229.

147: "Studies show that although the specific type of benzodiazepine has changed . . ." N. Sussman, pp. 44–50.

148: "Six different preparations of benzodiazepines . . ." Top 200 drugs of 1995, pp. 27–36.

148: "These drugs are safer to use . . ." D. V. Sheehan, Benzodiazepines in panic disorder and agoraphobia. *Journal of Affective Disorders*, 1987; 13:169–81.

149: "An estimated 1.6% of Americans are on long-term benzodiazepine therapy . . ." B. Jancin, How to break off a long-term relationship with a benzodiazepine. *Clinical Psychiatry News*, 1994, page 14. The author suggests these steps: treat the underlying condition with SSRI or tricyclic antidepressants, beta blockers, or other medications; or switch patient to long-acting from short-acting benzodiazepine and taper; avoid abrupt withdrawal.

149: "Indeed, studies have shown . . ." B. Jancin, p. 14.

150: "In an article in *Consumer Reports* . . ." Attributed to Dr. Stuart Yudofsky, in "High Anxiety," p. 21.

154: "In a 1990 study, 5 mg a day of Prozac . . ." F. Schneier et al., pp. 119–21.

160: "Studies show that these drugs can be very effective in the elderly . . ." G. Maletta et al., pp. 40–47.

163: "When used at high doses for long intervals . . . Xanax . . ." 1996 PDR, p. 2651.

163: "Even after relatively short-term use . . ." 1996 PDR, p. 2650.

177: "In one study Klonopin was effective in about 75% of the subjects . . ." J. Davidson et al., pp. 423–28. J. Davidson et al., 1991, pp. 16–20. N. Potts and J. Davidson, 1995, pp. 19–20.

177: "In a 1997 study of people with panic disorders, Klonopin . . ." J. Davidson, pp. 26–28.

Chapter 8. Sleep Medications

187: "In 1989, twenty million outpatient prescriptions . . ." D. K. Wysowski and C. Baum, pp. 1779–83.

188: "Almost 90% of people over age 60 . . ." R. F. Reynolds et al., pp. 9–12.

190: "Studies show that physicians often overprescribe . . ." D. Everitt and J. Avorn, pp. 357–62. D. I. Shorr and S. F. Bauwens, 1990, pp. 293–95. D. I. Shorr and S. F. Bauwens, 1992, pp. 78–82.

191: "Because of the finding of amnesia in two of our [7] subjects . . ." A. Kales et al., *Journal of Clinical Pharmacology*, 1976; p. 406.

192: "The new recommended adult dosage became 0.25 mg . . ." 1995 PDR, p. 2553.

194: "In our research we found that triazolam . . ." K. Adam and I. Oswald, *British Medical Journal*, 1993, p. 626.

194: "Considering the extent of use, reporting rates for triazolam [Halcion] . . ." D. K. Wysowski and D. Barash, *Archives of Internal Medicine*, 1991, p. 2003.

194: "The data reported herein show a . . ." D. K. Wysowski and D. Barash, *Archives of Internal Medicine*, 1991, p. 2006.

195: "Indeed, a 1993 study reported a rate of 44% . . ." M. Rathier and L. Korman, SA56.

195: "Upon discontinuing Halcion after prolonged usage withdrawal insomnia, according to *Conn's Current Therapy 1994*, 'is prompt and impressive.' " R. E. Rakel, p. 28.

195: "A 1995 report stated that Halcion's effects were enhanced . . ." S. M. Wolfe, March 1995, p. 10.

195: "That benzodiazepine hypnotics . . ." T. G. Dinan and B. E. Leonard, *British Medical Journal*, 1993, p. 1475.

195: "To ensure sleep during an overnight flight to Europe . . ." R. I. Shader and D. J. Greenblatt, *Journal of Clinical Psychopharmacology*, 1983, p. 273.

196: "Memory impairment and anterograde amnesia . . ." W. G. Clark et al., p. 269.

196: "We found that 30% of the prescriptions . . ." D. I. Shorr and S. F. Bauwens, *American Journal of Medicine*, 1992, p. 78.

196: "Use for more than 2–3 weeks requires reevaluation . . ." 1995 PDR, p. 2552.

197: "In one study, this dosage [0.25 mg Halcion] . . ." A. J. Bowen, pp. 337–42.

198: "When treatment is properly supervised . . ." M. B. Balter et al. The World Psychiatric Association Task Force on sedative hypnotics. *Eur-Psychiatry*, 1993, p. 45.

199: "Halcion's manufacturer recommends a dose of 0.125 mg . . ." 1997 PDR, p. 2095.

200: "One of the earliest and longest low-dose studies . . ." L. Merlotti et al., pp. 9–14.

200: "In conclusion, results of this study . . ." L. Merlotti et al., *Journal of Clinical Psychopharmacology*, 1989, p. 14.

200: "Not all studies demonstrated . . ." M. B. Scharf et al., 1990, p. 90.

200: "Efficacy, defined as significant difference from placebo . . ." G. Vogel et al., *Sleep Research*, 1988, p. 67.

200: "Ambien's package insert agrees . . ." 1996 PDR, p. 2416.

201: "It found 'remarkable similarity . . .' " J. M. Jonas et al., *Journal of Clinical Psychiatry*, 1992, p. 19.

201: "More recent reports have supported . . ." R. Cavallaro et al., pp. 374–75. L. M. Iruela et al., pp. 1495–96. M. Ansseau et al., p. 809.

201: "Indeed, a 1993 article comparing the side effects of Ambien and Halcion . . ." I. Berlin et al., pp. 100–106.

202: "While zolpidem [Ambien] . . ." R. W. Pies, *Journal of Clinical Psychiatry*, 1995, p. 35.

203: "The guidelines then state . . ." 1996 PDR, p. 2174.

204: "Flurazepam [Dalmane] 30 mg . . ." M. R. Salkind and T. Silverstone, *British Journal of Clinical Pharmacology*, 1975, pp. 223 and 225.

205: "The recommended usual adult dose is 30 mg before retiring. In some patients, 15 mg may be sufficient." 1993 PDR, p. 2119.

205: "While the recommended usual adult dose is 15 mg before retiring, 7.5 mg may be sufficient for some patients, and others may need 30 mg." 1994 PDR, p. 2070.

206: "Studies have further supported this fact." T. Roehrs et al., pp. 859–62. T. Roth et al., p. 123. Consensus conference, pp. 2410–14.

192: *1983:* 1983 PDR, pp. 2051.

1986: 1986 PDR, p. 1844.

1988: 1988 PDR, p. 2128.

Chapter 9. Smoking Cessation: Zyban (Bupropion)

209: "There is a chance that . . ." Zyban Product Information, 1997.

210: "The manufacturer's letter highlights a chart . . ." Zyban letter to physicians, August 1997.

211: "Another study cited in the Zyban package..." Zyban Product Information, 1997.

211: The results of this study at 52 weeks..." Correspondence, GlaxoWellcome, August 27, 1997.

211: "According to a 1996 report in the *American Journal of Psychiatry*..." H. I. Lief, p. 442.

211: Table 9.1. Zyban Product Information, 1997. Correspondence, GlaxoWellcome, August 27, 1997.

213: Zyban Product Information, 1997. Wellbutrin, 1997 PDR, p. 1179.

Chapter 10. Medications for Ulcers, Esophagitis, and Heartburn

225: "Tagamet, because of its effect on liver enzymes..." *Drug Facts and Comparisons*, 1993, p. 1609.

228: "Helicobacter can survive in dental plaque..." H. G. Desai et al., pp. 1205–8. K. Khandaker et al., p. 751. A. M. Nguyen et al., pp. 783–87.

231: "Smaller doses have been shown..." Glaxo Pharmaceuticals, Zantac Product Information, June 1993, p. 2. 1996 PDR, p. 1211.

231: "*Drug Facts and Comparisons*..." *Drug Facts and Comparisons*, 1993, p. 1609.

232: "Research, however, demonstrates..." American Society of Hospital Pharmacists, p. 1945.

232: "Thus, although Zantac..." E. W. Campion et al., pp. 945–47.

232: "If you are over 60..." S. M. Wolfe and R. E. Hope, p. 371.

234: "Lower doses, such as 100 mg h.s. [at bedtime]..." 1996 PDR, p. 1428.

237: "For example, a 1988 study..." S. Fiorucci et al., 1988, p. 1375.

240: "If you are over 60..." S. M. Wolfe and R. E. Hope, p. 369.

243: "The average reduction in omeprazole [Prilosec] clearance..." S. Landahl et al., p. 475.

243: "Another study examined several Prilosec dosages..." T. Lind et al., pp. 557–60.

Chapter 11. Cholesterol-Lowering Medications

250: "The first statin was Mevacor . . ." Top 200 drugs of 1995, pp. 27–36.

250: "In 1996, Zocor claimed the No. 21 position . . ." B. Buckley, pp. 27–45.

250: "Treatment alone costs more than $100 billion . . ." E. R. Gonzalez, p. 65.

250: "Patients with documented coronary heart disease . . ." E. R. Gonzalez, p. 65.

251: "A lot has been accomplished in a relatively short time . . ." J. I. Cleeman, pp. 1–7.

251: "In the group of 35- to 44-year-olds . . ." A. M. Gotto, pp. 1–7.

255: "The underused miracle drugs . . ." W. C. Roberts, p. 377.

255: "Mills's concern . . ." *Medical Letter on Drugs and Therapeutics*, page 67.

258: "Studies vary, but in one study 21% to 33% of patients . . ." B. Jacotot et al., pp. 257–63.

258: "Some physicians may consider this a waste of time . . ." D. L. Sprecher et al., pp. 537–43.

259: "In one study cholestyramine was used at a dose . . ." D. L. Sprecher et al., pp. 537–43.

259: "The authors commented: 'We have shown . . .' " D. L. Sprecher et al., pp. 537–43.

260: "Yet only one in four people who require treatment . . ." A. M. Gotto, pp. 377–88.

260: "According to a 1995 study, 'For every 10 percentage points . . .' " A. L. Gould et al., p. 2274.

262: "Mevacor, like other statin drugs . . ." C. D. Furberg et al., pp. 1679–87. D. Waters et al., pp. 2404–10.

262: "Up to 1995, this was the recommended starting dosage . . ." 1995 PDR, p. 1588.

262: "In the 1996 and 1997 PDRs . . ." 1997 PDR, p. 1746.

263: "A 1994 study published in the *Journal of the American Medical Association* . . ." M. Arca et al., pp. 453–59.

263: "A 1990 study showed its effectiveness in cardiac transplant patients." J. A. Kobashigawa et al., pp. IV281–83.

263: "The most impressive low-dose Mevacor study . . ." Rubenstein et al., pp. 1123–26.

263: "Achievement of desirable values of cholesterol . . ." Rubenstein et al., p. 1123.

265: "The highly respected *American Hospital Formulary Service* . . ." American Society of Hospital Pharmacists, 1996, p. 1260.

267: "Pravachol is an effective cholesterol- and LDL-C lowering drug . . ." B. Buckley, pp. 27–45.

267: "Multiple studies involving thousands of patients . . ." J. Shepherd et al., 1301–7. F. M. Sacks, pp. 1001–9. J. R. Crouse 3rd, pp. 455–59. M. Haria and D. McTavish, pp. 299–336. J. W. Jukema, pp. 2528–40.

267: "The manufacturer-recommended initial dose of Pravachol . . ." 1997 PDR, p. 774.

268: "A 6-fold range of interindividual variation . . ." 1997 PDR, p. 771.

268: "In a study published in *Cardiology* in 1994 . . ." E. Steinhagen-Thiessen, pp. 244–54.

268: "In another 1994 study of over 1,000 patients . . ." H. Sinzinger and C. Pirich, abstract.

268: "A 1991 study published in *Clinical Cardiology* . . ." P. H. Jones et al., pp. 146–51.

268: "More surprising, 'the 5 mg dose at bedtime . . .' " P. H. Jones et al., p. 150.

270: "The *American Hospital Formulary Service* drug reference . . ." American Society of Hospital Pharmacists, 1996, p. 1264.

271: "Multiple studies have confirmed that Zocor . . ."

271: "The manufacturer-recommended initial dose of Zocor . . ." 1997 PDR, p. 1825.

271: "Interestingly, although the 1997 PDR recommends Zocor . . ." 1997 PDR, p. 1822.

272: "Supporting these findings is a 1989 study in *Clinical Therapeutics* . . ." K. Saku et al., pp. 247–57.

272: "In one study, 11% of subjects . . ." J. Tuomilehto et al., pp. 941–9.

273: "In a 1990 study, elderly subjects . . ." J. F. Walker et al., pp. 53–56.

275: "However, two preliminary studies suggest that Lescol . . ." J. Herd et al., p. 222A. J. Herd et al., findings presented at American Heart Association Annual Meeting, New Orleans,

November 13, 1996, information on file, Sandoz Pharmaceutical Corporation.

275: "The 1996 *American Hospital Formulary Service* drug reference states . . ." American Society of Hospital Pharmacists, 1996, p. 1247.

276: "For example, in one study, 37% of subjects . . ." D. L. Sprecher et al., pp. 537–43.

276: "In another, 21% of subjects taking only *2.5 mg a day* . . ." B. Jacotot et al., pp. 257–63.

276: "For example, people with reduced liver function . . ." L. A. Jokubaitis, pp. 11–15.

277: "However, it also states: 'Elderly patients . . .' " Lescol Package Insert, November 1996.

252: Desirable and At-Risk Levels of LDL-C and Total Cholesterol. S. Grundy et al., p. 2330.

Chapter 12. Antihypertensive Medications

280: "The selected [antihypertensive] . . ." R. E. Rakel, *Conn's Current Therapy 1993*, p. 292.

280: "A 35-year-old man . . ." R. E. Rakel, *Conn's Current Therapy 1993*, p. 280.

282: "Blacks have a higher prevalence . . ." B. Sabella, p. 11.

285: "Reducing sodium intake . . ." M. R. Langenfeld and R. E. Schmieder, pp. 909–16.

286: "A 1997 study has shown . . ." P. K. Whelton et al., pp. 1624–32.

286: "The fact is that most of our patients . . ." Albert Einstein College of Medicine, Office of Continuing Medication. *Hypertension Management Today*, 1996, p. 4.

287: "A 1996 monograph from the Albert Einstein College of Medicine . . ." Albert Einstein College of Medicine, Office of Continuing Medication. *Hypertension Management Today*, 1996, p. 4.

289: "For the management of hypertension . . ." American Society of Hospital Pharmacists, 1996, p. 1900.

291: "The 1995 Joint National Committee . . ." E. D. Frohlich, pp. S48–52.

291: "A 1997 study found that thiazide diuretics . . ." J. S. Gottdiener et al., p. 2007–14.

291: "Tailored therapy is the preferred approach . . ." N. Curzen and H. Purcell, p. 154.

295: "The message should come loud and clear . . ." E. D. Frohlich, p. S51.

296: "The PDR descriptions for Esidrix . . ." 1997 PDR, p. 840 (Esidrix), p. 1719 (HydroDIURIL), p. 452 (Oretic).

299: "Indeed, the *AMA Drug Evaluations Annual 1994* . . ." American Medical Association, p. 593.

303: "A 1995 study found that people with hypertension . . ." B. M. Psaty et al., pp. 620–25.

303: "Studies published in 1990 and 1992 . . ." M. Pahor et al., pp. 493–97. M. Pahor et al., pp. 1061–65.

303: "For now, perhaps the best approach . . ." Safety of calcium-channel blockers, pp. 13–14.

306: "One drug reference cited a study . . ." R. E. Rakel, 1995, p. 274.

306: "Indeed, the manufacturer of Hytrin emphasizes . . ." 1997 PDR, p. 437.

Chapter 13. Aspirin (Acetylsalicylic Acid) and Tylenol (Acetaminophen)

313: "There are both theoretical and practical reasons . . ." J. Hirsh et al., p. 329S.

315: "According to a physician quoted in a 1997 issue of *Newsweek* . . ." S. Begley, p. 66.

315: "According to one journal article . . ." Hirsh et al., p. 330S.

315: "Using lower doses helps . . ." R. Stalnikowicz-Darvasi, pp. 13–16.

316: "Thus, the *AMA Drug Evaluations Annual 1995* warns . . ." American Medical Association, p. 752.

316: "As one leading drug reference put it . . ." K. L. Melmon et al., p. 500.

318: "According to the May 1994 *FDA Medical Bulletin* . . ." U.S. Government Food and Drug Administration (FDA), p. 8.

318: "Multiple studies have shown..." C. A. Silagy et al., pp. 84–89.

321: "Drugs such as aspirin, acetaminophen..." S. A. Cooper, 1984, p. 70.

321: "Tylenol and its generic, acetaminophen..." American Medical Association, 1995.

Chapter 14. Anti-Inflammatory Drugs

325: "Dosage of [all anti-inflammatory drugs]..." American Society of Hospital Pharmacists, 1994, p. 1159.

325: "Members include ibuprofen..." Top 200 drugs of 1995, pp. 27–36.

325: "More than 100 million prescriptions..." T. Mahmud, pp. 211–13.

328: "The incidence of side effects with anti-inflammatory medications..." *Meyler's Side Effects of Drugs*, E. Z. Dajani, 1996, pp. 835–36.

328: "Most side effects are gastrointestinal..." A. G. Gilman et al., p. 643.

328: "Gastrointestinal problems occur three times as often..." S. E. Gabriel et al., pp. 787–96. R. L. Savage, pp. 84–90. C. J. Shorrock and M. J. Langman, p. 3.

328: "The risk of hospitalization for gastrointestinal problems..." M. J. Langman et al., pp. 1075–78.

328: "A 1992 study of arthritis patients..." M. J. Parnham, pp. 37–39.

328: "A 1994 study produced similar findings..." A. S. Taha et al., 1994, pp. 891–95.

328: "A 1996 study agreed..." G. Singh et al., p. 1530.

328: "The onset of bleeding..." K. L. Melmon, p. 492.

328: "Indeed, the AMA states that..." *AMA Drug Evaluations Annual 1994*, page 115.

329: "A 1996 journal reported three cases of infertility..." M. Akil et al., pp. 76–78.

330: "In over 90% of studies..." E. Z. Dajani, 1996, 835–36.

330: "This includes the people who take aspirin daily..." R. Stalnikowicz-Darvasi, pp. 13–16.

332: "Studies, most of them involving dental surgery..." S. A.

Cooper et al., 1982, pp. 162–67. V. Minotti et al., pp. 177–83. H. J. McQuay et al., pp. 672–77. J. K. Petersen et al., pp. 637–40. H. Quiding et al., pp. 303–7.

332: "The evidence, although not conclusive . . ." P. S. Aisen, p. 83. W. F. Stewart, pp. 626–32.

334: "A 1996 article in the *American Journal of Orthopedics* . . ." R. W. Moskowitz, p. 4.

334: "Overall, many authorities agree that aspirin and Feldene . . ." D. Henry et al., pp. 1078–88.

334: "and perhaps Orudis." C. J. Grossman, pp. 253–57.

335: "However, a recent study found that sudden gastric bleeding . . ." G. Singh et al., pp. 1530–36.

335: "The reduced blood flow appears to be caused . . ." J. L. Wallace, pp. 98–102.

335: "Interestingly, animal studies utilizing cardiac drugs . . ." M. D. Barrachina et al., pp. R3–4. S. N. Elliott et al., pp. 524–30.

335: "Research is under way to synthesize NSAIDs . . ." G. Cirino et al., pp. 73–81. J. L. Wallace et al., pp. 249–55.

337: "The AMA agrees . . ." *AMA Drug Evaluations Annual 1994*, p. 115.

339: "It is estimated that between 25% and 40% . . ." A. S. Taha and R. I. Russell, pp. 580–83.

339: "the recommended strategy for initiating therapy . . ." 1997 PDR, p. 834.

342: "For example, the pain-relieving effect of 200 to 400 mg of Lodine . . ." 1995 PDR, pp. 2682–83.

342: "Large variations are possible in the response of individuals . . ." A. G. Gilman et al., p. 643.

345: "Patients over the age of 65 comprise about 12% . . ." A. J. Mazanec, p. 41.

345: "This is why some authorities recommend short-acting NSAIDs . . ." *United States Pharmacopeia, Drug Information (USP DI)*, p. 361.

351: "According to the manufacturer, Voltaren was the No. 1 . . ." Ciba-Geigy Corporation, July 1994.

352: "Diclofenac [Voltaren], like other NSAIDs . . ." 1997 PDR, p. 834.

353: "The results document the positive influence that B-vitamins contribute . . ." A. Kuhlwein et al., abstract.

356: "Doses of 25 mg were superior to placebo." 1997 PDR, p. 2875.

362: "Several studies have shown Lodine . . ." D. E. Griswold and J. L. Adams, pp. 181–206.

364: "Naprelan, like other NSAIDs . . ." 1997 PDR, p. 2862.

366: "The investigators concluded that diclofenac [Cataflam] . . ." T. G. Kantor, p. 66.

367: "Most studies show Clinoril . . ." J. L. Carson et al., pp. 1054–59.

368: "While banning Feldene has been hotly debated . . ." R. L. Savage et al., pp. 84–90.

370: "Diarrhea seems to be a problem for some taking Meclomen . . ." *AMA Drug Evaluations Annual 1994*, p. 1826.

373: "Many physicians tell me that the rate is far higher . . ." *Conn's Current Therapy 1994*, p. 949.

374: "Intermediary doses such as 200 mcg two or three times a day . . ." J. B. Raskin et al., pp. 344–50. I. Grazioli et al., pp. 289–94. W. W. Downie, pp. 1–6. J. Naves et al., p. 203.

374: "Indeed, in clinical studies doses as low as 25 mcg of Cytotec . . ." M. M. Cohen et al., pp. 605–11. E. Z. Dajani and C. H. Nissen, pp. 194S–200S.

374: "Similar protection was afforded by 50 mcg of Cytotec . . ." F. E. Silverstein et al., pp. 32–36. F. L. Lanza et al., pp. 633–36. G. C. Jiranek et al., pp. 656–61.

Chapter 15. Notes on Narcotic Pain Medications

379: "Narcotic pain relievers are frequently prescribed . . ." Top 200 drugs of 1995, pp. 27–36.

380: "Large doses [of narcotic pain medications] may be necessary . . ." Medical Board of California, page 4.

Chapter 16. Antihistamines

386: "The sixth most prevalent cause of chronic disease in the United States." University of Wisconsin Medical School, 1997, p. 1.

388: "Their [first-generation antihistamines] overall side effect rate . . ." M. N. Dukes, p. 98.

390: "Cases and fatalities continue to be reported to the FDA . . ." R. L. Woolsey et al., p. 1532.

391: "It is possible that those 1% to 2% with the lowest enzyme activity . . ." R. L. Woolsey et al., p. 1535.

393: "Thereby avoid this serious and potentially deadly complication." R. L. Woolsey et al., p. 1535.

393: "Serious cardiac effects also have been reported . . ." American Society of Hospital Pharmacists, 1993, p. 28.

393: "One tablet (60 mg) twice daily for adults and children 12 years and older." 1996 PDR, p. 1538.

395: "The data indicate that daily dosages of 60 mg . . ." M. L. Brandon and M. Weiner, pp. 74–75.

395: "Two years later, the same authors published another article . . ." M. L. Brandon and M. Weiner, pp. 1204–5.

395: "None of the terfenadine [Seldane] dosage schedules . . ." M. L. Brandon and M. Weiner, p. 1204.

396: "Apparently, the minimum effective dose which allowed . . ." Marion Merrill Dow, letter, November 6, 1993, p. 2.

397: "Indeed, a study published in 1977 suggested that 40 mg . . ." K. J. Huther et al., pp. 195–99.

398: "A 1992 study of healthy elderly and younger adults . . ." M. G. Eller et al., pp. 267–71.

398: "In contrast, a 1990 study found that 5 of 8 healthy elderly females . . ." K. J. Simons et al., pp. 540–47.

398: "Old age may also be a factor . . ." R. L. Woolsey et al., p. 1536.

400: "Dosage restriction [of Seldane is] . . ." R. L. Woolsey et al., p. 1532.

401: "in pre-release studies . . ." 1996 PDR, p. 2349.

401: "According to the 1997 PDR Supplement A . . ." 1997 PDR Supplement A, p. A288.

403: "In another study, the authors concluded . . ." C. J. Falliers et al., p. 257.

403: "Several measures of Zyrtec in blood levels . . ." 1997 PDR, p. 2054.

404: "In the elderly, the manufacturer notes that Zyrtec clearance . . ." 1997 PDR, p. 2054.

405: "Doses of 20 and 40 mg reduced allergic reactions..."
Hoechst Marion Roussel, 1996.

405: "In one study comparing doses of 40, 60, and 120 mg a
day ..." D. Tinkelman et al., p. 257.

407: "Benadryl's dosage recommendations also come with a
warning ..." 1996 PDR, p. 1899.

394: Table 16.1 Adapted from M. L. Brandon and M. Weiner,
1980, p. 73; and M. L. Brandon and M. Weiner, 1982, p. 1205.

Chapter 17. Motion Sickness Medications

412: "Among the antihistamines, the *AMA Drug Evaluations Annual 1994 ...*" American Medical Association, 1994.

414: "In one study exposing subjects to rough seas ..." L. G.
Schmitt and J. E. Shaw, pp. 258–62.

414: "The manufacturer recommends placing ..." 1995 PDR.

414: "However, one study suggested that placement ..." S. P.
Clissold and R. C. Heel, pp. 189–207.

416: "Some authorities believe ..." American Society of Hospital Pharmacists, 1994.

417: "Meant as a twenty-four-hour medication ..." American
Society of Hospital Pharmacists, 1994.

419: "Considerable interindividual variation may be seen ..."
1997 PDR, p. 2882.

Chapter 18. Other Medications

424: "In 1995, five antibiotics ranked within ..." Top 200 drugs
of 1995, pp. 27–36.

424: "In 1996, seven antibiotics ranked within ..." B. Buckley,
pp. 30, 45.

424: "For example, with Zithromax, the PDR tells us ..." 1997
PDR, supplement A, p. A255.

424: "Also, a 1993 study found ..." T. Mazzei et al., p. 57.

424: "While the manufacturer makes no specific recommendations ..." American Society of Hospital Pharmacists, 1996,
p. 231.

427: "In the March 1997 issue of the *Journal of Urology*..." M. D. Melekos et al., pp. 935–39.

431: "Among the standard treatments for fungal nails listed..." R. E. Rakel, p. 722.

431: "According to *Conn's Current Therapy 1995*..." R. E. Rakel, p. 722.

433: "A 1997 article in the *Journal of the American College of Cardiology*..." M. L. Slatton et al., p. 1206.

434: "In a 1994 article in *Clinical Psychiatry News*, it stated... Minidoses may give optimal neuroleptic results," p. 15.

434: "A report given by Dr. Robert Zipursky..." C. Sherman, pp. 1–2.

435: "Several studies have demonstrated that Asian patients..." K. M. Lin et al. 1988, pp. 195–201. K. M. Lin et al., 1989, pp. 1307–11.

436: "The manufacturer-recommended dosage of oral Zofran..." 1997 PDR, p. 1233.

437: "In these studies, 4 mg three times a day..." T. M. Beck, pp. 15–20. T. M. Beck et al., pp. 407–13. L. X. Cubeddu et al., 1990, pp. 810–6. L. X. Cubeddu et al., 1994, pp. 137–46.

437: "Indeed, in the 1995 PDR..." 1995 PDR, p. 862.

Chapter 19. Slow Responses to Serious Side Effects: The Coumadin Story

442: "In 1996, Coumadin ranked No. 10..." B. Buckley, pp. 27–45.

442: "They hemorrhage, as the PDR states..." 1994 PDR, p. 895.

444: "'As a result,' a 1989 article stated..." J. Hirsh et al. *Chest*, 1989, p. 7S.

444: "This change in responsiveness of thromboplastins..." J. Hirsh et al. *Chest*, 1989, p. 5S.

445: "The more than half a million Americans..." M. H. Eckman et al. *New England Journal of Medicine*, 1993, p. 696.

446: "Finally, in 1982 a study appeared in the *New England Jour-*

nal of Medicine . . .'' R. Hull et al. *New England Journal of Medicine*, 1982, 1676–81.

447: ''If the therapeutic ratio . . .'' J. Hirsh, D. Deykin, L. Poller, *Chest*, 1986, p. 11S.

447: ''In the wake of these developments, in 1984 the Committee . . .'' J. Hirsh, *Chest*, ACCP-NHLBI National Conference on Antithrombotic Therapy, 1986, 11s–15s.

448: ''Again it suggested . . .'' J. Hirsh and M. Levine. *Thrombosis and Haemostasis*, 1988, pp. 129–132.

448: ''For reasons that are difficult to explain . . .'' J. Hirsh, Oral Anticoagulant Drugs. *Drug Therapy*, 1991, p. 1869.

449: ''The present system . . .'' J. Hirsh, Oral Anticoagulant Drugs. *Drug Therapy*, 1991, pp. 1869.

449: In 1993, an article entitled . . . '' M. H. Eckman et al., p. 696.

449: ''This means that although two laboratories . . .'' M. H. Eckman et al. *New England Journal of Medicine*, 1993, p. 696.

449: ''*AMA Drug Evaluations Annual 1994*:'' Page 741.

Chapter 20. Solutions

455: ''The effectiveness of Effexor in long-term use . . .'' 1997 PDR, p. 2826.

456: ''Often, a commercial sponsor does not want . . .'' C. Peck, p. 117.

457: ''A thyroid hormone medication taken by millions . . .'' C. Clark, page B-3.

459: ''A 1990 journal article cited this problem . . .'' M. E. Kitler, pp. 236–37.

469: ''FDA's Tips for Taking Medicines . . .'' Food and Drug Administration, Department of Health and Human Services, pp. 1–6.

470: ''There was a lot of debate among the doctors . . .'' J. Mac-Donald, page A-10.

472: ''Clinical trials by physician-scientists . . .'' K. L. Melmon et al., page 942.

472: ''Traditionally, doctors have told . . .'' C. F. George, p. 1328.

475: ''Therapy as a science . . .'' A. G. Gilman et al., p. 65.

481: "As physicians feel under pressure . . ." G. Kolata, p. A-20.

483: *"Don't take over-the-counter painkillers like candy, experts warn . . ."* A. Gathright, p. A-18.

486: "Studies show that in regard to medications . . ." R. P. Ferguson et al., pp. 56–62.

Bibliography

General References

The following references have been used extensively. Rather than listing them in nearly every chapter, they are listed here. *JAMA* stands for the *Journal of the American Medical Association*.

American Medical Association. *AMA Drug Evaluations, Annual 1993, 1994, 1995, and 1996*. Chicago: American Medical Association, 1993–1996 editions.

American Society of Hospital Pharmacists. *American Hospital Formulary Service, Drug Information 1993, 1994, 1995, and 1996*. Gerald K. McEvoy, Editor. Bethesda, MD: 1993–1996.

Buckley, B. Top 200 drugs of 1996. *Pharmacy Times*, April 1997; 63(4):27–45.

Clark, W. G., D. C. Brater, and A. R. Johnson. *Goth's Medical Pharmacology*, 13th ed. St. Louis: C. V. Mosby, 1992.

Drug Facts and Comparisons. Facts and Comparisons, a Wolters Kluwer Company, St. Louis, 1993–1997.

Gilman, A. G., T. W. Rall, A. S. Nies, and P. Taylor. *Goodman and Gilman's The Pharmacological Basis of Therapeutics*. New York: Pergamon Press, 1990 and 1996.

Melmon, K. L., H. F. Morrelli, B. B. Hoffman, and D. W. Nierenberg. *Melmon and Morrelli's Clinical Pharmacology: Basic Principles in Therapeutics*, 3rd ed. New York: McGraw-Hill, 1993.

Physicians' Desk Reference, 47–51th eds. Montvale, N.J.: Medical
Economics Company, 1993–1997.

*Physicians GenRx: The Complete Drug Reference, 1994, 1995,
1996, and 1997*. Riverside, CT: Denniston Publishing, 1994–
1997.

Rakel, R. E. *Conn's Current Therapy 1993–1996*. Philadelphia:
W. B. Saunders Company, 1993–1996.

Silverman, H. M. *The Pill Book: The Illustrated Guide to the Most
Prescribed Drugs in the United States*, 7th rev. ed. New York:
Bantam Books, 1996.

Simonsen, L. Top 200 drugs of 1991, 1992, 1993, 1994. *Pharmacy Times*, April 1992, 1993, 1994, 1995, respectively.

Top 200 drugs of 1995. *Pharmacy Times*, April 1995, 27–36.

*United States Pharmacopeia, Drug Information (USP DI): Drug
Information for the Health Care Professional*. Taunton, MA:
Rand McNally, 1994.

Chapter 1. Side Effects—Why They Occur and How to Prevent Them

Callahan, A. M. The role of pharmacokinetics in optimizing drug
therapy. *Primary Psychiatry*, 1997; 4(7):31–4.

Cohen, J. S., and P. A. Insel, The *Physicians' Desk Reference*:
problems and possible improvements. *Archives of Internal Medicine*, 1996; 156:1375–80.

Connelly, D. P., E. C. Rich, S. P. Curley, and J. T. Kelly. Knowledge resource preferences of family physicians. *Journal of Family Practice,* 1990; 30(3) :353–59.

Dawling, S. Monitoring of tricyclic antidepressant therapy. *Clinical Biochemistry,* 1982, 15(1):56–61.

Ely, J. W., R. J. Burch, and D. C. Vinson. The information needs of family physicians: case-specific clinical questions. *Journal of Family Practice,* 1992; 35(3):265–69.

Faich, G. A. Adverse-drug-reaction reporting. *New England Journal of Medicine,* 1986; 14:1589.

Gilman, A. G., T. W. Rall, A. S. Nies, and P. Taylor. *Goodman and Gilman's The Pharmacological Basis of Therapeutics.* New York: Pergamon Press, 1990.

Griffin, J. P. and J. C. Weber. Voluntary systems of adverse reaction reporting—Part I. *Adverse Drug Reactions and Acute Poisoning Reviews,* 1985; 4(4):213–30.

Griffin, J. P. and J. C. Weber. Voluntary systems of adverse reaction reporting—Part II. *Adverse Drug Reactions and Acute Poisoning Reviews,* 1986; 5(1):23–55.

Guyatt, G., et al. Determining optimal therapy—randomized trials in individual patients. *New England Journal of Medicine,* 1986; 314(14):889–92.

Hsu, P., and A. R. Laddu. Analysis of adverse effects in a dose titration study. *Journal of Clinical Psychiatry,* 1994; 34:136–41.

Kahn, K. L. Above all, "do no harm." How shall we avoid errors in medicine? *JAMA,* 1995; 274(1):75–76.

Karch, F. E., and L. Lasagna. Toward the operational identification of adverse drug reactions. *Clinical Pharmacology and Therapeutics,* 1977; 21(3):247–54.

Leape, L. L., et al. Systems analysis of adverse drug events. ADE Prevention Study Group. *JAMA*, 1995; 274(1):35–43.

Martin, E. W. *Hazards of Medication: A Manual on Drug Interactions, Contraindications, and Adverse Reactions with Other Prescribing and Drug Information*, 2nd ed. Philadelphia: J. B. Lippincott Company, 1978.

Mullen, W. H., I. B. Anderson, S. Y. Kim, P. D. Blanc, and K. R. Olson. Incorrect overdose management advice in the *Physicians' Desk Reference. Annals of Emergency Medicine*, 1997; 29(2):255–61.

Peck, C., et al. Opportunities for integrating of pharmacokinetics, pharmacodynamics, and toxicokinetics in rational drug development. *Journal of Clinical Pharmacology*, 1994; 34:111–19.

Personal communication. Medical Economics Data Production Company (publishers of the PDR), September 12, 1994.

Price, P. L. A prescription for a prescription: the treatment of adverse drug reactions. *South Dakota Journal of Medicine*, 1994; 47(4):133–34.

Ross, D. and R. Bukata. Optimizing prescribing practices, Part 2. *Emergency Medicine and Acute Care Essays*, January 1993; 17(1):1–5.

Rowland, M., L. Sheiner, and J. Steimer. *Variability in Drug Therapy: Description, Estimation, and Control*. A Sandoz Workshop. New York: Raven Press, 1985.

Sheehan, D. V., and K. Hartnett-Sheehan. The role of SSRIs in panic disorder. *Journal of Clinical Psychiatry*, 1996; 517(10 suppl):51–58.

Slatton, M. L., et al. Does digoxin provide additional hemodynamic and autonomic benefit at higher doses in patients with mild to moderate heart failure and normal sinus rhythm? *Journal of the American College of Cardiology*, 1997; 29(6):1206–13.

Steel, K., P. M. Gertman, C. Crescenzi, and J. Anderson. Iatrogenic illness on a general medical service at a university hospital. *New England Journal of Medicine*, 1981 Mar 12, 304(11):638–42.

Sussman, N., and G. Stimmel. New dosing strategies for psychotropic drugs. *Primary Psychiatry*, 1997; 4(7):24–30.

Wernicke, J. F., et al. Low-dose fluoxetine therapy for depression. *Psychopharmacology Bulletin*, 1988; 24(1):183–188.

Chapter 2. The Scope of the Side Effect Problem

American Medical Association. *AMA Drug Evaluations, Annual 1993.* Chicago: American Medical Association, 1993.

Bates, D. W. et al. Incidence of adverse drug events and potential adverse drug events. Implications for prevention. ADE Prevention Study Group. *JAMA*, 1995; 274(1):29–34.

Clark, C. UCSD study says thyroid remedy weakens bones. *San Diego Union-Tribune*, April 27, 1994, B-3.

Cohen, J. S. Dosage titration issues [letter]. *Journal of Clinical Psychiatry*, 1996; 57(1):43.

Cohen, J. S., and P. A. Insel. The *Physicians' Desk Reference*: problems and possible improvements. *Archives of Internal Medicine*, 1996; 156:1375–80.

Dutch study attempts to qualify sexual dysfunction profiles among SSRIs. *Primary Psychiatry*, 1997; 4(7):22–23.

Faich, G. A., D. Knapp, M. Dreis, and W. Turner. National adverse drug reaction surveillance: 1985. *JAMA*, 1987; 257(15): 2068.

Fort Lauderdale Sun-Sentinel. Prescription drugs can be a problem. *San Diego Union-Tribune*, October 3, 1995, page A-6.

George, C. F. Adverse drug reactions and secrecy: knowledge is power; doctors should cede some of both to their patients. *British Medical Journal*, 1992; 304:1328.

Gibian, T. Rational drug therapy in the elderly, or how not to poison your elderly patients. *Australian Family Physician*, 1992; 21(12):1755–60.

Griffin, J. P., and J. C. Weber. Voluntary systems of adverse reaction reporting—Part I. *Adverse Drug Reactions and Acute Poisoning Reviews*, 1985; 4(4):213–30.

Griffin, J. P., and J. C. Weber. Voluntary systems of adverse reaction reporting—Part II. *Adverse Drug Reactions and Acute Poisoning Reviews*, 1986; 5(1):23–55.

Guyatt, G., et al. Determining optimal therapy—randomized trials in individual patients. *New England Journal of Medicine*, 1986; 314(14):889–92.

Hsu, P., and A. R. Laddu. Analysis of adverse effects in a dose titration study. *Journal of Clinical Psychiatry*, 1994; 34:136–41.

Hutchinson, T. A., et al. Frequency, severity and risk factors for adverse drug reactions in adult outpatients: a prospective study. *Journal of Chronic Diseases*, 1986; 39(7):533–42.

Jackson, J., J. Louwerens, F. Cnossen, and H. De Jong. Testing the effects of the imidazopyridine zolpidem on memory: an ecologically valid approach. *Human Psychopharmacology*, 1992; 7: 325–30.

Jacobsen, F. M. Fluoxetine-induced sexual dysfunction and an open trial of yohimbine. *Journal of Clinical Psychiatry*, 1992; 53(4):119–122.

Jancin, B. ''Simple'' fluoxetine dosage proves to be elusive. *Clinical Psychiatry News*, April 1994, pages 3, 17.

Jick, H. Adverse drug reactions: the magnitude of the problem. *Journal of Allergy and Clinical Immunology*, 1984; 74:555–557.

Kahn, K. L. Above all, "do no harm." How shall we avoid errors in medicine? *JAMA*, 1995; 274(1):75–76.

Karch, F. E., and L. Lasagna. Toward the operational identification of adverse drug reactions. *Clinical Pharmacology and Therapeutics*, 1977; 21(3):247–54.

Leape, L. L., et al. Systems analysis of adverse drug events. ADE Prevention Study Group. *JAMA*, 1995; 274(1):35–43.

Martin, E. W. *Hazards of Medication: A Manual on Drug Interactions, Contraindications, and Adverse Reactions with Other Prescribing and Drug Information*, 2nd ed. Philadelphia: J. B. Lippincott, 1978.

Martys, C. R. Adverse reactions to drugs in general practice. *British Medical Journal*, November 10, 1979, 2(6199):1194–97.

Merlotti, L., et al. The dose effects of zolpidem on the sleep of healthy normals. *Journal of Clinical Psychopharmacology*, 1989; 9(1):9–14.

Mullen, W. H., et al. Incorrect overdose management advice in the *Physicians' Desk Reference*. *Annals of Emergency Medicine*, 1997; 29(2):255–61.

Opie, L. ACE inhibitors: almost too good to be true. *Scientific American Science and Medicine*, July/August 1994, 14–23.

Orange, L. Welcome to the "new frontier" of psychopharmacology. *Clinical Psychiatry News*, 1993; 21(12):1, 20.

Personal communication. Medical Economics Data Production Company (publishers of the PDR), September 12, 1994.

Pies, R. W. Dose-related sensory distortions with zolpidem. *Journal of Clinical Psychiatry*, 1995; 56(1):35–36.

Pies, R. W. Dr. Pies replies [letter]. *Journal of Clinical Psychiatry*, 1996; 57(1):43.

Price, P. L. A prescription for a prescription: the treatment of adverse drug reactions. *South Dakota Journal of Medicine*, 1994; 47(4):133.

Recchia, A. G., and N. H. Shear. Organization and function of an adverse drug reaction clinic. *Journal of Clinical Psychiatry*, 1994; 34:68–79.

Ross, D., and R. Bukata. Optimizing prescribing practices, Part 2. *Emergency Medicine and Acute Care Essays*, January 1993; 17(1):1–5.

Slatton, M. L., et al. Does digoxin provide additional hemodynamic and autonomic benefit at higher doses in patients with mild to moderate heart failure and normal sinus rhythm? *Journal of the American College of Cardiology*, 1997; 29(6):1206–13.

Steel, K., P. M. Gertman, C. Crescenzi, J. Anderson. Iatrogenic illness on a general medical service at a university hospital. *New England Journal of Medicine*, March 12, 1981, 304(11):638–42.

Sussman, N., and G. Stimmel. New dosing strategies for psychotropic drugs. *Primary Psychiatry*, 1997; 4(7):24–30.

Venning, G. R. Identification of adverse reactions to new drugs. II: How were 18 important adverse reactions discovered and with what delays? *British Medical Journal Clinical Research Ed.*, 1983; 286(6361):289–92.

Venning, G. R. Identification of adverse reactions to new drugs. II (continued): How were 18 important adverse reactions discovered and with what delays? *British Medical Journal Clinical Research Ed.*, 1983; 286(6362):365–68.

Vogel, G., A. Thurmond, M. MacIntosh, and T. Clifton. The effects of zolpidem [Ambien] on transient insomnia. *Sleep Research*, 1988; 17:67.

Chapter 3. Why People Respond Differently to Medications and What to Do About It

Abrams, L. Matching drugs to patients: hypertension. *The Practitioner*, July 1994; 238:527–30.

Ambrosone, C. B., et al. Cigarette smoking, N-acetyltransferase 2 genetic polymorphisms, and breast cancer risk. *JAMA*, 1996; 276(18):1494–1501.

Batoosingh, K. Liability concerns exclude women from clinical trials. *Clinical Psychiatry News*, 1995; 23(3):9.

Buchwald, D., and D. Garrity. Comparison of patients with chronic fatigue syndrome, fibromyalgia, and multiple chemical sensitivities. *Archives of Internal Medicine*, 1994; 154:2049–53.

Callahan, A. M. The role of pharmacokinetics in optimizing drug therapy. *Primary Psychiatry*, 1997; 4(7):31–34.

Clark, W. G., D. C. Brater, and A. R. Johnson. *Goth's Medical Pharmacology*, 13th ed. St. Louis: C. V. Mosby, 1992.

Cooper, S. A. Comparative analgesic efficacies of aspirin and acetaminophen. *Archives of Internal Medicine*, 1981; 141(3 spec. no.):282–85.

Cooper, S. A. Five studies on ibuprofen for postsurgical dental pain. *American Journal of Medicine*, 1984, (7):70–77.

Ewing, J. A., B. A. Rouse, and R. M. Aderhold. Studies of the mechanism of Oriental hypersensitivity to alcohol. *Currents in Alcoholism*, 1979, 5:45–52.

Gender gap for pain. *Reader's Digest*, March 1997, 123–24.

Goedde, H. W., S. Harada, and D. P. Agarwal. Racial differences in alcohol sensitivity: a new hypothesis. *Human Genetics*, 1979; 51(3):331–34.

Grapefruit juice interactions with drugs. *The Medical Letter on Drugs and Therapeutics*, 1995; 37:73–74.

Harada, S., D. P. Agarwal, and H. W. Goedde. Isozyme variations in acetaldehyde dehydrogenase (e.c.1.2.1.3) in human tissues. *Human Genetics*, 1978; 44(2):181–85.

Jegalian, K. Cracking the code of custom drugs. *Science*, February, 1997, 17.

Lin, K. M., et al. Comparison of alprazolam plasma levels in normal Asian and Caucasian male volunteers. *Psychopharmacology*, 1988, 96(3):365–69.

Martin, E. W. *Hazards of Medication: A Manual on Drug Interactions, Contraindications, and Adverse Reactions with Other Prescribing and Drug Information*, 2nd ed. Philadelphia: J. B. Lippincott, 1978.

Meggs, W. Multiple chemical sensitivities—chemical sensitivity as a symptom of airway inflammation. *Clinical Toxicology*, 1995; 33(2):107–10.

Pajer, K. New strategies in the treatment of depression in women. *Journal of Clinical Psychiatry*, 1995; 56(suppl 2):30–37.

Rowland, M., L. B. Sheiner, and J. Steimer. *Variability in Drug Therapy: Description, Estimation, and Control. A Sandoz Workshop*. New York: Raven Press, 1985.

Rudorfer, M. Pharmacokinetics of psychotropic drugs in special populations. *Journal of Clinical Psychiatry*, 1993; 49 (9, suppl): 50–54.

Sabella, B. Hypertension in African-Americans. *Hypertension Management Today*, Albert Einstein College of Medicine, Office of Continuing Medication, 1997; 1(3):11–12.

Sachse, C., J. Brockmoller, S. Bauer, and I. Roots. Cytochrome P450 2D6 variants in a Caucasian population: allele frequencies and phenotypic consequences [see comments]. *American Journal of Human Genetics*, 1997; 60(2):284–95.

Shader, R., et al. The clinician and drug interactions: an update [editorial]. *Journal of Clinical Psychopharmacology*, 1996; 16: 197–201.

Shelton, R. C. Mechanisms of cytochrome P450 metabolism. *Brainwaves: The Clinician's Guide to Brain Research*. Memphis, TN: Physicians Postgraduate Press, January 1997.

Sindrup, S. H., K. Brosen, and L. F. Gram. Nonlinear kinetics of imipramine in low and medium plasma level ranges. *Therapeutic Drug Monitoring*, 1990; 12(5):445–49.

Sjoqvist, F., and L. Bertilsson. Clinical pharmacology of antide-pressant drugs: Pharmacogenetics. *Advances in Biochemical Psychopharmacology*, 1984; 39: 359–72.

Skjelbo, E., K. Brosen, J. Hallas, and L. F. Gram. The mephen-ytoin oxidation polymorphism is partially responsible for the N-demethylation of imipramine. *Clinical Pharmacology and Therapeutics*, 1991; 49(1):18–23.

Spector, R., et al. Diphenhydramine in Orientals and Caucasians. *Clinical Pharmacology and Therapeutics*, 1980; 28(2):229–34.

Tacke, U., et al. Debrisoquine hydroxylation phenotypes of pa-tients with high versus low to normal serum antidepressant con-centrations. *Journal of Clinical Psychopharmacology*, 1992; 12: 262–67.

Theoharides, T. C., editor. *Pharmacology*. Boston: Little, Brown, 1992.

Van Campen, S. Acetaldehyde syndrome and drug sensitivity. Un-published, 1990, 1–22.

Von Moltke, L., D. Greenblatt, J. Harmatz, and R. Shader. Cytochromes in psychopharmacology. Editorial. *Journal of Clinical Psychopharmacology*, 1994; 14(1):1–3.

Watkins, P. B. Drug metabolism by cytochromes P450 in the liver and small bowel. *Gastroenterology Clinics of North America*, 1992; 21(3):511–26.

Wolff, P. H. Ethnic differences in alcohol sensitivity. *Science*, January 1972; 449–50.

Zeiner, A., A. Paredes, and H. D. Christensen. The role of acetaldehyde in mediating activity to an acute dose of ethanol among different racial groups. *Alcoholism, Clinical and Experimental Research*, 1979; 3(1):11–18.

Chapter 4. Medication Sensitivities and Side Effects in the Elderly

Associated Press. Study: millions of elderly die from drug reactions. *North County Blade-Citizen*, 1995, 1.

Brawn, L. A., and C. M. Castleden. Adverse drug reactions. An overview of special considerations in the management of the elderly patient. *Drug Safety*, 1990; 5(6):421–35.

Cassel, C. K., D. E. Riesenberg, L. B. Sorenson, and J. R. Walsh. *Geriatric Medicine*, 1990, Springer-Verlag, New York.

Carbonin, P., et al. Cardiovascular therapy problems in the elderly patient. *Cardiologia*, 1991; 36(12 Suppl 1):275–79, Abstract.

Curzen, N., and H. Purcell. Matching the treatment to the patient in hypertension. *Practitioner*, 1997; 241(1572):152–56.

Elderly in special peril of medicine interactions. *San Diego Union-Tribune*, July 24, 1995, page B-1.

Feighner, J. P., and J. B. Cohn. Double-blind comparative trials of fluoxetine and doxepin in geriatric patients with major depressive disorder. *Journal of Clinical Psychiatry*, 1985; 46:20–25.

Ferguson, R. P., T. Wetle, D. Dubitzky, and D. Winsemius. Relative importance to elderly patients of effectiveness, adverse effects, convenience and cost of antihypertensive medications. A pilot study. *Drugs and Aging*, 1994; 4(1):56–62.

Ferry, M. E., P. Lamy, and L. Becker. Physicians' knowledge of prescribing for the elderly. *Journal of the American Geriatrics Society*, 1985; 33:616–25.

Foreman, M. D., S. L. Theis, and M. A. Anderson. Adverse events in the hospitalized elderly. *Clinical Nursing Research*, August 1993; 2(3):360–70.

Gibian, T. Rational drug therapy in the elderly, or how not to poison your elderly patients. *Australian Family Physician*, 1992; 21(12):1755–60.

Greenblatt, D. J., J. S. Harmatz, and R. I. Shader. Clinical pharmacokinetics of anxiolytics and hypnotics in the elderly. Therapeutic considerations (Part I). *Clinical Pharmacokinetics*, September 1991, 21(3):165–77.

Johnson, A. G., and R. O. Day. The problems and pitfalls of NSAID therapy in the elderly (Part I). *Drugs and Aging*, 1991; 1(2):130–43.

Karsh, J. Adverse reactions and interactions with aspirin. Considerations in the treatment of the elderly patient. *Drug Safety*, 1990; 5(5):317–27.

Kitler, M. E. Clinical trials in the elderly. Pivotal points. *Clinics in Geriatric Medicine*, 1990; 6(2):235–55.

Kolata, Gina (*New York Times* News Service). What ails elderly often prescribed. *San Diego Union-Tribune*, July 27, 1994, A-1, 20.

Kruse, W. H. Problems and pitfalls in the use of benzodiazepines in the elderly. *Drug Safety*, September–October 1990; 5(5):328–44.

Leslie, C., P. J. Scott, and F. I. Caird. Principal alterations to drug kinetics and dynamics in the elderly. *Medical Laboratory Sciences*, 1992; 49(4):319–25.

Lind, T., C. Cederberg, M. Olausson, and L. Olbe. Omeprazole in elderly duodenal ulcer patients: relationship between reduction in gastric acid secretion and fasting plasma gastrin. *European Journal of Clinical Pharmacology*, 1991; 40(6):557–60.

Lindley, C. M., M. P. Tully, V. Paramsothy, and R. C. Tallis. Inappropriate medication is a major cause of adverse drug reactions in elderly patients. *Age and Ageing*, July 1992; 21(4):294–300.

Llewellyn, J. G., and M. H. Pritchard. Influence of age and disease state in nonsteroidal anti-inflammatory drug associated gastric bleeding. *Journal of Rheumatology*, April 1988; 15(4):691–94.

Mazanec, D. J. Conservative treatment of rheumatic disorders in the elderly. *Geriatrics*, 1991; 46(5):41–45.

Nilsson-Ehle, I., and B. Ljungberg. Quinolone disposition in the elderly. Practical implications. *Drugs and Aging*, July–August 1991; 1(4):279–88.

Oh, V. M. Multiple medication: problems of the elderly patient. *International Dental Journal*, 1991; 41(6):348–58.

Recchia, A. G. and N. H. Shear. Organization and function of an adverse drug reaction clinic. *Journal of Clinical Psychiatry*, 1994; 34:68–79.

Schneider, J. K., L. C. Mion, and J. D. Frengley. Adverse drug reactions in an elderly outpatient population. *American Journal of Hospital Pharmacy*, January 1992; 49(1):90–96.

Sherman, D. S., J. Avorn, and E. W. Campion. Cimetidine use in nursing homes: prolonged therapy and excessive doses. *Journal of the American Geriatrics Society*, November 1987; 35(11): 1023–27.

Silagy, C. A., et al. Adverse effects of low-dose aspirin in a healthy elderly population. *Clinical Pharmacology and Therapeutics*, 1993; 54(1):84–89.

Smucker, W. D., and J. R. Kontak. Adverse drug reactions causing hospital admission in an elderly population: experience with a decision algorithm. *Journal of the American Board of Family Practice*, 1990; 3(2):105–109.

Stewart, R. B., et al. A longitudinal evaluation of drug use in an ambulatory elderly population. *Journal of Clinical Epidemiology*, 1991; 44(12):1353–59.

Van, J. (*Chicago Tribune*) Geriatric text uses common-sense approach to medical technology. *San Diego Union-Tribune*, July 26, 1995, page D-3.

Vernay, D., and G. Dordain. [The elderly and psychotropic drugs]. *Revue du Praticien*, 1990; 40(15):1385–89, Abstract.

Wolfe, S. M., and R. E. Hope. *Worst Pills, Best Pills II: The Older Adult's Guide to Avoiding Drug-Induced Death or Illness*. Washington, D.C.: Public Citizen's Health Research Group, 1993.

Zeeh, J., and D. Platt. Peculiarities of drug therapy in the elderly. *Fortschritte der Medizin*, January 30, 1993; 111(3):33–36. Abstract.

Chapter 5. The Uses and Limitations of Low-Dose Medication Therapy

Guyatt, G., et al. Determining optimal therapy—randomized trials in individual patients. *New England Journal of Medicine*, 1986; 314(14):889–92.

Chapter 6. Antidepressants

Altamura, A. C., S. A. Montgomery, and J. F. Wernicke. The evidence for 20 mg a day of fluoxetine as the optimal dose in the treatment of depression. *British Journal of Psychiatry*, 1988: 153(suppl 3), 109–12.

Altamura, A. C., M. Percudani, G. Guercetti, G. Invernizzi. Efficacy and tolerability of fluoxetine in the elderly: a double-blind study versus amitryptiline. *International Clinical Psychopharmacology*, 1989; 4(Suppl 1):103–6.

Aronson, T. A. A naturalistic study of imipramine in panic disorder and agoraphobia. *American Journal of Psychiatry*, 1987; 144:1014–19.

Anchors, M. Fluoxetine is a safer alternative to fenfluramine in the medical treatment of obesity. *Archives of Internal Medicine*, 1997; 157:1270.

Ayd, F. J. American College of Neuropsychopharmacology Report: Part II. Bupropion for cocaine use. *Psychiatric Times*, April 1995, 21.

Beasley, C. M., B. S. Bosomworth, and J. F. Wernicke. Fluoxetine: relationships among dose, response, adverse effects, and plasma concentrations in the treatment of depression. *Psychopharmacology Bulletin*, 1990; 26(1):18–24.

Bender, K. J. New antidepressants: a practical update. *Psychiatric Times*, February 1995; 12(1):2.

Bersani, G., et al. 5-HT2 receptor antagonism in dysthymic disorder: a double-blind placebo-controlled study with ritanserin. *Acta Psychiatrica Scandinavica*, 1991; 83(4):244–48.

Bhandary, A. N., J. Medicis, and P. S. Masand. Prescription patterns of newer antidepressants in a resident-managed adult psychiatric clinic. *Primary Psychiatry*, 1996; 3(5):59–63.

Brymer, C., and C. H. Winograd. Fluoxetine in elderly patients: is there cause for concern? *Journal of the American Geriatrics Society*, 1992; 40(9):902–5.

Buff, D. D., R. Brenner, S. S. Kirtane, and R. Gilboa. Dysrhythmia associated with fluoxetine treatment in an elderly patient with cardiac disease. *Journal of Clinical Psychiatry*, 1991; 52(4):174–76.

Cain, J. W. Poor response to fluoxetine: underlying depression, serotonergic overstimulation, or a "therapeutic window"? *Journal of Clinical Psychiatry*, 1992; 53(8):272–77.

Callahan, A. M. The role of pharmacokinetics in optimizing drug therapy. *Primary Psychiatry*, 1997; 4(7):31–34.

Cole, J. O., and J. A. Bodkin. Antidepressant drug side effects. *Journal of Clinical Psychiatry*, 1990; 51(1, suppl):21–26.

Coupland, N. J., C. J. Bell, and J. P. Potokar. Serotonin reuptake inhibitor withdrawal. *Journal of Clinical Psychopharmacology*, 1996; 16(5):356–62.

Daamen, M. J., and W. A. Brown. Single-dose fluoxetine in management of premenstrual syndrome. *Journal of Clinical Psychiatry*, 1992; 53(6):210–11.

Dawling, S. Monitoring of tricyclic antidepressant therapy. *Clinical Biochemistry*, 1982; 15(1):56–61.

Doogan, D. P. Toleration and safety of sertraline: experience worldwide. *International Clinical Psychopharmacology*, December 1991, 6 suppl 2:47–56.

Doogan, D. P., and C. J. Langdon. A double-blind, placebo-controlled comparison of sertraline and dothiepin in the treatment of major depression in general practice. *International Clinical Psychopharmacology*, 1994; 9(2):95–100.

Drugs for psychiatric disorders. *The Medical Letter on Drugs and Therapeutics*, 1997; 39:33–36.

Duerksen, S. Prozac taken during pregnancy hikes birth-defect risk, study shows. *San Diego Union-Tribune*, October 5, 1996, B-10.

Dunner, D. L., and G. C. Dunbar. Therapeutic considerations in treating depression in the elderly. *Journal of Clinical Psychiatry*, 1994; 55(12 suppl):48–58.

Dunner, D. L., and G. C. Dunbar. Optimal dose regimen for paroxetine. *Journal of Clinical Psychiatry*, 1992; 53(2, suppl):21–26.

Dutch study attempts to qualify sexual dysfunction profiles among SSRIs. *Primary Psychiatry*, 1997; 4(7):22–23.

Elliott, R. L., and S. D. Shillcutt. Using newer antidepressants in the medically ill: An update. *Primary Psychiatry*, 1996; 3(5): 42–56.

Fava, M., et al. Relapse in patients on long-term fluoxetine treatment: response to increased fluoxetine dose. *Journal of Clinical Psychiatry*, 1995; 56(2):52–55.

Feighner, J., et al. An overview of fluoxetine in geriatric depression. *British Journal of Psychiatry*, 1988; 153(suppl 3):105–108.

Fichter, C. G., T. H. Jobe, and B. G. Braun. Does fluoxetine have a therapeutic window? *Lancet*, 1991; 338(August 24):520–21.

Finlayson, R. Recognition and management of dysthymic disorder. *American Family Physician*, 1989; 40(4):229–38.

Fontaine, R., et al. A double-blind comparison of nefazodone, imipramine, and placebo in major depression. *Journal of Clinical Psychiatry*, 1994; 55(6):234–41.

Freeman, E. W., et al. Nefazodone in the treatment of premenstrual syndrome: a preliminary study. *Journal of Clinical Psychopharmacology*, 1994; 14(3):180–86.

Freyer, F. J. (Associated Press). Breakthrough smoking-cessation drug contains no nicotine. *San Diego Union-Tribune*, August 3, 1997, page D-3.

Gallagher, W. The DD's [dysthymic disorders]: Blues without end. *American Health*, 1988, 80–88.

Geracioti, T. D., Jr. Venlafaxine treatment of panic disorder: a case series. *Journal of Clinical Psychiatry*, 1995; 56(9):408–10.

Ginsburg, D. "Phen-Flu" for obesity. *Primary Psychiatry*, 1997; 4(7):17–20.

Gloger, S., et al. Panic attacks and agoraphobia: low dose clomipramine treatment. *Journal of Clinical Psychopharmacology*, 1989; 9(1):28–32.

Goldman, E. L. Ginkgo eases drug-induced sex dysfunction. *Clinical Psychiatry News*, 1997; 25(7):5.

Goodman, W. K., et al. Fluvoxamine in the treatment of obsessive-compulsive disorder and related conditions. *Journal of Clinical Psychiatry*, 1997; 58(suppl 5):32–49.

Goodnick, P. J., et al. Double-blind treatment of major depression with fluoxetine: use of pattern analysis and relation of HAM-D score to CGI change. *Psychopharmacology Bulletin*, 1987; 23(1): 162–63.

Greenblatt, D. J. Basic pharmacokinetic principles and their application to psychotropic drugs. *Journal of Clinical Psychiatry*, 1993; 54(suppl):8–13; discussion 55–56.

Harkness, R. (Knight-Ridder News Service). Ginkgo may counter

Prozac side effects. *San Diego Union-Tribune*, August 3, 1997, page D-6.

Hussein, S., and B. M. Kaufman. Bradycardia associated with fluoxetine in an elderly patient with sick sinus syndrome [letter]. *Postgraduate Medical Journal*, 1994; 70(819):56.

Jacobsen, F. M. Fluoxetine-induced sexual dysfunction and an open trial of yohimbine. *Journal of Clinical Psychiatry*, 1992; 53(4):119–22.

Jobson, K., M. Linnoila, J. Gillam, and J. L. Sullivan. Successful treatment of severe anxiety attacks with tricyclic antidepressants: A potential mechanism of action. *American Journal of Psychiatry*, 1978, 135; 7:863–64.

Kafka, M. P. Sertraline pharmacotherapy for paraphilias and paraphilia-related disorders: an open trial. *Annals of Clinical Psychiatry*, 1994; 6(3):189–95.

Katz, R. J., and M. Rosenthal. Adverse interaction of cyproheptadine with serotonergic antidepressants. *Journal of Clinical Psychiatry*, 1994; 55(7):314–15.

Kaye, N. S., and C. Dancu. Paroxetine and obsessive-compulsive disorder [letter]. *American Journal of Psychiatry*, October 1994; 151(10):1523.

Kerr, J. S., D. B. Fairweather, R. Mahendran, and I. Hindmarch. The effects of paroxetine, alone and in combination with alcohol on psychomotor performance and cognitive function in the elderly. *International Clinical Psychopharmacology*, November, 1992; 7(2):101–108.

Kirksey, D. F., and N. Harto-Truax. Private practice evaluation of the safety and efficacy of bupropion in depressed outpatients. *Journal of Clinical Psychiatry*, 1983; 44(5 Pt 2):143–47.

Kivela, S. L., and K. Pahkala. Dysthymic disorder in the aged in the community. *Psychiatry and Psychiatric Epidemiology*, 1989; 24(2):77–83.

Kline, M. D. Fluoxetine and anorgasmia. *American Journal of Psychiatry*, 1989; 146(6):804–805.

Kline, M. D., and S. Koppes. Acidophilus for sertraline-induced diarrhea [letter]. *American Journal of Psychiatry*, 1994; 151(10): 1521–2.

Kocsis, J. H., and A. J. Frances. A critical discussion of DMS—III dysthymic disorder. *American Journal of Psychiatry*, 1987; 144(12):1534–42.

LaFee, S. How mental illness adds up in United States, elsewhere. *San Diego Union-Tribune*, March 22, 1995; C-3.

Lillywhite, A. R., S. J., Wilson, and D. J. Nutt. Successful treatment of night terrors and somnambulism with paroxetine. *British Journal of Psychiatry*, April 1994; 164:551–54.

Louie, A. K., T. B. Lewis, and M. D. Lannon. Use of low-dose fluoxetine in major depression and panic disorder. *Journal of Clinical Psychiatry*, 1993; 54(1):435–38.

Lydiard, R. B., and J. C. Ballenger. Antidepressants in panic disorder and agoraphobia. *Journal of Affective Disorders*, 1987; 13: 153–68.

Maletta, G., K. M. Mattox, and M. Dysken. Guidelines for prescribing psychoactive drugs in the elderly: Part 1. *Geriatrics*, 1991; 46(9):40–47.

Markowitz, J. C., M. E. Moran, J. H. Kocsis, and A. J. Frances. Prevalence and comorbidity of dysthymic disorder among psychiatric outpatients. *Journal of Affective Disorders*, 1992; 24(2): 63–71.

McCall, W. V. Sertraline-induced stuttering. *Journal of Clinical Psychiatry*, 1994; 55(7):316.

McCue, R. Using tricyclic antidepressants in the elderly. *Clinics in Geriatric Medicine*, 1992; 8(2):323–34.

McElroy, S. L., P. E. Keck, and L. M. Friedman. Minimizing and managing antidepressant side effects. *Journal of Clinical Psychiatry*, 1995; 56(suppl 2):49–55.

Mendels, J., R. Johnston, J. Mattes, and R. Riesenberg. Efficacy and safety of b.i.d. [twice a day] doses of venlafaxine in a dose-response study. *Psychopharmacology Bulletin*, 1993; 29(2):169–74.

Metz, A., and R. I. Shader. Adverse interactions encountered when using trazodone to treat insomnia associated with fluoxetine. *International Clinical Psychopharmacology*, 1990; 5(3):191–94.

Mirtazapine—a new antidepressant. *The Medical Letter on Drugs and Therapeutics*, 1996; 38:113–14.

Musher, J. S. Anorgasmia with the use of fluoxetine. *American Journal of Psychiatry*, 1990; 147(7):948.

Nefazodone for depression. *The Medical Letter on Drugs And Therapeutics*, 1995; 37:33–34.

Newhouse, P. A. Use of serotonin selective reuptake inhibitors in geriatric depression. *Journal of Clinical Psychiatry*, 1996; 57(suppl 5):12–17.

Nierenberg, A. A., et al. Trazodone for antidepressant-associated insomnia. *American Journal of Psychiatry*, 1994; 151(7):1069–72.

Nolan, L., and K. O'Malley. Adverse effects of antidepressants in the elderly. *Drugs and Aging*, September–October 1992, 2(5):450–58.

Nurnberg, H. G., and E. F. Coccaro. Response of panic disorder and resistance of depression to imipramine. *American Journal of Psychiatry*, 1982, 139:1060–62.

Pearlstein, T. B., and A. B. Stone. Long-term fluoxetine treatment of late luteal phase dysphoric disorder. *Journal of Clinical Psychiatry*, 1994; 55(8):332–35.

Peck, P. Fluoxetine dramatically reduces premenstrual dysphoric. *Clinical Psychiatry News*, January 1995, p. 16.

Pies, R. W. Fluoxetine treatment of premenstrual syndrome. *Journal of Clinical Psychiatry*, 1990; 51(8):340.

Preskorn, S. Antidepressant response and plasma concentrations of bupropion. *Journal of Clinical Psychiatry*, 1983; 44(5 Pt 2): 137–39.

Preskorn, S. Comparison of the tolerability of bupropion, fluoxetine, imipramine, nefazodone, paroxetine, sertraline, and venlafaxine. *Journal of Clinical Psychiatry*, 1995; 56(suppl 6):12–21.

Preskorn, S. Pharmacokinetics of antidepressants: Why and how they are relevant to treatment. *Journal of Clinical Psychiatry*, 1993; 54 (9, suppl):14–34, discussion 55–56.

Preskorn, S. Targeted pharmacotherapy in depression management: comparative pharmacokinetics of fluoxetine, paroxetine and sertraline. *International Clinical Psychopharmacology*, 1994; suppl 3:13–19.

Reeves, R. R., and J. A. Bullen. Serotonin syndrome produced by paroxetine and low-dose trazodone [letter]. *Psychosomatics*, March–April 1995; 36(2):159–60.

Regalado, R. G. Anafranil in the management of long-term pain: a preliminary report. *Journal of Internal Medicine Research*, 1976; 4(suppl 2):54–55.

Reimherr, F. W., et al. Sertraline, a selective inhibitor of serotonin uptake, for the treatment of outpatients with major depressive disorder. *Psychopharmacology Bulletin*, 1988; 24(1): 200–205.

Rickels, K., et al. Nefazodone and imipramine in major depression: a placebo-controlled trial. *British Journal of Psychiatry*, 1994; 164(6):802–805.

Ringold, A. L. Paroxetine efficacy in social phobia [letter]. *Journal of Clinical Psychiatry*, August 1994; 55(8):363–64.

Rouillon, F. A study of panic disorder in general medicine; epidemiological data and treatment with clomipramine. *Encephale*, 1988; 14(5):371–78, abstract.

Roy, A., Sutton, M., and Pickar, D. Neuroendocrine and personality variables in dysthymic disorder. *American Journal of Psychiatry*, 1985; 142:94–97.

Roy, D., and S. Dawling. Application of an individually predicted dosage of amitriptyline to the treatment of depression. *International Clinical Psychopharmacology*, 1987; 2:307–15.

Rudorfer, M. Pharmacokinetics of psychotropic drugs in special populations. *Journal of Clinical Psychiatry*, 1993; 49 (9, suppl): 50–54.

Salzman, C. Practical considerations in the pharmacologic treatment of depression and anxiety in the elderly. *Journal of Clinical Psychiatry*, 1990; 51:1 (suppl) 40–43.

Schatzberg, A. F. Dosing strategies for antidepressant agents. *Journal of Clinical Psychiatry*, 1991; 52(5, suppl):14–20.

Schatzberg, A. F., et al. Current psychotropic dosing and monitoring guidelines. *Primary Psychiatry*, 1997; 4(7):35–63.

Schatzberg, A. F., et al. Recent studies on selective serotonergic antidepressants: trazodone, fluoxetine, and fluvoxamine. *Journal of Clinical Psychopharmacology*, 1987; 7(6):44S–49S.

Schneier, F., et al. Fluoxetine in panic disorder. *Journal of Clinical Psychopharmacology*, 1990; 10(2):119–21.

Sindrup, S. H., K. Brosen, and L. F. Gram. Pharmacokinetics of the selective serotonin reuptake inhibitor paroxetine: nonlinearity and relation to the sparteine oxidation polymorphism. *Clinical Pharmacology and Therapeutics*, 1992; 51(3):288–95.

Skop, B. P., et al. The serotonin syndrome associated with paroxetine, an over-the-counter cold remedy, and vascular disease. *American Journal of Emergency Medicine*, 1994; 12(6):642–44.

Spier, S. A., and M. A. Frontera. Unexpected deaths in depressed medical inpatients treated with fluoxetine [see comments]. *Journal of Clinical Psychiatry*, 1991; 52(9):377–82.

SSRI withdrawal syndrome. *Journal Watch for Psychiatry*, 1996; 2(12):93.

Stern, W. C., N. Harto-Truax, and N. Bauer. Efficacy of bupropion in tricyclic-resistant or intolerant patients. *Journal of Clinical Psychiatry*, 1983; 45(5, section 2):148–52.

Stewart, J. W., F. M. Quitkin, and D. F. Klein. The pharmacotherapy of minor depression. *American Journal of Psychotherapy*, 1992; 46(1):23–36.

Sussman, N., and G. Stimmel. New dosing strategies for psychotropic drugs. *Primary Psychiatry*, 1997; 4(7):24–30.

Tacke, U., et al. Debrisoquine hydroxylation phenotypes of patients with high versus low to normal serum antidepressant concentrations. *Journal of Clinical Psychopharmacology*, 1992; 12: 262–67.

Top 200 drugs of 1995. *Pharmacy Times*, April 1995, 27–36.

Uhde, T. W., and J. C. Nemiah. Chapter 18: Anxiety disorders (anxiety and phobic neuroses), in *Comprehensive Textbook of Psychiatry*, 6th ed. H. I. Kaplan and B. J. Sadock. Baltimore: Williams & Wilkins, 1993.

U.S. Government Food and Drug Administration (FDA). Fluoxetine-phenytoin interaction. *FDA Medical Bulletin*, May 1994.

Van der Kolk, B. A., et al. Fluoxetine in posttraumatic stress disorder. *Journal of Clinical Psychiatry*, 1994; 55(12):517–22.

Waldinger, M. D., M. W. Hengeveld, and A. H. Zwinderman. Paroxetine treatment of premature ejaculation: a double-blind, randomized, placebo-controlled study. *American Journal of Psychiatry*, 1994; 151(9):1377–79.

Wernicke, J. F., et al. Low-dose fluoxetine therapy for depression. *Psychopharmacology Bulletin*, 1988; 24(1):183–88.

Wolfe, S. M. *Public Citizen's Health Research Group Health Letter*, May 1994.

Wolfe, S. M., and R. E. Hope. *Worst Pills, Best Pills II: The Older Adult's Guide to Avoiding Drug-Induced Death or Illness*. Washington, D.C.: Public Citizen's Health Research Group, 1993.

Wood, A. J. Fluoxetine—reveal article. *New England Journal of Medicine*, 1994; 331(20):1354–61.

Zajecka, J., K. Tracy, and S. Mitchell. Discontinuation symptoms after treatment with serotonin reuptake inhibitors: a literature review. *Journal of Clinical Psychiatry*, 1997; 58(7):291–97.

Zinner, S. H. Panic attacks precipitated by sertraline [letter]. *American Journal of Psychiatry*, 1994; 151(1):147–48.

Zitrin, C. M., D. F. Klein, and M. G. Woerner. Behavior therapy, supportive psychotherapy, imipramine, and phobias. *Archives of General Psychiatry*, 1978; 35:307–16.

Chapter 7. Anti-Anxiety and Anti-Panic Medications

Aronson, T. A. A naturalistic study of imipramine in panic disorder and agoraphobia. *American Journal of Psychiatry*, 1987; 144:1014–19.

Ashton, H. Protracted withdrawal from benzodiazepines: the post-withdrawal syndrome. *Psychiatry Annals*, 1995; 25(3):174–76.

Ashton, H. Toxicity and adverse consequences of benzodiazepine use. *Psychiatric Annals*, 1995; 25(3):158–165.

Ayd, F. J. Biological psychiatry update: Triazolam/grapefruit juice. *Psychiatric Times*, November 1996; 13(11):42.

Ayd, F. J. Prescribing anxiolytics and hypnotics for the elderly. *Psychiatric Annals*, 1994; 24(2):91–97.

Ballenger, J. C. Panic disorder in the medical setting. *Journal of Clinical Psychiatry*, 1997; 58(suppl 2):13–17.

Bertilsson, L., and W. Kalow. Why are diazepam metabolism and polymorphic S-mephenytoin hydroxylation associated with each other in white and Korean populations but not in Chinese populations? [letter; comment]. *Clinical Pharmacology and Therapeutics*, May 1993; 53(5):608–10.

Boudoulas, H., and C. F. Wooley. Mitral valve prolapse syndrome. Evidence of hyperadrenergic state. *Postgraduate Medicine*, February 29, 1988, Spec No.: 152–62.

Cohen, J. S. Alprazolam treatment of panic attacks. *Journal of Clinical Psychiatry*, 1988; 49(8):325.

Coplan, J. D., L. Tiffon, and J. M. Gorman. Therapeutic strategies for the patient with treatment-resistant anxiety. *Journal of Clinical Psychiatry*, 1993; 54(suppl 5):69–77.

Davidson, J. Use of benzodiazepines in panic disorder. *Journal of Clinical Psychiatry*, 1997; 58(suppl 2): 26–28.

Davidson, J., S. Ford, R. Smith, and N. Potts. Long-term treatment of social phobia with clonazepam. *Journal of Clinical Psychiatry*, 1991; 52(suppl):16–20.

Davidson, J., et al. Treatment of social phobia with clonazepam and placebo. *Journal of Clinical Psychopharmacology*, 1993; 13: 423–28.

Dubovsky, S. L. Generalized anxiety disorder: new concepts and pharmacologic therapies. *Journal of Clinical Psychiatry*, 1990; 51 (suppl 1): 3–10.

Dukes, M. N. *Meyler's Side Effects of Drugs. An Encyclopedia of Adverse Reactions and Interactions*, 12th ed. New York: Elsevier Science Publishers, 1992, p. 98.

Freeman, E. W., K. Rickels, S. J. Sondheimer, and M. Polansky A double-blind trial of oral progesterone, alprazolam, and placebo in treatment of severe premenstrual syndrome. *JAMA*, 1995; 274(1): 51–57.

Geiselmann, B., and M. Linden. Prescription and intake patterns in long-term and ultra-long-term benzodiazepine treatment in primary care practice. *Pharmacopsychiatry*, 1991; 24:55–61.

Greenblatt, D. J., J. S. Harmatz, and R. I. Shader. Clinical pharmacokinetics of anxiolytics and hypnotics in the elderly. Therapeutic considerations (Part I). *Clinical Pharmacokinetics*, September 1991, 21(3):165–77.

Greenblatt, D. J., and C. E. Wright. Clinical pharmacokinetics of alprazolam. Therapeutic implications. *Clinical Pharmacokinetics*, 1993; 24(6):453–71.

Gorman, J. M., and L. A. Papp. Chronic anxiety: deciding the length of treatment. *Journal of Clinical Psychiatry*, 1990; 51(1 suppl):11–15.

High anxiety. *Consumer Reports*, January 1993; 19–24.

Hirschfeld, R. M. Panic disorder: diagnosis, epidemiology, a clinical course. *Journal of Clinical Psychiatry*, 1996; 517(10 suppl):3–8.

Jancin, B. How to break off a long-term relationship with a benzodiazepine. *Clinical Psychiatry News*, May 1994; 14.

Johnson, M. S. Response of ventricular arrhythmias to propranolol in mitral valve prolapse. *Alabama Medicine*, 1988; 58(3):14–16.

Kruse, W. H. Problems and pitfalls in the use of benzodiazepines in the elderly. *Drug Safety*, September–October 1990; 5(5):328–44.

Krystal, J. H., D. Deutsch, and D. Charney. The biological basis of panic disorder. *Journal of Clinical Psychiatry*, 1996; 517(10 suppl):23–31.

Lin, K. M., et al. Comparison of alprazolam plasma levels in normal Asian and Caucasian male volunteers. *Psychopharmacology*, 1988; 96(3):365–69.

Lydiard, R. B., and J. C. Ballenger. Antidepressants in panic disorder and agoraphobia. *Journal of Affective Disorders*, 1987; 13:153–68.

Lydiard, R. B., and S. A. Falsetti. Treatment options for social phobia. *Psychiatric Annals*, 1995; 25(9):570–76. Social phobias third most common lifetime psychiatric disorder in the U.S.

Maletta, G., K. M. Mattox, and M. Dysken. Guidelines for prescribing psychoactive drugs in the elderly: Part 1. *Geriatrics*, 1991; 46(9):40–47.

Markovitz, P. J. Treatment of anxiety in the elderly. *Journal of Clinical Psychiatry*, 1993; 54(suppl 5):64–68.

Marrou, C. My turn: Let me tell you a secret. *Newsweek*, June 24, 1996; 14.

Mavissakalian, M. R., and J. M. Perel. Imipramine dose-response relationship in panic disorder with agoraphobia. *Archives of General Psychiatry*, 1989; 46:127–31.

Miller, N. S. Liability and efficacy from long-term use of benzodiazepines: documentation and interpretation. *Psychiatric Annals*, 1995; 25(3):166–70.

Noyes, R., et al. Diazepam versus alprazolam for the treatment of panic disorder. *Journal of Clinical Psychiatry*, 1996; 57(8):349–55.

Nurnberg, H. G., and E. F. Coccaro. Response of panic disorder and resistance of depression to imipramine. *American Journal of Psychiatry*, 1982; 139:1060–62.

Potts, N. L., and J. R. Davidson. Epidemiology and pharmacotherapy of social phobia. *Psychiatric Times*, February 1995; 19–20.

Salzman, C. Practical considerations in the pharmacologic treatment of depression and anxiety in the elderly. *Journal of Clinical Psychiatry*, 1990, 51:1 (suppl) 40–43.

Schneider, L., Syapin, P., Pawluczyk, S. Seizures following triazolam withdrawal despite benzodiazepine treatment. *Journal of Clinical Psychiatry*, 1987; 48(10):418–19.

Schroeder, S. A., M. Krupp, L. Tierney, and S. McPhee. *Current Medical Diagnosis and Treatment 1990*. Norwalk, CT: Appleton and Lange, pp. 712–15.

Sheehan, D. V. Benzodiazepines in panic disorder and agoraphobia. *Journal of Affective Disorders*, 1987; 13:169–81.

Sheehan, D. V., and K. Hartnett-Sheehan. The role of SSRIs in panic disorder. *Journal of Clinical Psychiatry*, 1996; 517(suppl 10):51–58.

Snyder, D. W. Mitral valve prolapse. Recognizing and treating its manifestations and complications. *Postgraduate Medicine*, 1985; 77(5):281–84, 286–88.

Stoudemire, A., and M. G. Moran. Psychopharmacologic treatment of anxiety in the medically ill elderly patient: special considerations. *Journal of Clinical Psychiatry*, 1994; 54(5 suppl):27–33.

Sussman, N. Treating anxiety with minimizing abuse and dependence. *Journal of Clinical Psychiatry*, 1993; 54(5 suppl):44–50.

Top 200 drugs of 1995. *Pharmacy Times*, April 1995; 27–36.

Tucker, G. J. Treatment approaches to anxiety, depression, and aggression in the elderly. *Journal of Clinical Psychiatry*, 1994; 55(2 suppl):3–4.

Uhde, T. W., and J. C. Nemiah, eds. Chapter 18, "Anxiety Disorders (Anxiety and Phobic Neuroses)," by H. I. Kaplan and B. J. Sadock in the *Comprehensive Textbook of Psychiatry*, 6th ed. Baltimore: Williams & Wilkins: 1993.

Weiss, K. J. Management of anxiety and depression syndrome in the elderly. *Journal of Clinical Psychiatry*, 1994; 55(2 suppl):5–12.

Zitrin, C. M., D. F. Klein, and M. G. Woerner. Behavior therapy. *General Psychiatry*, 1978; 35:307–16.

Chapter 8. Sleep Medications

Adam, K., and I. Oswald. Small studies miss the difference (letter). *British Medical Journal*, 1993; 307:626.

Adam, K., and I. Oswald. Unpublished manufacturers research unfavorable (letter). *British Medical Journal*, 1993; 306(6890): 1475.

Ansseau, M., W. Pitchot, M. Hansenne, and A. Gonzalez Moreno. Psychotic reactions to zolpidem [letter]. *Lancet*, 1992; 339(8796): 809.

Ayd, F. J. Prescribing anxiolytics and hypnotics for the elderly. *Psychiatric Annals*, 1994; 24(2):91–97.

Ayd, F. J. Triazolam 0.25 mg: risks vs. benefits. *International Drug Therapy Newsletter*, 1992; 27(4): 13–16.

Ayd, F. J. Triazolam 0.25 mg: a reappraisal. *International Drug Therapy Newsletter*, 1992; 27(5):17–24.

Baker, M. I., and M. A. Oleen. The use of benzodiazepine hypnotics in the elderly. *Pharmacotherapy*, 1988; 8(4):241–47.

Balter, M. B., et al. The World Psychiatric Association Task Force on sedative hypnotics. *Eur-Psychiatry*, 1993; 8(1):45–49.

Berlin, I., et al. Comparison of the effects of zolpidem and triazolam on memory functions, psychomotor performances, and postural sway in healthy subjects. *Journal of Clinical Psychopharmacology*, April 1993; 13(2):100–106.

Bixler, E. O., et al. Next-day memory impairment with triazolam use. *Lancet*, 1991; 337:827–31.

Bowen, A. J. Comparative efficacy of triazolam, flurazepam, and placebo in out-patients insomniacs. *Journal of International Medical Research*, 1978; 6(4):337–42.

Brawn, L. A., and C. M. Castleden. Adverse drug reactions. An overview of special considerations in the management of the elderly patient. *Drug Safety*, 1990; 5(6):421–35.

Campion, E. W., J. Avorn, V. A. Reder, and N. J. Olins. Overmedication of the low-weight elderly. *Archives of Internal Medicine*, 1987; 147(5):945–47.

Carskadon, M. A., W. F. Seidel, D. J. Greenblatt, and W. C. Dement. Daytime carryover of triazolam and flurazepam in elderly insomniacs. *Sleep*, 1982; 5(4):361–71.

Cavallaro, R., M. G. Regazzetti, G. Covelli, and E. Smeraldi. Tolerance and withdrawal with zolpidem [letter]. *Lancet*, 1993; 342(8867):374–75.

Church, M. W., and L. C. Johnson. Mood and performance of poor sleepers during repeated use of flurazepam. *Psychopharmacology*, 1979; 61(3):309–16.

Cohen, J. S. Dosage titration issues [letter]. *Journal of Clinical Psychiatry*, 1996; 57(1):43.

Cohen, M. You don't have to be a neuroscientist to forget everything with triazolam—but it helps (letter). *JAMA*, 1988; 259(3): 352.

Consensus conference. Drugs and insomnia. The use of medications to promote sleep. *JAMA*, May 11, 1984; 251(18):410–14.

Cowley, G. More halcion headaches. *Newsweek*, March 7, 1994, 50–52.

De-Abajo, F. J., et al. Triazolam regulatory measures in Spain (abstract). *Lancet*, 1993; 341(8838):185.

Dement, W. C. The proper use of sleeping pills in the primary care setting. *Journal of Clinical Psychiatry*, 1992; 53:(12 suppl) 50–56.

Di Maio, L. You don't have to be a neuroscientist to forget everything with triazolam—but it helps (letter). *JAMA*, 1988; 259(3): 351.

Dinan, T. G., and B. E. Leonard. Triazolam: As safe as other benzodiazepines (letter). *British Medical Journal*, 1993; 306(6890): 1475.

Dominguez, R. A., B. J. Goldstein, A. F. Jacobson, and R. M. Steinbook. Comparative efficacy of estazolam, flurazepam, and placebo in outpatients with insomnia. *Journal of Clinical Psychiatry*, 1986; 47(7):362–65.

Elliott, W. J. You don't have to be a neuroscientist to forget everything with triazolam—but it helps (letter). *JAMA*, 1988; 259(3): 351.

Everitt, D., and J. Avorn. Clinical decision-making in the evaluation and treatment of insomnia. *American Journal of Medicine*, 1990; 89:357–362.

Ewing, J. A. You don't have to be a neuroscientist to forget every-thing with triazolam—but it helps (letter). *JAMA*, 1988; 259(3): 350.

Fairweather, D. B., J. S. Kerr, and I. Hindmarch. The effects of acute and repeated doses of zolpidem on subjective sleep, psychomotor performance and cognitive function in elderly volunteers. *European Journal of Clinical Pharmacology*, 1992; 43(6): 597–601.

Fillingim, J. M. Double-blind evaluation of temazepam, flurazepam, and placebo in geriatric insomniacs. *Clinical Therapeutics*, 1982; 4(5):369–80.

Greenblatt, D. J., J. S. Harmatz, and R. I. Shader. Clinical pharmacokinetics of anxiolytics and hypnotics in the elderly. Therapeutic considerations (Part I). *Clinical Pharmacokinetics*, September 1991; 21(3):165–77.

Greenblatt, D. J., and R. I. Shader. *Benzodiazepines in Clinical Practice*. New York: Raven Press, 1974.

Greenblatt, D. J., R. I. Shader, M. Divoll, and J. S. Harmatz. Adverse reactions to triazolam, flurazepam, and placebo in controlled clinical trials. *Journal of Clinical Psychiatry*, 1984; 45(5):192–95.

Hartmann, E., J. G. Lindsley, and C. Spinweber. Chronic insomnia: effects of tryptophan, flurazepam, secobarbital, and placebo. *Psychopharmacology*, 1983; 80(2):138–42.

Hartmann, P. M. Drug treatment of insomnia: indications and newer agents. *American Family Physician*, 1995; 51(1):191–94, 197–98.

Hypnotic drugs. *The Medical Letter on Drugs and Therapeutics*, 1996; 38:59–61.

Iruela, L. M., V. Ibanez-Rojo, and E. Baca. More on zolpidem side effects [letter]. *Lancet*, 1993; 342(8885):1495–96.

Jackson, J., J. Louwerens, F. Cnossen, and H. De Jong. Testing the effects of the imidazopyridine zolpidem on memory: an ecologically valid approach. *Human Psychopharmacology*, 1992; 7: 325–30.

Jick, H. Comparative studies with a new hypnotic under current investigation. *Current Therapeutic Research*, 1967; 9(7):355–57.

Jick, H. Evaluation of drug efficacy by a preference technic. *New England Journal of Medicine*, 1966; 275(25):1399–1403.

Jonas, J. M. Triazolam condemned by misinformation . . . (letter). *British Medical Journal*, 1993; 306(6890):1475.

Jonas, J. M., B. S. Coleman, A. Q. Sheridan, and R. W. Kalinske. Comparative clinical profiles of triazolam versus other shorter-acting hypnotics. *Journal of Clinical Psychiatry*, 1992; 53(12 suppl): 19–31.

Kales, A., E. O. Bixler, M. Scharf, and J. D. Kales. Sleep laboratory studies of flurazepam: a model for evaluating hypnotic drugs. *Clinical Pharmacology and Therapeutics*, 1976, 19(5): 576–83.

Kales, A., et al. Comparison of short and long half-life benzodiazepine hypnotics: triazolam and quazepam. *Clinical Pharmacology and Therapeutics*, 1986; 40:378–86.

Kales, A., et al. Hypnotic efficacy of triazolam: sleep laboratory evaluation of intermediate-term effectiveness. *Journal of Clinical Pharmacology*, 1976; 16:399–406.

Koshorek, G., et al. Dose effects of zolpidem on transient insomnia. *Sleep Research*, 1988; 17:47.

Kruse, W. H. Problems and pitfalls in the use of benzodiazepines in the elderly. *Drug Safety*, September–October 1990; 5(5):328–44.

Kummer, J., et al. Long-term polysomnographic study of the efficacy and safety of zolpidem in elderly psychiatric in-patients with insomnia. *Journal of International Medical Research*, 1993; 21(4):171–84.

Kushner, M. J. You don't have to be a neuroscientist to forget everything with triazolam—but it helps (letter). *JAMA*, 1988; 259(3):350.

Langtry, H. D., and P. Benfield. Zolpidem. A review of its pharmacodynamic and pharmacokinetic properties and therapeutic potential. *Drugs*, 1990; 40(2):291–313.

Leibowitz, M., and A. Sunshine. Long-term hypnotic efficacy and safety of triazolam and flurazepam. *Journal of Clinical Pharmacology*, 1978; 18(5–6):302–9.

Melatonin. *Medical Letter on Drugs and Therapeutics*, 1995; 24, 37(962):111–2.

Mendelson, W. B., et al. A clinical study of flurazepam. *Sleep*, 1982; 5(4):350–60.

Merlotti, L., et al. The dose effects of zolpidem on the sleep of healthy normals. *Journal of Clinical Psychopharmacology*, 1989; 9(1):9–14.

Morris, H. H., and M. L. Estes. Traveler's amnesia: transient global amnesia secondary to triazolam. *JAMA*, 1987; 258(7):945–46.

Morris, H. H., and M. L. Estes. You don't have to be a neuroscientist to forget everything with triazolam—but it helps (letter). *JAMA*, 1988; 259(3):351–52.

Neergaard, L. [Associated Press]. FDA seeks U.S. probe of Halcion sleeping pill. *San Diego Union-Tribune*, June 1, 1996; C1.

Picone, D. A., D. A. D'Mello, M. L. Foote, and B. Msibi. A review of the utilization of sedative-hypnotic drugs in a general hospital. *General Hospital Psychiatry*, 1993; 15: 51–54.

Pies, R. W. Dose-related sensory distortions with zolpidem. *Journal of Clinical Psychiatry*, 1995; 56(1):35–36.

Radack, H. B. You don't have to be a neuroscientist to forget everything with triazolam—but it helps (letter). *JAMA*, 1988; 259(3):351.

Rathier, M., and L. Korman. Triazolam use in older adults: patients' perceptions and physicians' practice. *Journal of the American Geriatric Society*, 1993; 41(10 suppl): SA56.

Reeves, R. L. Comparison of triazolam, flurazepam, and placebo as hypnotics in geriatric patients with insomnia. *Journal of Clinical Pharmacology*, 1977; 17(5–6):319–23.

Reynolds, C. F., D. J. Kupfer, C. C. Hoch, and D. E. Sewitch. Sleeping pills for the elderly: Are they ever justified? *Journal of Clinical Psychiatry*, 1985; 46(2 Pt 2):9–12.

Roche Products, Inc. Correspondence, February 7, 1995.

Roehrs, T., G. Vogel, W. Sterling, and T. Roth. Dose effects of temazepam in transient insomnia. *Arzneimittel-Forschung*, August 1990; 40(8):859–62.

Roger, M., P. Attali, and J. P. Coquelin. Multicenter, double-blind, controlled comparison of zolpidem and triazolam in elderly patients with insomnia. *Clinical Therapeutics*, 1993; 15(1):127–36.

Roth, T., G. Vogel, and W. Sterling. Effects of temazapam on transient insomnia. *Sleep Research*, 1987; 16:123.

Salkind, M. R., and T. Silverstone. A clinical and psychometric evaluation of flurazepam. *British Journal of Clinical Pharmacology*, 1975; 2(3):223–26.

Scharf, M. B., et al. Dose response effects of zolpidem in normal geriatric subjects. *Journal of Clinical Psychiatry*, 1991; 52(2):77–83.

Scharf, M. B., P. B. Roth, R. A. Dominguez, and J. C. Ware. Estazolam and flurazepam: a multicenter, placebo-controlled comparative study in outpatients with insomnia. *Journal of Clinical Pharmacology*, 1990; 30(5):461–67.

Scharf, M. B., et al. A polysomnagraphic comparison of temazepam 15 and 30 mg with triazolam 0.125 and 0.25 mg in chronic insomnia. *Current Therapeutic Research*, 1990; 48(3):555–67.

Scharf, M., G. Vogel, M. Kallaman, and R. Ochs. Dose-response of zolpidem in elderly patients with chronic insomnia. *Sleep Research*, 1991; 20:84.

Schneider, L., P. Syapin, and S. Pawluczyk. Seizures following triazolam withdrawal despite benzodiazepine treatment. *Journal of Clinical Psychiatry*, 1987; 48(10):418–19.

Shader, R. I., and D. J. Greenblatt. Triazolam and anterograde amnesia: all is not well in the Z-zone. *Journal of Clinical Psychopharmacology*, 1983; 3(5):273.

Shorr, D. I., and S. F. Bauwens. Diagnosis and treatment of outpatient insomnia by psychiatric and nonpsychiatric physicians. *American Journal of Medicine*, 1992; 93(1):78–82.

Shorr, D. I., and S. F. Bauwens. Effects of patient age and physician training in choice and dose of benzodiazepine-hypnotic drugs. *Archives of Internal Medicine*, 1990; 150: 293–95.

Top 200 drugs of 1995. *Pharmacy Times,* April 1995, 27–36.

Vogel, G., A. Thurmond, M. MacIntosh, and T. Clifton. The effects of zolpidem [Ambien] on transient insomnia. *Sleep Research*, 1988; 17:67.

Walsh, J., P. Schweitzer, J. Sugerman, and M. Muehlbach. Transient insomnia associated with a 3-hour phase advance of sleep time and treatment with zolpidem. *Journal of Clinical Psychopharmacology*, 1990; 10:184–89.

Wolfe, S. M. *Public Citizen's Health Research Group Health Letter*, March 1995; 11(3):1–14.

Wolfe, S. M., and R. Hope. *Worst Pills, Best Pills II: The Older Adult's Guide to Avoiding Drug-Induced Death or Illness*. Washington, D.C.: Public Citizen's Health Research Group, 1993.

Wysowski, D. K., and D. Barash. Adverse behavioral reactions attributed to triazolam in the Food and Drug Administration's spontaneous reporting system. *Archives of Internal Medicine*, 1991; 151:2003–8.

Wysowski, D. K., and C. Baum. Outpatient use of prescription sedative-hypnotic drugs in the United States, 1970 through 1989. *Archives of Internal Medicine*, 1991; 151:1779–83.

Chapter 9. Smoking Cessation: Zyban (Bupropion)

Correspondence: Zyban. GlaxoWellcome Medical Services. August 27, 1997.

Dalack, G. W., et al. Mood, major depression, and fluoxetine response in cigarette smokers. *American Journal of Psychiatry*, 1995; 152(3):398–403.

Ferry, L. H., and R. J. Burchette. Evaluation of bupropion versus placebo for treatment of nicotine dependence, in *New Research Program and Abstracts*, 147th Annual Meeting of the American Psychiatric Association. Washington, D.C., 1994, 199–200.

Ferry, L. H., et al. Enhancement of smoking cessation using the antidepressant bupropion hydrochloride (Abstract). *Circulation*, 1992; 86:671.

Freyer, F. J. (Associated Press). Breakthrough smoking-cessation drug contains no nicotine. *San Diego Union-Tribune*, August 3, 1997, page D-3.

Lief, H. I. Bupropion treatment of depression to assist smoking cessation. *American Journal of Psychiatry*, 1996; 153(3):442.

Zyban Sustained-Release Tablets (Bupropion). Package Insert, GlaxoWellcome, 1997.

Chapter 10. Medications for Ulcers, Esophagitis, and Heartburn

Babb, R. R. Cimetidine: clinical uses and possible side effects. *Postgraduate Medicine*, 1980; 68(6):87–93.

Berstad, A., et al. Treatment of duodenal ulcer with ranitidine, a new histamine H2-receptor antagonist. *Scandinavian Journal of Gastroenterology*, 1980; 15(5):637.

Blair, D. I., B. Kaplan, and J. Spiegler. Patient characteristics and lifestyle recommendations in the treatment of gastroesophageal reflux disease. *Journal of Family Practice*, 1997; 44(3):266–72.

Callaghan, J. T., A. Rubin, M. P. Knadler, and R. F. Bergstrom. Nizatidine, and H2-receptor antagonist: disposition and safety in the elderly. *Journal of Clinical Pharmacology*, 1987; 27(8):618–24.

Campion, E. W., J. Avorn, V. A. Reder, and N. J. Olins. Over-medication of the low-weight elderly. *Archives of Internal Medicine*, 1987; 147(5):945–47.

Cloud, M. L., W. W. Offen, and C. Matsumoto. Healing and subsequent recurrence of duodenal ulcer in a clinical trial comparing nizatidine 300-mg and 100-mg evening doses and placebo in the treatment of active duodenal ulcer. *Current Therapeutics and Research, Clinical Experience*, 1989; 45(3):359–67.

D'Alessandro, A., and S. Seri. Comparison of three different methods for evaluation of Helicobacter pylori (H.P.) in human dental plaque. *Bollettino—Societa Italiana Biologia Sperimentale*, 1992; 68(12):769–73; Abstract.

Desai, H. G., et al. Dental plaque: a permanent reservoir of Helicobacter pylori? *Scandinavian Journal of Gastroenterology*, 1991; 26(11):1205–8.

Dobrilla, G., et al. Placebo controlled studies with ranitidine in duodenal ulcer. *Scandinavian Journal of Gastroenterology*, 1981; 69(suppl):103–104.

Dobrilla, G., G. de Pretis, M. Felder, and F. Chilovi. Endoscopic double-blind controlled trial of ranitidine vs placebo in the short-term treatment of duodenal ulcer. *Hepato-Gastroenterology*, 1981; 28(1):49–52.

Drugs for treatment of peptic ulcers. *The Medical Letter on Drugs and Therapeutics*, 1997; 39(991):1–4.

Dyck, W. P., et al. Treatment of duodenal ulcers in the United States. *Scandinavian Journal of Gastroenterology*, 1987; 22(suppl 136):47–55.

Epstein, C. M. Histamine H2 antagonists and the nervous system. *American Family Physician*, 1985; 32(6):109–12.

Fiasse, R., et al. Omeprazole in the treatment of patients with severe reflux oesophagitis not responding to H2-receptor antagonists and ineligible for surgery. *Acta Gastroenterologica Belgica*, 1990; 53(5–6):573–84.

Fiorucci, S., et al. Do anticholinergics interact with histamine H2 receptor antagonists on night intragastric acidity in active duodenal ulcer patients? *American Journal of Gastroenterology*, 1988; 83(12):1371–75.

Fiorucci, S., et al. Effects of low and high doses of famotidine and ranitidine on nocturnal gastric pH. *Digestive Diseases and Science*, 1986; 31(suppl 10):393S.

Glaxo Pharmaceuticals. Zantac Product Information, June 1993.

Khandaker, K., et al. DNA fingerprints of Helicobacter pylori from mouth and antrum of patients with chronic ulcer dyspepsia [letter]. *Lancet*, 1993; 342(8873):751.

Kolata, G. (New York Times News Service). What ails elderly often prescribed. *San Diego Union-Tribune*, July 27, 1994, A-20.

Kurata, J. H., A. N. Nogawa, Y. K. Chen, and C. E. Parker. Dyspepsia in primary care: perceived causes, reasons for improvement, and satisfaction with care. *Journal of Family Practice*, 1997; 44(3):281–88.

Landahl, S., et al. Pharmacokinetic study of omeprazole in elderly healthy volunteers. *Clinical Pharmacokinetics*, 1992; 23(6):469–76.

Langman, J. S., D. A. Henry, G. Bell, and A. Ogilvie. Cimetidine and ranitidine in duodenal ulcer. *British Medical Journal*, 1980; 281(6238):473–74.

Langman, J. S., D. A. Henry, and A. Ogilvie. Ranitidine and cimetidine for duodenal ulcer. *Scandinavian Journal of Gastroenterology*, 1981; (suppl);69:115–17.

Lauritsen, K., et al. Effect of 10 mg and 20 mg omeprazole daily on duodenal ulcer: double-blind comparative trial. *Alimentary Pharmacology and Therapeutics*, February 1989; 3(1):59–67.

Lauritsen, K., et al. Omeprazole 20 mg three days a week and 10 mg daily in prevention of duodenal ulcer relapse; double-blind comparative trial. *Gastroenterology*, 1991; 100(3):663–69.

Lind, T., C. Cederberg, M. Axelson, and L. Olbe. Long-term acid inhibitory effect of different daily doses of omeprazole 24 hours after dosing. *Scandinavian Journal of Gastroenterology*, 1986; 21(suppl 118):137–8.

Lind, T., C. Cederberg, M. Olausson, and L. Olbe. Omeprazole in elderly duodenal ulcer patients: relationship between reduction in gastric acid secretion and fasting plasma gastrin. *European Journal of Clinical Pharmacology*, 1991; 40(6):557–60.

Metz, D. C., et al. Currently used doses of omeprazole in Zollinger-Ellison symdrome are too high. *Gastroenterology*, 1992; 103:1498–1508.

Nguyen, A. M., et al. Detection of Helicobacter pylori in dental plaque by reverse transcription-polymerase chain reaction. *Journal of Clinical Microbiology*, 1993; 31(4):783–87.

Porro, G. B., and F. Parente. Nature of non-ulcer dyspepsia and related conditions. *Baillieres Clinical Gastroenterology*, 1995; 9(3):549–62.

Regardh, C. G. Pharmacokinetics and metabolism of omeprazole in man. *Scandinavian Journal of Gastroenterology*, 1986; 118(suppl):99–104.

Robinson, M., et al. Effect of different doses of omeprazole on 24-hour oesophageal acid exposure in patients with gastro-oesophageal reflux. *Alimentary Pharmacology and Therapeutics*, 1991; 5:645–51.

Samanta, A., D. Nahass, and S. Habba. Efficacy of nizatidine: a new H2 receptor antagonist in the treatment of duodenal ulcer; a dose response study. *American Journal of Gastroenterology*, 1986; 81(9):852.

Savarino, V., et al. Low bedtime doses of H2-receptor antagonists for acute treatment of duodenal ulcers. *Digestive Diseases and Sciences*, 1989; 34(7):1043–46.

Sherman, D. S., J. Avorn, and E. W. Campion. Cimetidine use in nursing homes: prolonged therapy and excessive doses. *Journal of the American Geriatrics Society*, 1987; 35(11):1023–27.

Simonsen, L. Top 200 drugs of 1993. *Pharmacy Times*, April 1994.

Smallwood, R. A., et al. Safety of acid-suppressing drugs. *Digestive Diseases and Sciences*, 1995; 40(2 Suppl):63S–80S.

Smith, J. L. Clinical pharmacology of famotidine. *Digestion*, 1985; 32(suppl 1):15–23.

Top 200 drugs of 1995. *Pharmacy Times*, April 1995, 27–36.

Wolfe, S. M., and R. E. Hope. *Worst Pills, Best Pills II: The Older Adult's Guide to Avoiding Drug-Induced Death or Illness*. Washington, D.C.: Public Citizen Health Research Group, 1993.

Young, M. D., et al. Determining the optimal dosage regimen for H2-receptor antagonist therapy—a dose validation approach. *Alimentary Pharmacology and Therapeutics*, 1989; 3:47–57.

Zakim, D., and T. D. Boyer. *Hepatology: A Textbook of Liver Disease*, 2nd ed. Philadelphia: W. B. Saunders, 1990.

Chapter 11. Cholesterol-Lowering Medications

Arca, M., G. L. Vega, and S. M. Grundy. Hypercholesterolemia in postmenopausal women: metabolic defects and response to low-dose lovastatin. *JAMA*, 1994; 271(6):453–59.

Bach, L. A., M. E. Cooper, R. C. O'Brien, and G. Jerums. The use of simvastatin, an HMG CoA reductase inhibitor, in older patients with hypercholesterolemia and atherosclerosis. *Journal of the American Geriatric Society*, 1990; 38:10–14.11.

Baseline serum cholesterol and treatment effect in the Scandinavian Simvastatin Survival Study (4S) [see comments]. *Lancet*, 1995; 345(8960):1274–75.

Behounek, B. D., et al. A multinational study of the effects of low-dose pravastatin in patients with non-insulin-dependent diabetes mellitus and hypercholesterolemia. Pravastatin Multinational Study Group for Diabetes. *Clinical Cardiology*, 1994; 17(10): 558–62.

Berger, G. M., et al. Treatment of hypercholesterolemia with the

HMG CoA reductase inhibitor, simvastatin. *Cardiovascular Drugs and Therapy*, 1989; 3:219–27.

Byington, R. P., et al. Pravastatin, lipids, and atherosclerosis in the carotid arteries (PLAC-II). *American Journal of Cardiology*, 1995; 76(9):54C–59C.

Byington, R. P., et al. Reduction in cardiovascular events during pravastatin therapy. Pooled analysis of clinical events of the Pravastatin Atherosclerosis Intervention Program. *Circulation*, 1995; 92(9):2419–25.

The Canadian Coronary Atherosclerosis Intervention Trial. *Circulation*, 1994; 89(3):959–68.

Choice of lipid-lowering drugs. *The Medical Letter on Drugs and Therapeutics*, 1996; 38:67–69.

Cleeman, J. I. Educating professionals and the general public about cholesterol. *Lipid Management in Clinical Practice: Report from the National Lipid Educated Council*, 1996; 1(2):1–3.

Crouse, J. R. 3rd, et al. Pravastatin, lipids, and atherosclerosis in the carotid arteries (PLAC-II). *American Journal of Cardiology*, 1995; 75(7):455–59.

Expert Panel on Detection, Evaluation, and Treatment of High Blood Cholesterol in Adults. Summary of the second report of the National Cholesterol Education Program Expert Panel on Detection, Evaluation, and Treatment on High Blood Cholesterol in Adults (Adult Treatment Panel II). *JAMA*, 1993; 269:3015–23.

Furberg, C. D., et al. Effect of lovastatin on early carotid atherosclerosis and cardiovascular events. Asymptomatic Carotid Artery Progression Study (ACAPS) Research Group [see comments]. *Circulation*, October 1994; 90(4):1679–87.

Gonzalez, E. R. The pharmacist's role in lipid reduction therapy. *Pharmacy Times*, April 1997; 63(4):65–70.

Gotto, A. M. Coronary heart disease in the United States: the scope of the problem. *Lipid Management in Clinical Practice: Report from the National Lipid Educated Council*, 1996; 1(2):4.

Gould, A. L., et al. Cholesterol reduction yields clinical benefit. A new look at old data. *Circulation*, 1995; 91(8):2274–82.

Grundy, S. M., et al. Guide to primary prevention of cardiovascular diseases. A statement for healthcare professionals from the Task Force on Risk Reduction. American Heart Association Science Advisory and Coordinating Committee. *Circulation*, 1997; 95(9):2329–31.

Haria, M., and D. McTavish. Pravastatin. A reappraisal of its pharmacological properties and clinical effectiveness in the management of coronary heart disease. *Drugs*, 1997; 53(2):299–336.

Herd, J., et al. Beneficial effects of fluvastatin on clinical cardiac and all fatal events in patients with mild cholesterol elevations. *Journal of Investigative Medicine*, 1997; 45(3):222A.

Herd, J., et al. The effect of fluvastatin on coronary atherosclerosis: the lipoprotein and coronary atherosclerosis study (LCAS). Findings presented at American Heart Association Annual Meeting, New Orleans, November 13, 1996. Information on file, Sandoz Pharmaceutical Corporation, East Hanover, NJ.

Jacotot, B., J. D. Banga, P. Pfister, and M. Mehra. Efficacy of a low dose-range of fluvastatin (XU 62–320) in the treatment of primary hypercholesterolaemia. A dose-response study in 431 patients. The French-Dutch Fluvastatin Study Group. *British Journal of Clinical Pharmacology*, September 1994; 38(3):257–63.

Jokubaitis, L. A. Development and pharmacology of fluvastatin. *British Journal of Clinical Practice [Symposium Supplement]*, 1996; 77A:11–15.

Jones, P. H., et al. Once-daily pravastatin in patients with primary hypercholesterolaemia: a dose-response study. *Clinical Cardiology*, February 1991; 14(2):146–51.

Jukema, J. W., et al. Effects of lipid lowering by pravastatin on progression and regression of coronary artery disease in symptomatic men with normal to moderately elevated serum cholesterol levels. The Regression Growth Evaluation Statin Study (REGRESS). *Circulation*, 1995; 91(10):2528–40.

Kobashigawa, J. A., et al. Low-dose lovastatin safely lowers cholesterol after cardiac transplantation. *Circulation*, 1990; 82(5 Suppl):IV281–3.

Lansberg, P. J., et al. Long-term efficacy and tolerability of simvastatin in a large cohort of elderly hypercholesterolemic patients. *Atherosclerosis*, 1995; 116(2):153–62.

Lescol Package Insert, Sandoz Pharmaceuticals Corporation, East Hanover, NJ, November 1996.

Mevacor Package Insert, Merck & Co., West Point, PA, September 1996.

Mol, J. T., et al. Effects of synvinolin (MK-733) [simvastatin] on plasma lipids in familial hypercholesterolemia. *Lancet*, 1986; 2: 936–39.

Nash, D. T. Meeting national cholesterol education goals in clinical practice—a comparison of lovastatin and fluvastatin in primary prevention. *American Journal of Cardiology*, 1996; 78(6A): 26–31.

National Cholesterol Education Program: second report of the National Cholesterol Education Program Expert Panel on Detection, Evaluation, and Treatment on High Blood Cholesterol in Adults (Adult Treatment Panel II). *Circulation*, 1994; 89:1329–1445.

Plosker, G. L., and A. J. Wagstaff. Fluvastatin: a review of its pharmacology and use in the management of hypercholesterolaemia. *Drugs*, 1996; 51(3):433–59.

Randomised trial of cholesterol lowering in 4444 patients with coronary heart disease: the Scandinavian Simvastatin Survival Study (4S). *Lancet*, 1994; 344(8934):1383–89.

Roberts, W. C. The underused miracle drugs: the statin drugs are to atherosclerosis what penicillin was to infectious disease [editorial]. *American Journal of Cardiology*, 1996; 78:377–78.

Rubinstein, A., Y. Lurie, I. Groskop, and M. Weintrob. Cholesterol-lowering effects of a 10 mg daily dose of lovastatin in patients with initial total cholesterol levels 200 to 240 mg/dl (5.18 to 6.21 mmol/liter). *American Journal of Cardiology*, 1991; 68(11):1123–26.

Sacks, F. M., et al. The effect of pravastatin on coronary events after myocardial infarction in patients with average cholesterol levels. Cholesterol and Recurrent Events Trial investigators. *New England Journal of Medicine*, 1996; 335(14):1001–9.

Saku, K., J. Sasaki, and K. Arakawa. Low-dose effect of simvastatin on serum lipids, lipoproteins, and apolipoproteins in patients with hypercholesterolemia. *Clinical Therapeutics*, 1989; 11(2):247–57.

Shepherd, J., et al. Prevention of coronary heart disease with pravastatin in men with hypercholesterolemia. West of Scotland Coronary Prevention Study Group. *New England Journal of Medicine*, 1995; 333(20):1301–7.

Sherman, D. S., J. Avorn, and E. W. Campion. Cimetidine use in nursing homes: prolonged therapy and excessive doses. *Journal of the American Geriatrics Society*, 1987; 35(11):1023–27.

Sinzinger, H., and C. Pirich. The RED-LIP study—pravastatin in primary isolated hypercholesterolemia—an open, prospective, multicenter trial. *Wiener Klinische Wochenschrift*, 1994; 106(23):721–27; Abstract.

Sprecher, D. L., et al. Low-dose combined therapy with fluvastatin and cholestyramine in hyperlipidemic patients [see comments]. *Annals of Internal Medicine*, 1994; 120(7):537–43.

Steinhagen-Thiessen, E. Comparative efficacy and tolerability of 5 and 10 mg simvastatin and 10 mg pravastatin in moderate primary hypercholesterolemia. Simvastatin Pravastatin European Study Group. *Cardiology*, 1994; 85(3–4):244–54.

Top 200 drugs of 1995. *Pharmacy Times*, April 1995, 27–36.

Tuomilehto, J., et al. Dose-response of simvastatin in primary hypercholesterolemia. *Journal of Cardiovascular Pharmacology*, 1994; 24(6):941–49.

Walker, J. F., R. A. Pingeon, and D. A. Shapiro. Efficacy and tolerability of simvastatin in the elderly. *Drug Investigation*, 1990; 2(suppl. 2):53–56.

Walker, J. F., and J. A. Tobert. The clinical efficacy of lovastatin and MK-733 [simvastatin]—an overview. *European Heart Journal*, 1987; 8(Suppl. E):93–96.

Waters, D., et al. Effects of cholesterol lowering on the progression of coronary atherosclerosis in women. A Canadian Coronary Atherosclerosis Intervention Trial (CCAIT) substudy. *Circulation*, November 1, 1995; 92(9):2404–10.

Waters, D., et al. Effects of monotherapy with an HMG-CoA reductase inhibitor on the progression of coronary atherosclerosis as assessed by serial quantitative arteriography.

Yoshida, H., et al. Effect of low-dose simvastatin on cholesterol levels, oxidative susceptibility, and antioxidant levels of low-density lipoproteins in patients with hypercholesterolemia: a pilot study. *Clinical Therapeutics*, May–June 1995; 17(3):379–89.

Yoshino, G., et al. Comparison of the effects of pravastatin and simvastatin in hypercholesterolemic subjects. *Current Therapeutic Research*, 1990; 48(2):259–67.

Zocor Package Insert, Merck & Co., West Point, PA, December 1996.

Chapter 12. Antihypertensive Medications

Abrams, L. Matching drugs to patients: hypertension. *The Practitioner*, July 1994; 238:527–30.

Albert Einstein College of Medicine, Office of Continuing Medication. *Hypertension Management Today*, 1997; 1(3):1–14.

Albert Einstein College of Medicine, Office of Continuing Medication. *Hypertension Management Today*, 1996; 1(1):1–14.

Burt, V. L., et al. Prevalence of hypertension in the U.S. adult population. Results from the Third National Health and Nutrition Examination Survey, 1988–1991. *Hypertension*, 1995; 25(3):305–13.

Burt, V. L., et al. Trends in the prevalence, awareness, treatment, and control of hypertension in the adult U.S. population. Data from the health examination surveys, 1960 to 1991. *Hypertension*, 1995; 26(1):60–69.

Carr, A. A., L. M. Prisant, and P. B. Bottini. Hypertension: not solely a blood pressure problem. *Postgraduate Medicine*, 1994; 95(6):79–86.

Chrysant, S. G. Antihypertensive effectiveness of low-dose lisinopril-hydrochlorothiazide combination. A large multicenter study. Lisinopril-Hydrochlorothiazide Group. *Archives of Internal Medicine*, 1994; 154(7):737–43.

Correspondence, Dr. Michael Ziegler, February 7, 1995, pages 1–3.

Clobass Study Group. Low-dose clonidine administration in the treatment of mild or moderate essential hypertension: results from a double-blind placebo-controlled study (Clobass). *Journal of Hypertension*, 1990; 8(6):539–46.

Corea, L., et al. Verapamil 240 SR versus verapamil 120 SR in arterial hypertension. A randomized double-blind, placebo-controlled study with 24-hour ambulatory blood pressure monitoring. *Cardiovascular Drugs and Therapy*, 1990; 4(6):1501–7.

Crespo, C. J., C. M. Loria, and V. L. Burt. Hypertension and other cardiovascular disease risk factors among Mexican Americans, Cuban Americans, and Puerto Ricans from the Hispanic Health and Nutrition Examination Survey. *Public Health Reports*, 1996; 111 Suppl 2:7–10.

Curzen, N., and H. Purcell. Matching the treatment to the patient in hypertension. *Practitioner*, 1997; 241(1572):152–56.

Cushman, W. C. Systolic hypertension in the elderly. Safe treatment with low-dose thiazide diuretics. *Postgraduate Medicine*, 1993; 94(2):143–48, 151.

Cushman, W. C., et al. Treatment of hypertension in the elderly. III. Response of isolated systolic hypertension to various doses of hydrochlorothiazide: results of a Department of Veterans Affairs cooperative study. *Archives of Internal Medicine*, 1991; 151(10): 1954–60.

Ding, Y. A., T. C. Chou, and K. C. Lin. Effects of long-acting propranolol and verapamil on blood pressure, platelet function, metabolic and rheological properties in hypertension. *Journal of Human Hypertension*, 1994; 8(4):273–78.

Ferguson, R. P., T. Wetle, D. Dubitzky, and D. Winsemius. Relative importance to elderly patients of effectiveness, adverse effects, convenience and cost of antihypertensive medications. A pilot study. *Drugs and Aging*, 1994; 4(1):56–62.

The fifth report of the Joint National Committee on Detection, Evaluation, and Treatment of High Blood Pressure (JNC V). *Archives of Internal Medicine*, 1993; 153(2):154–83.

Fletcher, A., and C. Bulpitt. Quality of life and antihypertensive drugs in the elderly. *Aging*, 1992; 4(2):115–23.

Fogari, R., et al. Fixed combination of benazepril and very low dose hydrochlorothiazide in the treatment of mild to moderate essential hypertension: evaluation by 24-hour noninvasive ambulatory blood pressure monitoring. *International Journal of Clinical Pharmacology and Therapeutics*, 1994; 32(11):606–11.

Frohlich, E. D. Continuing advances in hypertension: the Joint National Committee's fifth report. *American Journal of the Medical Sciences*, 1995; 310(suppl 1):S48–52.

Furberg, C. D., B. M. Psaty, and J. V. Meyer. Nifedipine. Dose-related increase in mortality in patients with coronary heart disease. *Circulation*, 1995; 92(5):1326–31.

Gottdiener, J. S., et al. Effect of single-drug therapy on reduction of left ventricular mass in mild to moderate hypertension: comparison of six antihypertensive agents. The Department of Veterans Affairs Cooperative Study Group on Antihypertensive Agents. *Circulation*, 1997; 95(8):2007–14.

Hart, W. Lisinopril-hydrochlorothiazide combination compared with the monocomponents in elderly hypertensive patients. *Journal of Human Hypertension*, 1991; 5(suppl 2):85–89.

Holzgreve, H., et al. Hydrochlorothiazide and verapamil in the treatment of hypertension. The Verapamil Versus Diuretic (VERDI) Trial Research Group. *Journal of Cardiovascular Pharmacology*, 1991; 18(suppl 6):S33–37.

Houghton, J. L., et al. Racial differences in myocardial ischemia and coronary flow reserve in hypertension. *Journal of the American College of Cardiology*, 1994; 23(5):1123–29.

Ishikawa, K., et al. Short-acting nifedipine and diltiazem do not reduce the incidence of cardiac events in patients with healed myocardial infarction. Secondary Prevention Group. *Circulation*, May 20, 1997; 95(10):2368–73.

Ishizaki, T., et al. A dose ranging study of atenolol in hypertension: fall in blood pressure and plasma renin activity, beta-blockade and steady-state pharmacokinetics. *British Journal of Clinical Pharmacology*, 1983; 16(1):17–25.

Jaattela, A., S. Baandrup, J. Houtzagers, and G. Westergren. The efficacy of low dose metoprolol CR/ZOK in mild hypertension and in elderly patients with mild to moderate hypertension. *Journal of Clinical Pharmacology*, 1990; 30(suppl 2):S66–71.

Jachuck, S. J., H. Brierly, S. Jachuck, and P. Willcox. The effect of hypotension drugs on the quality of life. *Journal of the Royal College of General Practitioners*, 1982; 32:103–5.

Kaplan, N. M. Guidelines for the treatment of hypertension: an American view. Fifth Joint National Committee. *Journal of Hypertension*, 1995; 13(suppl 2):S113–17.

Kelly, J. L., and L. L. Hart. Hydrochlorothiazide dosage in hypertension. *Dicp*, 1990; 24(2):157–58.

Knauf, H. The role of low-dose diuretics in essential hypertension. *Journal of Cardiovascular Pharmacology*, 1993; 22(suppl 6):S1–7.

Kochar, M. S., K. M. Landry, and S. M. Ristow. Effects of reduction in dose and discontinuation of hydrochlorothiazide in patients with controlled essential hypertension. *Archives of Internal Medicine*, 1990; 150(5):1009–11.

Lang, H. The results of a large multicentre study comparing low-dose lisinopril-hydrochlorothiazide with the monocomponents. *Journal of Human Hypertension*, 1991; 5(suppl 2):73–6.

Langenfeld, M. R., and R. E. Schmieder. Salt and left ventricular hypertrophy: what are the links? *Journal of Human Hypertension*, 1995; 9(11):909–16.

Lewin, A. J., M. C. Lueg, S. Targum, and P. Cardenas. A clinical trial evaluating the 24-hour effects of bisoprolol/hydrochlorothiazide 5 mg/6.25 mg combination in patients with mild to moderate hypertension. *Clinical Cardiology*, 1993; 16(10):732–36.

Marshall, A. J., D. W. Barritt, S. Heaton, and J. D. Harry. Dose response for blood pressure and degree of cardiac beta-blockade with atenolol. *Postgraduate Medical Journal*, 1979; 55(646):537–40.

Middlemost, S. J., R. Tager, J. Davis, and P. Sareli. Effectiveness of enalapril in combination with low-dose hydrochlorothiazide versus enalapril alone for mild to moderate systemic hypertension in black patients. *American Journal of Cardiology*, 1994; 73(15): 1092–97.

Neaton, J. D., et al. Treatment of mild hypertension study: final results. *JAMA*, 1993; 207:713–24.

Opie, L. ACE inhibitors: almost too good to be true. *Scientific American Science and Medicine*, July/August 1994, 14–23.

Pahor, M., et al. Calcium-channel blockade and incidence of cancer in aged populations. *Lancet*, 1996; 348(9026):493–97.

Pahor, M., et al. Risk of gastrointestinal haemorrhage with calcium antagonists in hypertensive persons over 67 years old. *Lancet*, 1996; 347(9008):1061–65.

Pogue, V. A., C. Ellis, J. Michel, and C. K. Francis. New staging system of the fifth Joint National Committee report on the detection, evaluation, and treatment of high blood pressure (JNC-V) alters assessment of the severity and treatment of hypertension. *Hypertension*, 1996; 28(5):713–18.

Prisant, L. M., et al. Low-dose drug combination therapy: an alternative first-line approach to hypertension treatment. *American Heart Journal*, 1995; 130(2):359–66.

Psaty, B. M., et al. The risk of myocardial infarction associated with antihypertensive drug therapies. *JAMA*, 1995; 274(8):620–25.

Rappelli, A. Controlling hypertension: lisinopril-hydrochlorothiazide vs captopril-hydrochlorothiazide. An Italian multicentre study. *Journal of Human Hypertension*, 1991; 5(suppl 2):55–57.

Rappelli, A., et al. Evaluation of the safety and efficacy of the lisinopril + hydrochlorothiazide and captopril + hydrochlorothiazide combinations in the treatment of essential arterial hypertension. *Minerva Medica*, 1992; 83(1–2):57–64, Abstract.

Rutledge, D. R. Race and hypertension. What is clinically relevant? *Drugs*, 1994; 47(6):914–32.

Rutledge, D. R., Y. Sun, and E. A. Ross. Polymorphisms within the atrial natriuretic peptide gene in essential hypertension. *Journal of Hypertension*, 1995; 13(9):953–55.

Sabella, B. Hypertension in African-Americans. *Hypertension Management Today*, Albert Einstein College of Medicine, Office of Continuing Medication, 1997; 1(3):11–12.

Safety of calcium-channel blockers. *The Medical Letter on Drugs and Therapeutics*, 1997; 39:13–14.

Sambol, N. C., and L. B. Sheiner. Population dose versus response of betaxolol and atenolol: a comparison of potency and variability [see comments]. *Clinical Pharmacology and Therapeutics*, 1991; 49(1):24–31.

Sambol, N. C., A. Bostrom, and R. L. Williams. Effect of hydrochlorothiazide 25 mg/day on essential hypertension. *Clinical Pharmacy*, 1990; 9(11):873–75.

Stein, C. M., P. Neill, and T. Kusemamuriwo. Antihypertensive effects of low doses of hydrochlorothiazide in hypertensive black Zimbabweans. *International Journal of Cardiology*, 1992; 37(2):231–35.

Venter, C. P. Low-dose thiazide diuretics in primary hypertension [letter]. *South African Medical Journal*, 1992; 81(8):437.

Weber, M. A., and J. H. Laragh. Hypertension: steps forward and steps backward. The Joint National Committee fifth report. *Archives of Internal Medicine*, 1993; 153(2):149–52.

Weir, M. R., et al. A dose escalation trial comparing the combination of diltiazem SR and hydrochlorothiazide with the monotherapies in patients with essential hypertension. *Journal of Human Hypertension*, 1992; 6(2):133–38.

Whelton, P. K., et al. Effects of oral potassium on blood pressure. Meta-analysis of randomized controlled clinical trials. *JAMA*, 1997; 28, 277(20):1624–32.

Zhang, Z. J., W. W. Cheng, and Y. M. Yang. Low dose of processed rhubarb in preventing pregnancy induced hypertension. *Chung-Hua Fu Chan Ko Tsa Chih Chinese Journal of Obstetrics and Gynecology*, 1994; 29(8):463–64, 509. Abstract.

Ziegler, M. G., E. Lernhardt, and V. Solt-Buzsaki. Dose response to hydrochlorothiazide in hypertensives receiving a calcium channel blocker. *Clinical and Experimental Hypertension—Theory and Practice*, 1988; A10(5):791–800.

Chapter 13. Aspirin (Acetylsalicylic Acid) and Tylenol (Acetaminophen)

Batkin, S., S. J. Taussig, and J. Szekerezes. Antimetastatic effect of bromelain with or without its proteolytic and anticoagulant activity. *Journal of Cancer Research and Clinical Oncology*, 1988; 114(5):507–8.

Begley, S. Jagged little pill. *Newsweek*, August 18, 1997, 66.

Brune, K. The pharmacological profile of non-opioid (OTC) analgesics: aspirin, paracetamol (acetaminophen), ibuprofen, and *Agents and Actions*, 1988; 25(suppl):9–19.

Buerke, M., W. Pittroff, J. Meyer, and H. Darius. Aspirin therapy: optimized platelet inhibition with different loading and maintenance doses. *American Heart Journal*, 1995; 130(3 Pt 1):465–72.

Cappelleri, J. C., J. Lau, B. Kupelnick, and T. C. Chalmers. Efficacy and safety of different aspirin dosages on vascular diseases in high-risk patients. A metaregression analysis. *Online Journal of Current Clinical Trials*, 1995; Doc No 174:[6442].

Col, N. F., et al. Does aspirin consumption affect the presentation or severity of acute myocardial infarction? *Archives of Internal Medicine*, 1995; 155(13):1386–89.

Cooper, S. A. Comparative analgesic efficacies of aspirin and acetaminophen. *Archives of Internal Medicine*, 1981; 141(3 spec No):282–85.

Cooper, S. A. Five studies on ibuprofen for postsurgical dental pain. *American Journal of Medicine*, 1984; July: 70–77.

Cooper, S. A., et al. Evaluation of oxycodone and acetaminophen in treatment of postoperative dental pain. *Oral Surgery, Oral Medicine, and Oral Pathology*, 1980; 50(6):496–501.

Dalen, J. E., and R. J. Goldberg. Prophylactic aspirin and the elderly population. *Clinics in Geriatric Medicine*, 1992; 8(1):119–26.

Day, L., and M. Barnfield. Who should be taking daily aspirin? *Practitioner*, 1995; 239(1552):426–30.

Faich, G. A. Analgesic risks and pharmacoepidemiology [editorial]. *JAMA*, 1986; 256(13):1788.

Faulkner, G., P. Prichard, K. Somerville, and M. J. Langman. Aspirin and bleeding peptic ulcers in the elderly. *British Medical Journal*, 1988; 297(6659):1311–13.

Gathright, A. Don't take over-the-counter painkillers like candy, experts warn. *San Diego Union-Tribune*, January 26, 1995, A-18.

Haney, D. Q. (Associated Press.) Heavy use of drugs like Tylenol found to put kidneys, liver at risk. *San Diego Union-Tribune*, December 23, 1994, A-27.

Heinicke, R. M., et al. Effect of bromelain on human platelet aggregation. *Experimentia*, 1972; 28:844–45.

Hirsh, J., et al. Aspirin and other platelet-active drugs. The relationship between dose, effectiveness, and side effects. *Chest*, 1992; 102(suppl 4):327S–336S.

Hoffmann, W., et al. Reevaluation of the Cottbus Reinfarction Study with 30 mg aspirin per day 4 years after the end of the study. *Prostaglandins, Leukotrienes, and Essential Fatty Acids*, 1991; 42(2):137–39.

Johnson, A. G., and R. O. Day. The problems and pitfalls of NSAID therapy in the elderly (Part I). *Drugs and Aging*, 1991; 1(2):30–43.

Karsh, J. Adverse reactions and interactions with aspirin. Considerations in the treatment of the elderly patient. *Drug Safety*, 1990; 5(5):317–27.

Kaufman, D. W., et al. Nonsteroidal anti-inflammatory drug use in relation to major upper gastrointestinal bleeding. *Clinical Pharmacology and Therapeutics*, April 1993; 53(4):485–94.

Kelly, G. S. Bromelain: a literature review and discussion of its therapeutic application. *Alternative Medicine Review*, 1996; 1(4): 243–57.

Lotz-Winter, H. On the pharmacology of bromelain: an update with special regard to animal studies on dose-dependent effects. *Planta Medica*, 1990; 56(3):249–53.

McAnally, L. E., C. R. Corn, and S. F. Hamilton. Aspirin for the prevention of vascular death in women. *Annals of Pharmacotherapy*, 1992; 26(12):1530–4.

McQuay, H. J., et al. A multiple dose comparison of combinations of ibuprofen and codeine and paracetamol, codeine and caffeine after third molar surgery. *Anaesthesia*, 1992; 47(8):672–7.

Montalescot, G., G. Drobinski, and D. Thomas. [What dose of aspirin should be prescribed in patients with coronary disease?] *Annales de Cardiologie et D'Angeiologie*, 1995; 44(8):469–72, Abstract.

Morita, A. H., et al. Chromatographic fractionation and characterization of the active platelet aggregation inhibitory factor of bromelain. *Archives of Internal Pharmacology and Therapeutics*, 1979; 239:340–50.

Naschitz, J. E., et al. Overt gastrointestinal bleeding in the course of chronic low-dose aspirin administration for secondary prevention of arterial occlusive disease. *American Journal of Gastroenterology*, 1990; 85(4):408–11.

Oren, R., et al. Gastroduodenal injury associated with intake of 100–325 mg aspirin daily. *Postgraduate Medical Journal*, 1993; 69(815):712–14.

Pendergrass, P. B., J. N. Scott, L. J. Ream, and M. A. Agna. Effect of small doses of aspirin and acetaminophen on total menstrual loss and pain of cramps and headache. *Gynecologic and Obstetric Investigation*, 1985; 19(1):32–37.

Perneger, T. V., P. K. Whelton, and M. J. Klag. Risk of kidney failure associated with the use of acetaminophen, aspirin, and nonsteroidal antiinflammatory drugs. *New England Journal of Medicine*, 1994; 331(25):1675–79.

Petersen, J. K., F. Hansson, and S. Strid. The effect of an ibuprofen-codeine combination for the treatment of patients with pain after removal of lower third molars. *Journal of Oral and Maxillofacial Surgery*, 1993; 51(6):637–40.

Piletta, P., H. C. Porchet, and P. Dayer. Central analgesic effect of acetaminophen but not of aspirin. *Clinical Pharmacology and Therapeutics*, 1991; 49(4):350–54.

Quiding, H., et al. Ibuprofen plus codeine, ibuprofen, and placebo in a single- and multidose cross-over comparison for coxarthrosis pain. *Pain*, September 1992; 50(3):303–7.

Ridker, P. M., et al. The effect of chronic platelet inhibition with low-dose aspirin on atherosclerotic progression and acute thrombosis: clinical evidence from the Physicians' Health Study. *American Heart Journal*, 1991; 122(6):1588–92.

Settipane, G. A. Adverse reactions to aspirin and related drugs. *Advances in Inflammation Research*, 1984; 6:189–201.

Silagy, C. Aspirin and the elderly. Current status. *Drugs and Aging*, 1993; 3(4):301–7.

Silagy, C. A., et al. Adverse effects of low-dose aspirin in a healthy elderly population. *Clinical Pharmacology and Therapeutics*, 1993; 54(1):84–89.

Skoglund, L. A., P. Skjelbred, and G. Fyllingen. Analgesic efficacy of acetaminophen 1000 mg, acetaminophen 2000 mg, and the combination of acetaminophen 1000 mg and codeine phosphate 60 mg versus placebo in acute postoperative pain. *Pharmacotherapy*, 1991; 11(5):364–69.

Slattery, J., C. P. Warlow, C. J. Shorrock, and M. J. Langman. Risks of gastrointestinal bleeding during secondary prevention of vascular events with aspirin—analysis of gastrointestinal bleeding during the UK-TIA trial. *Gut*, 1995; 37(4):509–11.

Stalnikowicz-Darvasi, R. Gastrointestinal bleeding during low-dose aspirin administration for prevention of arterial occlusive events. A critical analysis. *Journal of Clinical Gastroenterology*, 1995; 21(1):13–16.

Swedish Aspirin Low-Dose Trial (SALT) of 75 mg aspirin as secondary prophylaxis after cerebrovascular ischaemic events. The SALT Collaborative Group. *Lancet*, 1991; 338(8779): 1345–49.

Taussig, S. J., and S. Batkin. Bromelain, the enzyme complex of pineapple (*Ananas comosus*) and its clinical application. An update. *Journal of Ethnopharmacology*, 1988; 22(2):191–203.

Urquhart, E. Analgesic agents and strategies in the dental pain model. *Journal of Dentistry*, 1994; 22(6):336–34.

U.S. Government Food and Drug Administration (FDA). *FDA Medical Bulletin*, May 1994, 8–9.

van Gijn, J. Aspirin: dose and indications in modern stroke prevention. *Neurologic Clinics*, 1992; 10(1):193–207; discussion 208.

Vellini, M., et al. Possible involvement of eicosanoids in the pharmacological action of bromelain. *Arzneimittel-Forschung*, 1986; 36(1):110–12.

Weil, J., et al. Prophylactic aspirin and risk of peptic ulcer bleeding. *British Medical Journal*, 1995; 310(6983): 827–30.

Chapter 14. Anti-Inflammatory Drugs

Aabakken, L. NSAID-associated gastrointestinal damage: methodological considerations and a review of the experience with enteric coated naproxen. *European Journal of Rheumatology and Inflammation*, 1992; 12(2):9–20.

Aisen, P. S. Inflammation and Alzheimer disease. *Molecular and Chemical Neuropathology*, 1996; 28(1–3):83–88.

Akil, M., R. S. Amos, and P. Stewart. Infertility may sometimes be associated with NSAID consumption. *British Journal of Rheumatology*, 1996; 35(1): 76–78.

Barrachina, M. D., et al. Transdermal nitroglycerin prevents nonsteroidal anti-inflammatory drug gastropathy. *European Journal of Pharmacology*, 1995; 281(2):R3–4.

Bloomfield, S. S., J. Mitchell, G. Bichlmeir, and T. P. Barden. Low dose ibuprofen and aspirin analgesia for postpartum uterine cramps. *Clinical Pharmacology and Therapeutics*, 1983; 33(2): 194.

Bernhard, G. C. Worldwide safety experience with nabumetone. *Journal of Rheumatology*, 1992; 19 (suppl 36):48–57.

Brawn, L. A., and C. M. Castleden. Adverse drug reactions. An overview of special considerations in the management of the elderly patient. *Drug Safety*, 1990; 5(6):421–35.

Brooks, C. D., et al. Ibuprofen and aspirin in the treatment of rheumatoid arthritis: a cooperative double-blind trial. *Rheumatology and Physical Medicine*, 1970; 10(suppl): 48–63.

Brown, J. F., P. J. Hanson, and B. J. Whittle. Nitric oxide donors increase mucus gel thickness in rat stomach. *European Journal of Pharmacology*, 1992; 223(1):103–4.

Brune, K. The pharmacological profile of non-opioid (OTC) analgesics: aspirin, paracetamol (acetaminophen), ibuprofen, and phenazones. *Agents and Actions*, 1988; Supplements. 25: 9–19.

Caldwell, J. R., and S. H. Roth. A double-blind study comparing the efficacy and safety of enteric coated naproxen to naproxen in the management of NSAID intolerant patients with rheumatoid arthritis and osteoarthritis. Naproxen EC Study Group. *Journal of Rheumatology*, 1994; 21(4):689–95.

Carson, J. L., et al. The association of nonsteroidal anti-inflammatory drugs with uppergastrointestinal tract bleeding. *Archives of Internal Medicine*, 1987; 147(1):85–88.

Carson, J. L., et al. The relative gastrointestinal toxicity of the nonsteroidal anti-inflammatory drugs. *Archives of Internal Medicine*, 1987; 147(6):1054–59.

Cassel, C. K., D. E. Riesenberg, L. B. Sorenson, and J. R. Walsh, *Geriatric Medicine*. New York: Springer-Verlag, 1990.

Chalmers, T. M. Clinical experience with ibuprofen in the treatment of rheumatoid arthritis. *Annals of the Rheumatic Diseases*, 1969; 28:513–17.

Chiang, S. T., et al. Oxaprozin dose proportionality. *Journal of Clinical Pharmacology*, November–December 1984; 24(11–12): 515–22.

Ciccolunghi, S. N., H. A. Chaudri, and B. I. Schubiger. The value and results of long-term studies with diclofenac sodium (Voltarol). *Rheumatology and Rehabilitation*, 1979 (suppl 2):100–15.

Ciccolunghi, S. N., H. A. Chaudri, B. I. Schubiger, and R. Reddrop. Report on a long-term tolerability study of up to two years with diclofenac sodium (Voltaren). *Scandinavian Journal of Rheumatology*, 1978; 22 (suppl):86–96.

Cipollone, F., et al. Effects of nabumetone on prostanoid biosynthesis in humans. *Clinical Pharmacology and Therapeutics*, 1995; 58(3):335–41.

Cirino, G., et al. Flurbinitroxybutylester: a novel anti-inflammatory drug has enhanced antithrombotic activity. *Thrombosis Research*, 1995; 79(1):73–81.

Cohen, M. M., L. Clark, L. Armstrong, and J. D'Souza. Reduction of aspirin-induced fecal blood loss with low-dose misoprostol tablets in man. *Digestive Diseases and Sciences*, 1985; 30(7):605–11.

Cooper, S. A. Five studies on ibuprofen for postsurgical dental pain. *American Journal of Medicine*, 1984; (7):70–77.

Cooper, S. A. The relative efficacy of ibuprofen in dental pain. *Compendium of Continuing Education in Dentistry*, 1987; 8(8): 578–97.

Cooper, S. A., et al. Analgesic efficacy of an ibuprofen-codeine combination. *Pharmacotherapy*, 1982; 2(3):162–7.

Dajani, E. Z. Prostaglandins, NSAIDS, and GI mucosal integrity:

can we identify patients at risk of NSAID-induced gastric injury? [editorial; comment]. *American Journal of Gastroenterology*, 1996; 91(5):835–36.

Dajani, E. Z., and N. M. Agrawal. Prevention and treatment of ulcers induced by nonsteroidal anti-inflammatory drugs: an update. *Journal of Physiology and Pharmacology*, 1995; 46(1):3–16.

Dajani, E. Z., and C. H. Nissen. Gastrointestinal cytoprotective effects of misoprostol. Clinical efficacy overview. *Digestive Diseases and Sciences*, 1985; 30(11 suppl):194S–200S.

Distel, M., C. Mueller, E. Bluhmki, and J. Fries. Safety of meloxicam: a global analysis of clinical trials. *British Journal of Rheumatology*, 1996; 35 (suppl 1):68–77.

Downie, W. W. Diclofenac/misoprostol. A review of the major clinical trials evaluating its clinical efficacy and upper gastrointestinal tolerability in rheumatoid arthritis and osteoarthritis. *Drugs*, 1993; 45 (suppl 1): 1–6; discussion 36–37.

Drug watch. *Reader's Digest*, July 1996, 132.

Duerrigl, T., M. Vitaus, I. Pucar, and M. Miko. Diclofenac sodium (Voltaren): results of a multi-centre comparative trial in adult-onset rheumatoid arthritis. *Journal of International Medical Research*, 1975; 3:139–44.

Elliott, S. N., W. McKnight, G. Cirino, and J. L. Wallace. A nitric oxide-releasing nonsteroidal anti-inflammatory drug accelerates gastric ulcer healing in rats. *Gastroenterology*, 1995; 109(2):524–30.

Friedel, H. A., H. D. Langtry, and M. M. Buckley. Nabumetone. A reappraisal of its pharmacology and therapeutic use in rheumatic diseases. *Drugs*, 1993; 45(1):131–56.

Fries, J. F. Selective cyclooxygenase inhibition: promise for future

NSAID therapy? *Scandinavian Journal of Rheumatology*, 1996; 102(suppl):1–2.

Fries, J. Toward an understanding of NSAID-related adverse events: the contribution of longitudinal data. *Scandinavian Journal of Rheumatology. Supplement*, 1996; 102:3.

Fries, J. F., et al. Toward an epidemiology of gastropathy associated with nonsteroidal anti-inflammatory drug use. *Gastroenterology*, 1989; 96:647–55.

Gabriel, S. E., L. Jaakkimainen, and C. Bombardier. Risk for serious gastrointestinal complications related to use of nonsteroidal anti-inflammatory drugs. A meta-analysis. *Annals of Internal Medicine*, 1991; 115(10):787–96.

Garcia-Gonzalez, A., and M. H. Weisman. The arthritis of familial Mediterranean fever. *Seminars in Arthritis and Rheumatism*, December 1992; 22(3):139–50.

Gathright, A. Don't take over-the-counter painkillers like candy, experts warn. *San Diego Union-Tribune*, January 26, 1995, A-18.

Geczy, M., L. Peltier, and R. Wolbach. Naproxen tolerability in the elderly: a summary report. *Journal of Rheumatology*, 1987; 14(2):348–54.

Gibian, T. Rational drug therapy in the elderly, or How not to poison your elderly patients. *Australian Family Physician*, 1992; 21(12):1755–60.

Graham, D. Y., et al. Long-term nonsteroidal antiinflammatory drug use and Helicobacter pylori infection. *Gastroenterology*, 1991; 100(6): 1653–57.

Grazioli, I., et al. Multicenter study of the safety/efficacy of misoprostol in the prevention and treatment of NSAID-induced gastroduodenal lesions. *Clinical and Experimental Rheumatology*, 1993; 11(3):289–94.

Griswold, D. E., and J. L. Adams. Constitutive cyclooxygenase (COX-1) and inducible cyclooxygenase (COX-2): rationale for selective inhibition and progress to date. *Medicinal Research Reviews*, 1996; 16(2):181–206.

Grossman, C. J., et al. Inhibition of constitutive and inducible cyclooxygenase activity in human platelets and mononuclear cells by NSAIDs and Cox 2 inhibitors. *Inflammation Research*, 1995; 44(6):253–57.

Hawkey, C. J. Non-steroidal anti-inflammatory drug gastropathy: causes and treatment. *Scandinavian Journal of Gastroenterology*, 1996; 220(suppl):124–27.

Helzner, E. C., J. Fricke, and B. G. Cunningham. An evaluation of ibuprofen 200 mg, ibuprofen 400 mg and naproxen 200 mg and 400 mg in postoperative oral surgery pain. *Clinical Pharmacology and Therapeutics*, 1992; 51(2):122.

Henriksson, K., A. Uribe, B. Sandstedt, and C. E. Nord. Helicobacter pylori infection, ABO blood group, and effect of misoprostol on gastroduodenal mucosa in NSAID-treated patients with rheumatoid arthritis. *Digestive Diseases and Sciences*, 1993; 38(9):1688–96.

Henry, D., A. Dobson, and C. Turner. Variability in the risk of major gastrointestinal complications from nonaspirin nonsteroidal anti-inflammatory drugs. *Gastroenterology*, 1993; 105(4):1078–88.

Henry, D., et al. Variability in risk of gastrointestinal complications with individual non-steroidal anti-inflammatory drugs: results of a collaborative meta-analysis. *British Medical Journal*, 1996; 312(7046):1563–66.

Hingorani, K. Double-blind crossover trial comparing ibuprofen with flufenamic acid in rheumatoid arthritis. *Rheumatology and Physical Medicine*, 1970; 10(suppl):76–82.

Hyneck, M. L. An overview of the clinical pharmacokinetics of nabumetone. *Journal of Rheumatology*, 1992; 19(suppl 36):20–24.

Ingemanson, C. A., B. Carrington, B. Sikstrom, and R. Bjorkman. Diclofenac in the treatment of primary dysmenorrhoea. *Current Therapeutic Research*, 1981; 30(5):632–39.

Jiranek, G. C., et al. Misoprostol reduces gastroduodenal injury from one week of aspirin: an endoscopic study. *Gastroenterology*, 1989; 96(2 Pt 2 suppl):656–61.

Johnson, A. G., and R. O. Day. The problems and pitfalls of NSAID therapy in the elderly (Part I). *Drugs and Aging*, 1991; 1(2):130–43.

Jung, D., and K. E. Schwartz. Steady-state pharmacokinetics of enteric-coated naproxen tablets compared with standard naproxen tablets. *Clinical Therapeutics*, 1994; 16(6):923–29.

Kantor, T. G. Use of diclofenac in analgesia. *American Journal of Medicine*, 1986; (suppl 4B):64–69.

Karsh, J. Adverse reactions and interactions with aspirin. Considerations in the treatment of the elderly patient. *Drug Safety*, 1990; 5(5):317–27.

Kaufman, D. W., et al. Nonsteroidal anti-inflammatory drug use in relation to major upper gastrointestinal bleeding. *Clinical Pharmacology and Therapeutics*, 1993; 53(4):485–94.

Kendall, M. J., et al. A pharmacokinetic study of the active metabolite of nabumetone in young healthy subjects and older arthritis patients. *European Journal of Clinical Pharmacology*, 1989; 36(3):299–305.

Kimmey, M. B. NSAID, ulcers, and prostaglandins. *Journal of Rheumatology*, 1992; (Nov. 19 suppl) 36:68–73.

Kot, T. V., R. O. Day, and P. M. Brooks. Preventing acute gout when starting allopurinol therapy. Colchicine or NSAIDs? *Medical Journal of Australia*, August 2, 1993; 159(3):182–84.

Kuhlwein, A., H. J. Meyer, and C. O. Koehler. Reduced diclofenac administration by B vitamins: results of a randomized double-blind study with reduced daily doses of diclofenac (75 mg diclofenac versus 75 mg diclofenac plus B vitamins) in acute lumbar vertebral syndromes. *Klinische Wochenschrift*, 1990; 68(2):107–15, Abstract.

Langman, M. J. Non-steroidal anti-inflammatory drugs and peptic ulcer. *Hepato-Gastroenterology*, 1992; 39(suppl 1):37–39.

Langman, M. J., et al. Risks of bleeding peptic ulcer associated with individual non-steroidal anti-inflammatory drugs [published erratum appears in *Lancet* May 21, 1994; 343(8908):1302]. *Lancet*, April 30, 1994; 343(8905):1075–78.

Langman, M. J. S. Epidemiologic evidence on the association between peptic ulceration and antiinflammatory drug use. *Gastroenterology*, 1989; 96: 640–46.

Lanza, F. L., et al. A double-blind placebo-controlled comparison of the efficacy and safety of 50, 100, and 200 micrograms of misoprostol QID in the prevention of ibuprofen-induced gastric and duodenal mucosal lesions and symptoms. *American Journal of Gastroenterology*, 1989; 84(6):633–6.

Lee, M. Prevention and treatment of nonsteroidal anti-inflammatory drug-induced gastropathy. *Southern Medical Journal*, 1995; 88(5):507–13.

Linden, B., M. Distel, and E. Bluhmki. A double-blind study to compare the efficacy and safety of meloxicam 15 mg with piroxicam 20 mg in patients with osteoarthritis of the hip. *British Journal of Rheumatology*, 1996; 35(suppl 1):35–38.

Llewellyn, J. G., and M. H. Pritchard. Influence of age and disease state in nonsteroidal antiinflammatory drug associated gastric bleeding. *Journal of Rheumatology*, 1988; 15(4):691–94.

Machtey, I. Diclofenac in the treatment of painful joints and traumatic tendinitis (including strains and sprains): a brief review. *Seminars in Arthritis and Rheumatism*, 1985; 15(2 suppl 1):87–92.

Mahmud, T., D. L. Scott, and I. Bjarnason. A unifying hypothesis for the mechanism of NSAID related gastrointestinal toxicity. *Annals of the Rheumatic Diseases*, 1996; 55(4):211–13.

Mazanec, D. J. Conservative treatment of rheumatic disorders in the elderly. *Geriatrics*, May 1991, 46(5):41–5.

McMahon, F. G., R. Vargas, J. R. Ryan, and D. A. Fitts. Nabumetone kinetics in the young and elderly. *American Journal of Medicine*, 1987; 83(4B):92–95.

Meyler's Side Effects of Drugs, 12th ed. New York: Elsevier Science Publishers, 1992.

Millaire, A., et al. Treatment of recurrent pericarditis with colchicine. *European Heart Journal*, January 1994; 15(1):120–24.

Minotti, V., et al. Double-blind evaluation of analgesic efficacy of orally administered diclofenac, nefopam, and acetylsalicylic acid (ASA) plus codeine in chronic cancer pain. *Pain*, February 1989, 36(2):177–83.

Mitchell, J. A., et al. Selectivity of nonsteroidal antiinflammatory drugs as inhibitors of constitutive and inducible cyclooxygenase. *Proceedings of the National Academy of Sciences of the United States of America*, December 15, 1993; 90(24):11693–7.

Moskowitz, R. W. The appropriate use of NSAIDs in arthritic conditions. *American Journal of Orthopedics*, 1996; 25(9 suppl): 4–6.

Mutru, O., et al. Diclofenac sodium (Voltaren) and indomethacin in the ambulatory treatment of rheumatoid arthritis: a double-blind multicentre study. *Scandinavian Journal of Rheumatology*, 1978; (suppl)22:51–56.

Nabumetone—a new NSAID. *The Medical Letter on Drugs and Therapeutics*, April 17, 1992; 34(868):38–40.

Naves, J., R. Santoyo, and I. Morales. [Prophylactic effect of Misoprostol on gastric lesions induced by aspirin (ASA) in healthy subjects]. *Revista de Gastroenterologia de Mexico*, 1989; 54(4): 203–6.

Neustater, B. R., and J. S. Barkin. Non-steroidal anti-inflammatory drugs (NSAID) cause gastrointestinal ulcers mainly in Helicobacter pylori carriers. *Gastrointestinal Endoscopy*, 1995; 41(2):186–87.

New findings on the risks of common NSAIDs. *Sports Medicine Digest*, September 1996, 18(9):104.

Nuutinen, L. S., E. Wuolijoki, and I. T. Pentikainen. Diclofenac and oxycodone in treatment of postoperative pain: a double-blind trial. *Acta Anaesthesiologica Scandinavica*, 1986; 30(8):620–24.

Oxaprozin for arthritis. *The Medical Letter on Drugs and Therapeutics*, February 19, 1993; 35(890):15–16.

Parnham, M. J. Meeting Report on the Joint International Meeting of the 3rd Meeting on Side Effects of Anti-Inflammatory Drugs and 13th European Workshop on Inflammation. *Agents and Actions*, 1992; 35:37–39.

Porro, G. B., et al. Gastroduodenal tolerability of nabumetone versus naproxen in the treatment of rheumatic patients. *American Journal of Gastroenterology*, 1995; 90(9):1485–88.

Publig, W., C. Wustinger, and C. Zandl. Non-steroidal anti-inflammatory drugs (NSAID) cause gastrointestinal ulcers mainly in Helicobacter pylori carriers. *Wiener Klinische Wochenschrift*, 1994; 106(9):276–9.

Rainsford, K. D. Mechanisms of NSAID-induced ulcerogenesis: structural properties of drugs, focus on the microvascular factors, and novel approaches for gastro-intestinal protection. *Acta Physiologica Hungarica*, 1992; 80(1–4):23–38.

Rask, M. R. Colchicine use in 6,000 patients with disk disease and other related resistantly-painful spinal disorders. *Journal of Neurological and Orthopedic Medicine and Surgery*, 1989; 10(4): 291–98.

Raskin, J. B., et al. Misoprostol dosage in the prevention of nonsteroidal anti-inflammatory drug-induced gastric and duodenal ulcers: a comparison of three regimens. *Annals of Internal Medicine*, 1995; 123(5):344–50.

Revell, S., and L. Fenney. Impossible to state which NSAID is safer [letter; comment]. *British Medical Journal*, 1995; 311(6996): 54–55.

Rodriguez de la Serna, A., and M. Diaz-Rubio. Multicenter clinical trial of zinc acexamate in the prevention of nonsteroidal antiinflammatory drug induced gastroenteropathy. Spanish Study Group on NSAID Induced Gastroenteropathy Prevention. *Journal of Rheumatology*, 1994; 21(5): 927–33.

Roth, S. H. Nabumetone: a new NSAID for rheumatoid arthritis and osteoarthritis. *Orthopaedic Review*, 1992; 21(2):223–27.

Roth, S. H. NSAID gastropathy. A new understanding. *Archives of Internal Medicine*, 1996; 156(15):1623–28.

Sabata, S., et al. Lipoxygenase inhibitor and colchicine as antiarthritic agents in the rat. *Prostaglandins, Leukotrienes and Medicine*, July 1986; 23(1):95–102.

Sager, D. S., and R. M. Bennett. Individualizing the risk/benefit ratio of NSAIDs in older patients. *Geriatrics*, 1992; 47(8):24–31.

Savage, R. L., P. W. Moller, C. L. Ballantyne and J. E. Wells. Variation in the risk of peptic ulcer complications with nonsteroidal antiinflammatory drug therapy. *Arthritis and Rheumatism*, 1993; 36(1):84–90.

Schattenkirchner, M. Long-term safety of ketoprofen in an elderly population of arthritic patients. *Scandinavian Journal of Rheumatology*, 1991; 91(suppl):27–36.

Seattle Times. Warning issued on ibuprofen [Motrin], chicken pox. *San Diego Union-Tribune*, January 27, 1995, A-11.

Seideman, P., B. Fjellner, and A. Johannesson. Psoriatic arthritis treated with colchicine. *Journal of Rheumatology*, 1987; 14:777–79.

Shapiro, S. S., and K. Diem. The effects of ibuprofen in the treatment of dysmenorrhea. *Current Therapeutic Research*, 1981; 30(3):327–34.

Shorrock, C. J. and M. J. Langman. Nonsteroidal anti-inflammatory drug-induced gastric damage: epidemiology. *Digestive Diseases*, 1995; 13(suppl 1):3–8.

Siegmeth, W., and P. Placheta. Long-term comparative study: diclofenac (Voltaren) and naproxen (Proxen) in arthritis. *Journal Suisse de Medecine*, 1978; 108(9):349–353, Abstract.

Silverstein, F. E., et al. Gastric protection by misoprostol against 1,300 mg of aspirin. An endoscopic dose-response study. *American Journal of Medicine*, 1987; 27, 83(1A):32–36.

Simon, L. S., and T. Goodman. NSAID-induced gastrointestinal toxicity. *Bulletin on the Rheumatic Diseases*, 1995; 44(3):1–5.

Singh, G. et al. Gastrointestinal tract complications of nonsteroidal anti-inflammatory drug treatment in rheumatoid arthritis. A prospective observational cohort study. *Archives of Internal Medicine*, 1996; 156(14):1530–56.

Skeith, K. J., M. Wright, and P. Davis. Differences in NSAID tolerability profiles. Fact or fiction? *Drug Safety*, 1994; 10(3):183–95.

Smalley, W. E., W. A. Ray, J. R. Daugherty, and M. R. Griffin.

Nonsteroidal anti-inflammatory drugs and the incidence of hospitalizations for peptic ulcer disease in elderly persons. *American Journal of Epidemiology*, 1995; 141(6):539–45.

SmithKline Beecham Pharmaceuticals. Correspondence [Relafen], August 30, 1993.

Stewart, W. F., C. Kawas, M. Corrada and E. J. Metter. Risk of Alzheimer's disease and duration of NSAID use. *Neurology*, 1997; 48(3):626–32.

Stroehmann, I., M. Fedder, and H. Zeidler. German drug monitoring studies with nabumetone. *Drugs*, 1990; (40 suppl)5:38–42.

Syntex Laboratories Inc. Correspondence, July 13, 1994.

Taha, A. S., et al. Chemical gastritis and Helicobacter pylori related gastritis in patients receiving non-steroidal anti-inflammatory drugs: comparison and correlation with peptic ulceration. *Journal of Clinical Pathology*, 1992; 45(2):135–39.

Taha, A. S., et al. Effect on gastric and duodenal mucosal prostaglandins of repeated intake of therapeutic doses of naproxen and etodolac in rheumatoid arthritis. *Annals of the Rheumatic Diseases*, 1990; 49(6):354–58.

Taha, A. S., et al. Gastric and duodenal mucosal blood flow in patients receiving non-steroidal anti-inflammatory drugs—influence of age, smoking, ulceration and Helicobacter pylori. *Alimentary Pharmacology and Therapeutics*, 1993; 7(1):41–5.

Taha, A. S., et al. Predicting NSAID related ulcers—assessment of clinical and pathological risk factors and importance of differences in NSAID. *Gut*, 1994; 35(7):891–95.

Taha, A. S., and R. I. Russell. Helicobacter pylori and nonsteroidal anti-inflammatory drugs: uncomfortable partners in peptic ulcer disease. *Gut*, 1993; 34(5):580–3.

Taha, A. S., R. D. Sturrock, and R. I. Russell. Mucosal erosions in long-term non-steroidal anti-inflammatory drug users: predisposition to ulceration and relation to Helicobacter pylori. *Gut*, March 1995; 36(3):334–6.

Thompson, M., and D. Bell. Further experience with ibuprofen in the treatment of arthritis. *Rheumatology and Physical Medicine*, 1970; 10(suppl):100–103.

Upjohn Company. Motrin Package Insert, September 1992.

Valtonen, E. J. A comparative short-term trial with Voltaren (diclofenac sodium) and naproxen in soft-tissue rheumatism. *Scandinavian Journal of Rheumatology*, 1978; (suppl)22:69–73.

von Schrader, H. W., et al. Nabumetone—a novel anti-inflammatory drug: bioavailability after different dosage regimens. *International Journal of Clinical Pharmacology, Therapy, and Toxicology*, December 1984; 22(12):672–76.

Walker, J. S. NSAID: an update on their analgesic effects. *Clinical and Experimental Pharmacology and Physiology*, 1995; 22(11): 855–60.

Wallace, J. L. Gastric ulceration: critical events at the neutrophil—endothelium interface. *Canadian Journal of Physiology and Pharmacology*, January 1993; 71(1):98–102.

Wallace, J. L., and D. N. Granger. Pathogenesis of NSAID gastropathy: are neutrophils the culprits? *Trends in Pharmacological Sciences*, April 1992; 13(4):129–31.

Wallace, J. L., B. K. Reuter, and G. Cirino. Nitric oxide-releasing nonsteroidal anti-inflammatory drugs: a novel approach for reducing gastrointestinal toxicity. *Journal of Gastroenterology and Hepatology*, 1994; 9(suppl 1):S40–44.

Wallace, J. L., et al. A diclofenac derivative without ulcerogenic properties. *European Journal of Pharmacology*, 1994; 257(3): 249–55.

Willkens, R. F. An overview of the long-term safety experience of nabumetone. *Drugs*, 1990; 40(suppl 5):34–37.

Wilson, D. E., and P. C. Wilson. Effects of misoprostol on histamine-related gastric secretion in man. *Journal of the Association for Academic Minority Physicians*, 1989; 1(1):16–18.

Wolfe, S. Call to ban popular arthritis drug: Feldene. *Public Citizen's Health Research Group Health Letter*, January 1995, p. 4.

Wolfe, S. Toradol (Ketorolac), a killer painkiller, revisited. *Public Citizen's Health Research Group Health Letter*, November 1994, p. 8.

Chapter 15. Notes on Narcotic Pain Medications

Forbes, J. A., C. J. Kehm, C. D. Grodin, and W. T. Beaver. Evaluation of ketorolac, ibuprofen, acetaminophen, and anacetaminophen-codeine combination in postoperative oral surgery pain. *Pharmacotherapy*, 1990; 10(6 (Pt 2)):94S–105S.

Hellman, M., U. Ahlstrom, L. Andersson, and S. Strid. Analgesic efficacy of an ibuprofen-codeine combination in patients with pain after removal of lower third molars. *European Journal of Clinical Pharmacology*, 1992; 43(4):347–50.

Medical Board of California. A statement by the medical board. *Medical Board of California Action Report*, July 1994, pages 4–5.

Quiding, H., et al. Ibuprofen plus codeine, ibuprofen, and placebo in a single-and multidose cross-over comparison for coxarthrosis pain. *Pain*, 1992; 50(3):303–7.

Torabinejad, M., et al. Effectiveness of various medications on postoperative pain following root canal obturation. *Journal of Endodontics*, 1994; 20(9):427–31.

Walton, G. M., and J. P. Rood. A comparison of ibuprofen and ibuprofen-codeine combination in the relief of post-operative oral surgery pain [see comments]. *British Dental Journal*, 1990; 169(8):245–417.

Windle, M. L., L. A. Booker, and W. F. Rayburn. Postpartum pain after vaginal delivery; a review of comparative analgesic trials. *Journal of Reproductive Medicine*, 1989; 34(11):891–95.

Chapter 16. Antihistamines

Allegra package insert. Hoechst Marion Roussel, Inc. Kansas City, Missouri, July, 1996.

Associated Press. Allergy medicine faces loss of FDA approval. *San Diego Union-Tribune*, January 14, 1997, A-7.

Brandon, M. L., and M. Weiner. Clinical studies of terfenadine [Seldane] in seasonal allergic rhinitis. *Arzneimittel-Forschung/Drug Research*, 1982; 32(11):1204–5.

Brandon, M. L., and M. Weiner. Clinical investigation of Terfenadine, a non-sedating antihistamine. *Annals of Allergy*, 1980; 44: 71–75.

Brobyn, R. D. Astemizole in maintenance therapy of chronic allergic rhinitis. In *Histamine and Allergic Disease*. M. B. Emanuel, ed. Oxford, United Kingdom: The Medicine Publishing Foundation, 1983, pp. 16–17.

Cetirizine—a new antihistamine. *The Medical Letter on Drugs and Therapeutics*, 1996; 38:21–23.

Correspondence: Allegra. Hoechst Marion Roussel, June 20, 1997.

DuBuske, L. Dose-ranging comparative evaluation of cetirizine in patients with seasonal allergic rhinitis. *Annals of Allergy, Asthma, and Immunology*, 1995; 74(4):345–54.

Dukes, M. N. *Meyler's Side Effects of Drugs. An Encyclopedia of*

Adverse Reactions and Interactions, 12th ed. New York: Elsevier Science Publishers, 1992.

Eller, M. G., et al. Pharmacokinetics of terfenadine in healthy elderly subjects. *Journal of Clinical Pharmacology*, 1992; 32(3): 267–71.

Falliers, C. J., et al. Double-blind comparison of cetirizine and placebo in the treatment of seasonal rhinitis. *Annals of Allergy*, 1991; 66(3):257–62.

Fexofenadine. *The Medical Letter on Drugs and Therapeutics*, 1996; 38:95–96.

Fexofenadine HCl. *Pharmacy Times*, 1997; 63(3):71–72.

Hannuksela, M., et al. Dose ranging study: cetirizine in the treatment of atopic dermatitis in adults. *Annals of Allergy*, 1993; 70(2): 127–33.

Hoechst Marion Roussel, Inc. Allergra package insert. Kansas City, Missouri, July, 1996.

Honig, P. K., D. C. Wortham, A. Lazarev, and L. R. Cantilena. Grapefruit juice alters the systemic bioavailability and cardiac repolarization of terfenadine in poor metabolizers of terfenadine. *Journal of Clinical Pharmacology*, 1996; 36(4):345–51.

Huther, K. J., G. Renftle, J. T. Burke, and J. Koch-Weser. Inhibitory activity of terfenadine on histamine-induced skin wheals in man. *European Journal of Clinical Pharmacology*, 1977; 12:195–199.

Marion Merrill Dow. Correspondence, November 6, 1993.

Rihoux, J. P., and S. Mariz. Cetirizine. An updated review of its pharmacological properties and therapeutic efficacy. *Clinical Reviews in Allergy*, 1993; 11(1):65–88.

Roth, T., et al. Sedative effects of antihistamines. *Journal of Allergy and Clinical Immunology*, 1987; 80(1):94–98.

Schweitzer, P. K., M. J. Muehlbach, and J. K. Walsh. Sleepiness and performance during three-day administration of cetirizine or diphenhydramine. *Journal of Allergy and Clinical Immunology*, 1994; 94(4):716–24.

Seldane Patient Information. Marion Merrill Dow, May, 1993.

Simons, K. J., T. J. Martin, W. T. Watson, and F. E. Simons. Pharmacokinetics and pharmacodynamics of terfenadine and chlorpheniramine in the elderly. *Journal of Allergy and Clinical Immunology*, 1990; 85(3):540–47.

Tinkelman, D., et al. Efficacy and safety of fexofenadine in fall seasonal allergic rhinitis. *Journal of Allergy and Clinical Immunology*, 1996; 97(1):1009.

University of Wisconsin Medical School. Sedation and safety issues. *Dialogues in redefining allergy*, 1997; 1(2):1–16.

Walsh, G. M. The anti-inflammatory effects of cetirizine. *Clinical and Experimental Allergy*, 1994; 24:81–85.

Wolfe, S. Do not use: terfenadine (Seldane) or astemizole (Hismanal). *Worst Pills, Best Pills News*, 1997; 3(3):9, 12.

Woolsey, R. L., Y. Chen, J. P. Freiman, and R. A. Gillis. Mechanism of the cardiotoxic actions of terfenadine. *JAMA*, 1993; 269(12), 1532–36.

Chapter 17. Motion Sickness Medications

Ciba Consumer Pharmaceuticals. Correspondence, March 2, 1995.

Clissold, S. P., and R. C. Heel. Transdermal hyoscine (scopolamine): a preliminary review of its pharmacodynamic properties and therapeutic efficacy. *Drugs*, 1985; 29:189–207.

Parrott, A. C., and R. Jones. Effects of transdermal scopolamine upon psychological test performance at sea. *European Journal of Clinical Pharmacology*, 1985; 28:419–23.

Price, N. Transdermal delivery of scopolamine for prevention of motion-induced nausea in rough seas. *Clinical Therapeutics*, 1979; 2(4):258–62.

Schmitt, L. G., and J. E. Shaw. Transdermal delivery of scopolamine for prevention of motion-induced nausea in rough seas. *Clinical Therapeutics*, 1979; 2(4):258–262.

Shaw, J., and J. Urquhart. Programmed, systemic drug delivery by the transdermal route. ALZA Corporation, Palo Alto, CA. Unpublished.

Chapter 18. Other Medications

Beck, T. M. Efficacy of ondansetron tablets in the management of chemotherapy-induced emesis: review of clinical trials. *Seminars in Oncology*, 1992; 19(6 suppl 15):20–25.

Beck, T. M., et al. Efficacy of oral ondansetron in the prevention of emesis in outpatients receiving cyclophosphamide-based chemotherapy. *Annals of Internal Medicine*, 1993; 118(6):407–13.

Coccaro, E., and R. Kavoussi. Biological and pharmacological aspects of borderline personality disorder. *Hospital Community Psychiatry*, 1991; 42(10):1029–33.

Cubeddu, L. X., I. S. Hoffmann, N. J. Fuenmayor, and A. L. Finn. Efficacy of ondansetron (GR 38032F) and the role of serotonin in cisplatin-induced nausea and vomiting [see comments]. *New England Journal of Medicine*, 1990; 322(12):810–16.

Cubeddu, L. X., et al. Efficacy of oral ondansetron, a selective antagonist of 5-HT3 receptors, in the treatment of nausea and vomiting associated with cyclophosphamide-based chemotherapies. *American Journal of Clinical Oncology*, 1994; 17(2):137–46.

Lin, K. M., R. E. Poland, J. K. Lau, and R. T. Rubin. Haloperidol and prolactin concentrations in Asians and Caucasians. *Journal of Clinical Psychopharmacology*, 1988; 8(3):195–201.

Lin, K. M., et al. A longitudinal assessment of haloperidol doses and serum concentrations in Asian and Caucasian schizophrenic patients. *American Journal of Psychiatry*, 1989; 146(10):1307–11.

Mazzei, T., et al. Pharmacokinetics of azithromycin in patients with impaired hepatic function. *Journal of Antimicrobial Chemotherapy*, 1993; suppl E:57–63.

McIntyre, C., and G. Simpson. How much neuroleptic is enough? *Psychiatric Annals*, 1995; 23(3):135–39.

Melekos, M. D., et al. Post-intercourse versus daily ciprofloxacin prophylaxis for recurrent urinary tract infections in premenopausal women. *Journal of Urology*, 1997; 157(3):935–39.

"Minidoses" may give optimal neuroleptic results. *Clinical Psychiatry News*, 1994; 22(7):15.

Sherman, C. Haloperidol curbs early psychosis in low doses. *Clinical Psychiatry News*, 1997; 25(7):1–2.

Slatton, M. L., et al. Does digoxin provide additional hemodynamic and autonomic benefit at higher doses in patients with mild to moderate heart failure and normal sinus rhythm? *Journal of the American College of Cardiology*, 1997; 29(6):1206–13.

Systemic antifungal drugs. *The Medical Letter on Drugs and Therapeutics*, 1996; 38:10–12.

Terbinafine for onychomycosis. *The Medical Letter on Drugs and Therapeutics*, 1996; 38:72–74.

Yoshikawa, T., and D. Norman. *Antimicrobial Therapy in the Elderly Patient*. New York: Marcel Dekker, 1994.

Chapter 19. Slow Responses to Serious Side Effects: The Coumadin Story

Altman, R., et al. Comparison of two levels of anticoagulant therapy in patients with substitute heart valves. *Journal of Thoracic Cardiovascular Surgery*, 1991; 101:427–431.

American College of Chest Physicians and the National Heart, Lung, and Blood Institute National Conference on Antithrombotic Therapy (summary). *Archives of Internal Medicine*, 1986; 146: 462–71.

Bailey, E. L., T. A. Harper, and P. H. Pinkerton. Therapeutic range of one-stage prothrombin time in the control of oral anticoagulant therapy. *Canadian Medical Association Journal*, 1971; 94.

Bern, M. M., et al. Prophylaxis against central vein thrombosis with low-dose warfarin. *Surgery*, 1986; 99:216–20.

Conley, C. L., and W. I. Morse. Thromboplastic factors in the estimation of prothrombin concentration. *American Journal of Medical Science*, 1948; 215:158–69.

Dalen, J. E. Atrial fibrillation: Reducing stroke risk with low-dose anticoagulation. *Geriatrics*, 1994; 49(5):24–32.

Eckman, M. H., H. J. Levine, and S. G. Pauker. Effect of laboratory variation in the prothrombin-time ratio on the results of oral anticoagulant therapy. *New England Journal of Medicine*, 1993; 329 (10):696–70.

Gogstad, G. O., et al. Utility of a modified calibrational model for reliable conversion of thromboplastin times to international normalized ratios. *Thrombosis Haemostasis*, 1986; 56:178–82.

Hirsh, J. Is the dose of warfarin prescribed by American physicians unnecessarily high? *Archives of Internal Medicine*, 1987; 147(1):769–71.

Hirsh, J. Oral anticoagulant drugs. *Drug Therapy*, 1991; 324(26): 1865–75.

Hirsh, J., D. Deykin, and L. Poller. "Therapeutic range" for oral anticoagulant therapy. *Chest*, 1986; 89(2):11S–15S.

Hirsh, J., and M. Levine. Confusion over the therapeutic range for monitoring oral anticoagulant therapy in North America. *Thrombosis and Haemostasis*, 1988; 59(2):129–32.

Hirsh, J., et al. Optimal therapeutic range for oral anticoagulants. *Chest*, 1989; 95(2):5S–11S.

Hirsh, J., et al. Aspirin and other platelet active drugs, relationship among dose, effectiveness, and side effects. *Chest*, 1989; 95(2): 12S–18S.

Hull, R., et al. Different intensities of anticoagulation in the long-term treatment of proximal venous thrombosis. *New England Journal of Medicine*, 1982; 307:1676–81.

Hyers, T. M., R. D. Hull, and J. G. Weg. Antithrombotic therapy for venous thromboembolic disease. *Chest*, ACCP-NHLBI National Conference on Antithrombotic Therapy, 1986; 89(2):26S–32S.

Kirkwood, T. B. L. Calibration of reference thromboplastins and standardizations of the prothrombin time ratio. *Thrombosis Haemostasis*, 1983; 49:238–44.

Levine, M. N., G. Raskob, and J. Hirsh. Hemorrhagic complications of long-term anticoagulant therapy. *Chest*, 1989; 95(2):26S–36S.

Loeliger, E. A. ICSH/ICTH recommendations for reporting prothrombin time in oral anticoagulant control. *Thrombosis Haemostasis*, 1985; 54:155–156.

Moschos, C. F., P. C. Wong, and H. S. Sise. Controlled study of the effective level of long-term anticoagulation. *JAMA*, 1964; 190:799–805.

Poller, L. Progress in standardization in anticoagulant control. *Hematology Review*, 1987; 1:225–41.

Poller, L., et al. Fixed minidose warfarin: a new approach to prophylaxis against venous thrombosis after major surgery. *British Medical Journal*, 1987; 295:1309–12.

Poller, L., and D. A. Taberner. Dosage and control of oral anticoagulants: an international collaborative survey. *British Journal of Haematology*, 1982; 51:479–85.

Poller, L., and J. M. Thomson. The Manchester comparative reagent, in H. C. Hemker, E. A. Loeliger, Velkamp, eds. *Human Blood Coagulation*. New York: Springer, 1969: 290–95.

Resnekov, L., J. Chediak, J. Hirsh, and D. Lewis. Antithrombotic agents in coronary artery disease. *Chest*, ACCP-NHLBI National Conference on Antithrombotic Therapy, 1986; 89(2):54S–65S.

Taberner, D. A., L. Poller, J. M. Thomson, and K. V. Darby. The effect of the international sensitivity index of thromboplastin on the precision of international normalised ratios. *Journal of Clinical Pathology*, 1989; 42:92–96.

Turpie, A. G., et al. Randomised comparison of two intensities of oral anticoagulant therapy after tissue heart valve replacement. *Lancet*, 1988; 1:1242–45.

Wright, I. S. Recent developments in antithrombotic therapy. *Annals of Internal Medicine*, 1969; 71(4):823–31.

Wright, I. S., D. F. Beck, and C. D. Marple. Myocardial infarction and its treatment with anticoagulants. Summary of findings in 1031 cases. *Lancet*, 1954; 92–97.

Zucker, S., M. H. Cathey, P. J. Sox, and E. C. Hallec. Standardization of laboratory tests for controlling anticoagulant therapy. *American Journal of Clinical Pathology*, 1970; 53:348–54.

Chapter 20. Solutions

Blair, D. I., B. Kaplan, and J. Spiegler. Patient characteristics and lifestyle recommendations in the treatment of gastroesophageal reflux disease. *Journal of Family Practice*, 1997; 44(3):266–72.

Cicinelli, E., F. Savino, I. Cagnazzo, and P. Scorcia. Comparative study of progesterone plasma levels after nasal spray and intramuscular administration of natural progesterone in menopausal women. *Gynecologic and Obstetric Investigation*, 1993, 35(3): 172–74.

Clark, C. The power of suggestion: placebos seem to work, but the experts can't explain how they do it. *San Diego Union-Tribune*, March 9, 1994, E-1, 3.

Cohen, J. S., and P. A. Insel. The *Physicians' Desk Reference*: problems and possible improvements. *Archives of Internal Medicine*; 1996; 156:1375–80.

Correspondence. Department of Health and Human Services, Food and Drug Administration (FDA), March 7, 1994.

Donahue, J. G., et al. Inhaled steroids and the risk of hospitalization for asthma. *JAMA*, 1997; 277(11): 887–91.

Donovan, S., et al. Duration of antidepressant trials: clinical and research implications. *Journal of Clinical Psychopharmacology*, 1994; 14(1):64–66.

Faich, G. A., et al. Reassurance about generic drugs? *New England Journal of Medicine*, 1987; 316(23):1473–75.

Ferguson, R. P., T. Wetle, D. Dubitzky, and D. Winsemius. Relative importance to elderly patients of effectiveness, adverse effects, convenience and cost of antihypertensive medications. A pilot study. *Drugs and Aging*, 1994; 4(1):56–62.

Food and Drug Administration, Department of Health and Human Services. FDA's tips for taking medicines: How to get the most benefits with the fewest risks. Publication No. (FDA) 96-3221. U.S. Government Printing Office, February 1996, 1–6.

Fritz, S. Patients seldom pick their treatment, professor finds. *Los Angeles Times*, December 15, 1993, A29.

Gathright, A. Don't take over-the-counter painkillers like candy, experts warn. *San Diego Union-Tribune*, January 26, 1995, A-18.

George, C. F. Adverse drug reactions and secrecy: knowledge is power; doctors should cede some of both to their patients. *British Medical Journal*, 1992; 304:1328.

Grapefruit juice interactions with drugs. *The Medical Letter*, 1995; 37:73–74.

Guyatt, G., et al. Determining optimal therapy—randomized trials in individual patients. *New England Journal of Medicine*, 1986; 314(14):889–92.

Houghton, W. Would Freud do 15-minute med checks? *Psychiatric Times*, June 1994: 23–25.

Jick, H. Adverse drug reactions: the magnitude of the problem. *Journal of Allergy and Clinical Immunology*, 1984, 74, 555–57.

Kessler, D. A. Communicating with patients about their medicines. *New England Journal of Medicine*, 1991; 325:1650–52.

Kitler, M. E. Clinical trials in the elderly: Pivotal points. *Clinics in Geriatric Medicine*, 1990; 6(2):235–55.

Kolata, G. (New York Times News Service). What ails elderly

often prescribed. *San Diego Union-Tribune*, July 27, 1994, A-1, 20.

Kuhlwein, A., H. J. Meyer, and C. O. Koehler. Reduced diclofenac administration by B vitamins: results of a randomized double-blind study with reduced daily doses of diclofenac (75 mg diclofenac versus 75 mg diclofenac plus B vitamins) in acute lumbar vertebral syndromes. *Klinische Wochenschrift*, 1990; 68(2): 107–15, Abstract.

Lindley, C. M., M. P. Tully, V. Paramsothy, and R. C. Tallis. Inappropriate medication is a major cause of adverse drug reactions in elderly patients. *Age and Ageing*, July 1992; 21(4):294–300.

Long, J. W. *The Essential Guide to Prescription Drugs*. New York: Harper Perennial, 1992.

Martin, E. W. *Hazards of Medication: A Manual on Drug Interactions, Contraindications, and Adverse Reactions with Other Prescribing and Drug Information*, 2nd ed. Philadelphia: J. B. Lippincott Company, 1978.

MacDonald, J. (Associated Press) Technician's hunch led to diet drug study: heart authorities might be linked to use of fen-phen. *San Diego Union-Tribune*, July 23, 1997, A10.

Miracle drugs or media drugs: when drug companies manipulate the news, you can't believe what you read, watch, or hear. *Consumer Reports*, February 1992, 142–46.

Mullen, W. H., et al. Incorrect overdose management advice in the *Physicians' Desk Reference*. *Annals of Emergency Medicine*, 1997; 29(2):255–61.

Peck, C., et al. Opportunities for integrating of pharmacokinetics, pharmacodynamics, and toxicokinetics in rational drug development. *Journal of Clinical Pharmacology*, 1994; 34:111–9.

Peskin, T., et al. Malpractice, patient satisfaction, and physician-patient communication. *JAMA*, 1995; 274(1):22.

Price, P. L. A prescription for a prescription: the treatment of adverse drug reactions. *South Dakota Journal of Medicine*, 1994; 47(4):133–34.

Pushing drugs to doctors. *Consumer Reports*, February 1992, 87–94.

Rowland, M., L. Sheiner, and J. Steimer. *Variability in Drug Therapy: Description, Estimation, and Control*. A Sandoz Workshop. New York: Raven Press, 1985.

Sedgwick, J. The booming self-care market makes health care cheaper and more accessible—but is all of this good for us? *Self*, April 1993, 121–25, 184–88.

Sheiner, L., S. Beal, and N. Sambol. Study designs for dose-ranging. *Clinical Pharmacology and Therapeutics*, 1989; 46(1): 63–77.

Slatton, M. L., et al. Does digoxin provide additional hemodynamic and autonomic benefit at higher doses in patients with mild to moderate heart failure and normal sinus rhythm? *Journal of the American College of Cardiology*, 1997; 29(6):1206–13.

Solomon, J. With or without you: forget Washington, Wall Street is reforming health care. *Newsweek*, August 15, 1994, 58–59.

Turri, M., and G. Stein. The determining of practically useful doses of new drugs: some methodological considerations. *Statistics in Medicine*, 1986; 5:449–57.

Uhlman, M. [Knight-Ridder News Service]. Medicine revolution is brewing. *San Diego Union-Tribune*, May 8, 1994, I1–2.

Wernicke, J. F., et al. Low-dose fluoxetine therapy for depression. *Psychopharmacology Bulletin*, 1988; 24(1):183–88.

Weyrauch, K. F. Malpractice, patient satisfaction, and physician-patient communication. *JAMA*, 1995; 274(1):22–23; discussion 23–24.

Young, M. Globalization of the pharmaceutical industry: the physician's role in optimizing drug use. *Journal of Clinical Psychopharmacology*, 1990; 30:990–93.

Acknowledgments

First and foremost, my deepest thanks go to my wife, Barbara, for her unwavering support of this full-time, financially unsupported project that began in 1990—and for her willingness to read and reread the manuscript in its many drafts over the years.

Also deserving of my gratitude are Audrey Wolf, my agent, who guided *Make Your Medicine Safe* to the right publisher. Ann McKay Thoroman at Avon Books provided invaluable guidance and encouragement in shaping the book into its finished form. My working relationship with these talented professionals was everything a writer could desire.

Dr. Larry Romane gets extra credit for reading several drafts of the manuscript and offering many helpful suggestions, medical and otherwise. Thanks also to Drs. Tony Weisenberger, Lee Kaplan, Denny Cook, and Dan Gardner for their medical input and overall encouragement. A special thanks to Dr. Paul Insel for imparting his expertise in writing a research-based work and for his integral involvement in our 1996 journal article, "The *Physicians' Desk Reference*: Problems and Possible Improvements," which was an unexpected offshoot of this project. And a general thank-you to the many other physicians, nurses, health professionals, and other people who readily shared their experiences, knowledge, and suggestions.

I would also like to thank the staff at the Biomedical Library at the University of California, San Diego, especially Barbara Slater, for their frequent and cheerful assistance in obtaining articles from distant sources.

A word of gratitude is also due for the many pharmaceutical companies that provided me with considerable verbal and written input, as well as studies relevant to many medications in this book. I hope that my criticisms of some pharmaceutical industry methodologies are understood to be just that—criticisms of methods, not of the industry as a whole. My intention is that some of these criticisms may lead to changes that will provide benefits for patients, physicians, and the pharmaceutical industry itself.

Because of physical disabilities, I have written the entire manuscript of *Make Your Medicine Safe*, as well as collected approximately 2,000 pages of data and notes, with a voice-run computer. The voice program also allowed me to spend hundreds of hours scanning the entire medical library reference system (Medline) while barely lifting a finger. Without this computer technology, I could not have completed this work.

General Index

A

ACE inhibitors, 300–302
  effectiveness of, 301
  listing of, 301–302
  side effects, 301
Acetaldehyde syndrome, 50–51
Addiction
  meaning of, 92
  Wellbutrin and drug craving
    reduction, 123
  See also Dependency
Advertising, and nonprescription
    drug use, 483–484
African-Americans
  and drug response, 49
  and hypertension, 281–282
Age
  and dose response, 56–57
  See also Elderly
Agoraphobia, medications for,
    137, 141, 154
Alcohol use
  acetaldehyde syndrome, 50–51
  and anti-inflammatory drugs,
    337–338
Alcohol withdrawal, medications
    for, 170, 178
Aldactazide, 298
Allegra, 404–406, 466–467
  and elderly, 405
  low-dose, 405, 406
  side effects, 404–405

Allergies
  antihistamines, 385–410
  multiple chemical sensitivity
    syndrome (MCSS), 54–56
Alpha receptor blockers, 306–
    307
  listing of, 307
  mechanism of action, 306
  side effects, 306
AMA Drug Evaluations Annual,
    477
Ambien, 199–202
  dosage guidelines, 202
  and elderly, 201–202
  low-dose, 200–201
  side effects, 201
*American Hospital Formulary
    Service, Drug Information*,
    477
*American Medical Association
    Drug Evaluations*, 16
Amnesia
  and Halcion, 191–192, 193–
    194, 196
  and Valium, 170
Anafranil, 127–128
  dosage guidelines, 128
Antacids, 229
Anti-anxiety drugs, 143–184
  antidepressants, 144, 154–155
  Atarax, 182–183
  Ativan, 174–176

605

Drug Index

JAY SYLVAN COHEN lives in Del Mar, California, with his wife, Barbara, his son, Rory, and two cats and two dogs.

Dr. Cohen graduated cum laude and as a Chapter Scholar (his college's equivalent to Phi Beta Kappa) from Ursinus College in 1967. He obtained his medical degree at Temple University in 1971.

He first worked as a general medical physician at the student health department at San Diego State University. In 1973 he joined David Bresler's pain research team in the Department of Anesthesiology at the University of California, Los Angeles, Medical School. In 1974, he entered a residency in the Department of Psychiatry at the University of California, San Diego, and is presently an associate professor there.

From 1977 through 1990, Dr. Cohen practiced psychiatry and psychopharmacology (the specialty of psychiatric medications and their interactions with the central nervous system). On staff at the Naval Regional Medical Center, Balboa Hospital, San Diego, he was a frequent lecturer to interns and residents.

Dr. Cohen began writing *Make Your Medicine Safe* in 1990 with the expectation of finishing the book by 1992 or 1993. However, in 1990 he sustained the first of a series of pain syndromes that was finally diagnosed in 1997 as reflex sympathetic dystrophy (RSD), a disease of the nervous system. RSD is a little-known, yet not uncommon affliction that may involve the spinal cord and central nervous system. As his disabilities grew, this project was halted many times and nearly abandoned. It was only with the help and encouragement of many others that he was able, at a pace that his physical handicaps allowed, to gradually complete the project in 1997.

Dr. Cohen is currently involved in a personal as well as professional search for new, effective methods of treatment of reflex sympathetic dystrophy.

Expertly detailed, pharmaceutical guides
can now be at your fingertips
from U.S. Pharmacopeia

THE USP GUIDE TO MEDICINES
78092-5/$6.99 US/$8.99 Can

- More than 2,000 entries for both prescription and non-prescription drugs
- Handsomely detailed color insert

THE USP GUIDE TO HEART MEDICINES
78094-1/$6.99 US/$8.99 Can

- Side effects and proper dosages for over 400 brand-name and generic drugs
- Breakdown of heart ailments such as angina, high cholesterol and high blood pressure

THE USP GUIDE TO VITAMINS AND MINERALS
78093-3/$6.99 US/$8.99 Can

- Precautions for children, senior citizens and pregnant women
- Latest findings and benefits of dietary supplements

Complete and Authoritative
Health Care Sourcebooks
from Avon Books

EMERGENCY CHILDCARE:
A Pediatrician's Guide   by Peter T. Greenspan M.D.
77635-9/$5.99 US/$7.99 Can   and Suzanne Le Vert

A HANDBOOK OF NATURAL
FOLK REMEDIES   by Elena Oumano Ph. D.
78448-3/$5.99 US/$7.99 Can

ESTROGEN: Answers to
All Your Questions   by Mark Stolar, M.D.
79076-9/$5.99 US/$7.99 Can

MIGRAINES: Everything You
Need to Know About Their
Cause and Cure   by Arthur Elkind, M.D.
79077-7/$5.99 US/$7.99 Can

HGH: The Promise of
Eternal Youth   by Suzanne Le Vert
78885-3/$5.99 US/$7.99 Can

HELP AND HOPE FOR
HAIR LOSS   by Gary S. Hitzig, M.D.
78710-5/$6.50 US/$8.50 Can

MAXIMIZE THE BENEFITS
MINIMIZE THE RISKS

- Do you take aspirin, or any other over-the-counter pain medication on a regular basis?
- Are you experiencing jitteriness, or episodes of panic or insomnia after using an antidepressant drug?
- Have sleep medications produced unpleasant side effects?
- Do you suspect your hypertension medication may be too strong?
- Do nonprescription antihistamines make you drowsy?
- Do you know the differences between the various allergy and motion sickness medications and how to choose the one that's right for you?
- Are you aware that the side effects of some drugs are grossly understated by the manufacturer?
- Do you know which medications are highly addictive?

FOR YOUR HEALTH,
COMFORT, AND SAFETY
DISCUSS ALL MEDICATIONS
WITH YOUR DOCTOR